Surviving Cancer

Surviving Cancer

*The Use of Complementary
and Alternative Methods in the
Treatment of Breast Cancer*

A Case Study and Scientific Analysis

Joseph E. Bosiljevac, Jr.,
MD, PhD, FACS

To order additional copies of this book, contact:
Xlibris Corporation
1-888-795-4274
www.Xlibris.com
Orders@Xlibris.com
84160

Contents

SECTION I

Introduction

While in private practice I have listened to and observed many of my patients who found relief in complementary and alternative methods (including chiropractic treatments, vitamins, and supplements), EDTA chelation, oxidative therapy with hydrogen peroxide, and prolozone/prolotherapy for joint and soft-tissue injections. I saw the tunnel vision of conventional (allopathic) medicine, which is well-versed to treat established disease and cover symptoms with medication or surgery. However, over the course of my first career, I became frustrated, realizing that the causative factors many times were not being addressed. In addition, various idiopathic diseases can be considered in a catch-all term meaning "we do not know the cause."

Donna came to me as a patient with breast cancer in 1994 and subsequently developed a local chest wall recurrence within a year. Textbooks would give her a very poor chance at survival in five years (less than 10 %). As related in Donna's story, she became disillusioned with the treatment proposed by conventional medicine and elected to try alternative methods. She approached me to see if I would supervise and follow her at intervals with whatever methods she elected. The experience with Donna over the years, accompanied by additional observations with other patients, increased my curiosity about complementary and alternative methods.

I had the opportunity to participate in several medical missions in third world countries. This allowed me to witness lifestyle and health at other levels and in other environments. Despite the technology available to me in the United States, I found that I could perform successful surgery with basic tools. Observing the lifestyles and natural foodstuffs in these "lesser" countries I saw a good healing ability, tolerance of pain, and immunity that overshadows our own.

I became impressed at how "the Guy upstairs" put us together and realized the body has a tremendous ability to heal itself if we do the proper groundwork and it continues to fight back and attempts to survive even if we trash it. After a while it gives out. I honestly feel most people lose thirty more good years of living.

In the midst of a busy practice, I pursued a doctoral degree in natural medicine. Two years of didactic study pursued during evening hours and weekends was followed by a full year performing the research involved for my dissertation. This resulted in friends calling me Doctor-Doctor. I also worked with the Cenegenics Medical and Research Institute in Las Vegas, Nevada, helping patients initiate a wellness program based on metabolic and hormonal balance.

Basically, I look at the overall human organism as a "human machine" and try to identify what part might have broken down to allow a disease to develop. Curiosity led me along further paths and I explore the postulate as presented by Moritz (2008) that cancer is a survival mechanism with the body attempting to develop a line of cells to survive in a toxic environment.

Although I believe that there is a place for conventional surgery, radiotherapy, and chemotherapy in the treatment of cancer, I also believe that the areas of nutrition and detoxification are relatively ignored. Not only are we exposed to many more chemicals in our present environment, but also currently accepted nutritional guidelines promoted to the public are not clear and easily misunderstood. Individual variability is ignored by the health-care industry directed clinical guidelines attempting to make one size fit all. I believe that the practice of medicine today is about 20% science and 80% good judgment. A case in point would be trying to quantify and identify the quality of spirituality and its importance in promoting health.

The initial part entitled "The Journey Begins" summarizes my thoughts in lay terms and also gives an idea of my professional opinion that has developed after experience with Donna and others during my career. A good way of approaching this book is to first look at this section which can be used as an overview prior to the sections.

The next part of this book presents Donna's story in her own words. Not only does this show her progress as she tries various alternative methods, but it also displays the psychosocial aspects as she fights for her life. This is a portrayal of her private life with which many can identify.

I then follow this very personal story with my doctoral dissertation. This gives my medical version of Donna's illness as a case study and an update after that reported in her personal story.Presenting the original dissertation afterward gives a scientific background and references to the line of thinking used in studying Donna's particular case. My extensive experience with conventional medicine and surgery and my doctoral degree in natural medicine allows me to give an educated, unbiased, and balanced view with an attempt at a scientific explanation. The original purpose of the dissertation attempted to identify the effectiveness of the various methods used by Donna. The focus of the paper changed as it developed, supporting a holistic approach to her recovery. Chapter Four, "Results and Findings" and chapter Five, "Conclusions" give a good summary of the data collected and reviewed in the scientific analysis of Donna's illness.

It may be helpful to then look at the section "The Journey Begins" another time. Basically, not only does this serve as a summary but I hope will also spark curiosity. Curiosity is felt to be an integral characteristic of the clinician-scientist. Using this trait, serial observation over the years leads to experience. Good judgment comes from experience.

I hope the spark of curiosity will be ignited in patients and medical professionals that may look at this material. General ideas can then be expounded in looking at other cases and the overall picture of health. Conventional medicine does not need to compete with complementary and alternative methods. Neither is all encompassing or complete on its own. Basically, the road to good health involves both sides of the fence.

The Journey Begins

The first thing I would admit is that I do not know all the answers or that I am an expert. What I offer with the information presented in this book is a view from a small window about cancer survival and healthy living. My conventional (allopathic) experience includes medical school, a rotating internship in a large charity hospital, five years of surgical training, several medical missions to third world countries, and thirty years in private practice. I then add my doctoral training and personal adventures with patients using natural medicine alternatives. This section contains opinions based on my studies, observations, and experience. I feel they are unbiased, developed from a wide background, and initiated by curiosity. In this summary, I plan to cover a wide range of material with no specific references since the information provided is widely available. It is by no means comprehensive but presented in a general sense and in the manner I approach patients using lay terms.

One purpose of this book is to present a remarkable story about defeating cancer. This is not about "percent response to therapy" with eventual recurrence that is quoted in the medical literature regarding accepted cancer treatments. Donna has quality survival with no current evidence of gross active disease, either locally in the chest wall or in other parts of the body (metastatic). She provides inspiration for dealing with one of the situations in life that is quite scary. Donna continues working inside and outside the home and interacting with her family while she deals with the fear of losing a body part, and potentially, her life.

This story is about observations and experiences that may or may not be able to be proven scientifically, but minimally should arouse curiosity and encourage thinking beyond conventional wisdom. My dissertation attempts to perform a scientific analysis of her survival. However, I am not able to identify any "magic bullet" or remarkable cancer cure. A holistic view of the overall human organism is portrayed.

Another purpose of this book is to introduce how to fit healthy living into an individual lifestyle. My approach with patients is realistic. There is a perfect world and there is a real world. The ideal world is living in a monastery in the Himalayas. This is not realistic for most people. Rigid routines would not be followed if it took all the fun out of living. The key word here is balance.

The word physician means two things to me. The first is "healer" and the second is "teacher."A healer has the patient foremost as a goal. This means listening to patients' concerns and fears. It also means understanding their lifestyle and habits. A healer uses the wide variety of information available for promoting health. One of the advantages of my position is that I have experience on both sides of the fence. Neither allopathic medicine nor natural medicine provides a complete picture/answer for the patient. With information that is currently available on the Internet, patients spend time reading about complementary aspects outside the boundaries of conventional medicine. They may have had experience with a relative or friend who benefited from one of these alternative methods. Out of respect for their physician, many patients will not say anything or argue whatever alternative method is discouraged. However, they have their own thoughts and feelings, which may or may not be medically valid but are still an integral part of their own healing process.

The traditional Greek word from which physician is derived means "teacher." As such, the doctor must be able to provide information and direction for the patient to make decisions on their own level. I discourage the use of scientific and medical terms that may be confusing for the lay person. Treatment and lifestyle changes need to be acceptable for compliance.

Quality of life needs to be preserved. I know my father spent the last six months of his life going back and forth for cancer treatments and finally told me one day "this is not worth it." A large percentage of the health-care budget is spent on patients in the last months of their life. Expensive treatment modalities are available to attempt to deal with things that are broken. If the patient understands the basics about what should be accomplished, they are in a better position to implement any changes for their own particular lifestyle. To prescribe so many pills that need to be taken so many times a day discourages compliance, besides changing the underlying chemical balance. To spend the last few months of life receiving toxic chemotherapy is not sensible if the horse is out of the barn and quality of life is not maintained.

A third purpose is to arouse curiosity about complementary and alternative methods. For this we need to briefly discuss natural medicine. Conventional medicine is disease based. In other words, treatment involves approaching an established illness or treating the resultant symptoms. Basically, an acute illness or symptoms are the body's response to disease. Natural medicine encourages the body to heal itself. I have patients who tell me they are glad that I am now using natural techniques. If they have a sore throat they ask, "What herb do I take?" No no no! They are missing the boat. The real question is: Why did the machine break down, and you developed a sore throat?

There are various components that comprise "natural medicine." Among these are Chinese medicine, Ayurvedic, chiropractic, homeopathy, naturopathy, yoga, acupuncture, and iridology. Physical therapy in conventional medicine does not usually include massage or deep tissue manipulation, such as Rolfing. Various treatments used in these areas that are not approved by conventional third-party payers include chelation, oxidative therapy (hydrogen peroxide), and prolotherapy/prolozone.

Look at the long history of natural health spas that were originally started in Europe. The basis of most of these institutions consists of rest, fresh air, whole food nutrition, and clean water. They rely on the ability of the body to heal itself. Natural herbs are used rather than purified or manufactured medications. However, the primary modalities are those mentioned above. There is a lot written in the current scientific literature regarding chronic inflammation in the development of many pathologic processes, such as autoimmune disease, atherosclerosis, diabetes, and cancer. The methods used in these health spas aim to diminish inflammation and improve resistance.

There are many people who suffer from allergies, and they do not want to be outdoors because of a runny nose and itchy eyes. Natural medicine points out that lack of fresh air and staying in a climate-controlled environment inside a building or car may worsen allergy symptoms. Many ventilation systems contain dust and molds. Fresh air and daily exposure to allergens improve resistance.

A natural technique to improve allergies is to ingest a teaspoon of *local* honey daily. Witchcraft? The honey contains pollen of many plants that cause allergy symptoms. The use of a small amount every day is similar to desensitization with allergy shots. There is no immediate effect, but I have seen many patients with improved symptoms after using *local* honey on a daily basis for one year.

Used in both conventional as well as natural medicine, nutrition is one of the most important aspects in prolonging health. It is hard to give a specific diet as a general guideline. Genetics, chemical balance, lifestyle, and potential compliance need to be considered. My general comments to patients about nutrition concern whole foods. In other words, when you are in the checkout line at the grocery store there should be no boxes, no bottles, and no cans. I have also received feedback like, "Gee, Doc, then I will not have any groceries." Packaged and processed food contains preservatives and other chemicals. Carbonated beverages and fruit drinks loaded with high-fructose corn syrup are killers, although some will consider these their daily serving of fruit. High fructose corn syrup may contribute to increased body stores of mercury. Many diet drinks or foods contain potentially harmful sweeteners.

Although there has been a lot of interest regarding cholesterol and fat, the real factor in nutritional health is sugar. Sugar causes insulin spikes even if a person is not diabetic. This also occurs with starches since these are comprised of many sugar molecules hooked together that break apart with digestion. Insulin is chemically closely related to growth hormone. As such, it may tie up growth hormone receptors on cells and interfere with the hormone axis. Ingestion of fat or protein at the same time blunts this insulin spike, but avoiding refined sugar and starches is one of the most important aspects of prolonging health.

In my opinion, the food pyramid is upside down. The American diet should comprise 40%-50% fats, 30% protein, and 20% carbohydrates in an ideal world. Obviously, the fats need to be good fats, such as nuts, seeds, and olive oil, with the avoidance of oxygenating good fats during cooking at high temperatures. Some saturated fats, such as the short chain butyric acid found in butter, have good effects. Butyric acid has clearly been shown to reduce cancer risk. However, this does not mean eating tons of butter is healthy. What I want to point out is that natural sources are preferred and generally more healthful than products presented to us after processing. Margarine is chemically very close to plastic.

Protein intake needs to be high-quality protein, and there does not need to be only chicken and fish with exclusion of red meat. The ideal world would use lean wild game since this should be void of the hormones and chemicals fed to livestock in preparation for the market. Dairy products may also contain hormones and antibiotics. Range-fed cattle can be exposed to pesticides and other chemicals depending on weed control where they are raised, which theoretically, could also affect wild game. Toxins are stored in animal fat. Keep this in mind when detoxification is covered.

The carbohydrates should be mostly vegetables with a few fruits. Vegetables promote an alkaline environment, which is important for chemical balance. We function better if our system is alkaline. Fruits tend to provide more sugar and an acid environment. Variety is the key. Simple carbohydrates and starches obtained from processed grain have lost most of their nutritional value as well as fiber content. I feel it is a real travesty when bread or other packaged food states "vitamin fortified"—in other words, putting back what was taken out.

Vegetables are more nutritious when eaten raw or lightly steamed. This is due to active enzymes, which help our body assimilate the nutrients. When patients say that they have had a remarkable improvement with one agent, such as Acai, or some other juice extract, this likely has more to do with the fact that they are receiving active enzymes that have not been destroyed during pasteurization. These patients were probably severely deficient in these enzymes, and thus note a rapid- and short-term benefit. I do not believe in magic bullets.

There has been an overemphasis on the danger of cholesterol to our health. It is important to recognize that cholesterol is an essential nutrient. It serves as a precursor in the synthesis of vitamin D, a precursor to sex hormones, and an essential component in the formation of every cell wall. It is incorporated into the myelin sheath, which surrounds nerves and may affect transmission of nerve impulses in the brain or peripheral nerves. It is also a component of bile salts, which are used for digestion. Perhaps the response of the body if there is a deficiency in one of these areas would be to elevate the cholesterol level.

To simply throw a pill at a high number without looking at the underlying cause is an example of a disease or symptom-oriented system. When statins are used to treat high cholesterol, a deficiency of CoQ10 can subsequently occur since its synthesis in the liver follows the same pathway and is also blocked by these drugs. CoQ10 is used by mitochondria in cells to produce energy. Lack of CoQ10 may decrease the energy production in cells to the point where it could affect the pumping ability of the heart. Now more drugs need to be given because the patient develops congestive heart failure. Another domino in the line falls. CoQ10 deficiency can affect other muscles, causing weakness and muscle pain. CoQ10 can be given as a supplement but the cost is not covered by insurance. This doesn't make sense.

A high-glycemic (sugar) diet disrupts the hormone axis and plays a major role in altered lipid (fat) metabolism, elevating cholesterol and triglyceride levels. The ratio of good and bad cholesterol is adversely affected by a high-glycemic diet. It also promotes an acid environment. Oxidation of fat that occurs with cooking or frying is more detrimental than overall fat intake in the development of hardening of the arteries. Fats are necessary for health, but the chemistry is quite complex and it is not as simple as avoiding fat in the diet to prevent deposits inside the arteries.

I feel that whether a whole food is organic is not as important as using whole foods. Yes, there will be exposure to pesticides and chemicals in the nonorganic variety. I am not convinced that the organic foods are entirely toxin free since there is no guaranteed control. Food from the local farmer's market or someone's garden may be helpful. However, despite precautions, we are still exposed to many environmental toxins. Consider the neighbor who puts fertilizer and pesticides on the lawn—we are still exposed on our side of the fence. There may be run off during a rainstorm, or the water source may be contaminated. Grapes, cherries, strawberries, apples, pears, and peaches are some of the worst sources of fruits loaded with toxins. Companion planting uses lemon balm, chives, and rose bushes next to fruit trees to control pests instead of using chemicals.

Even if pure apple or grape juice with no sugar added was chosen as healthy, there can be a concentration of toxins in the product. So from the nutritional aspect, I look at eating whole foods, and then consider detoxification. These were the main aspects of Donna's program. Her multiple supplements had a lot of detox properties.

Many types of detoxification methods are available, including various liver and bowel cleanses. A formal initial extensive detoxification followed by a regular routine may be helpful. The most important daily measure includes eating whole raw vegetables while avoiding processed and fast food. Fresh, raw garlic and onions can help detoxify the liver. Milk thistle (silymarin) and dandelion root extract can also be used for this.

Chelator means "claw" and represents an agent that will grab onto and hold tightly another molecule. Substances harmful to health then can be eliminated from body stores using chelating agents. Chlorophyll is an excellent chelator of organic substances and some heavy metals. Cilantro chelates mercury. Vitamin C is an antioxidant, as well as a natural chelator. Lactic acid produced by anaerobic exercise serves as a chelator. Chlorella is a good general system cleanser. Weight loss can release toxins stored in fat and cause symptoms. Feeling lousy during diet programs may be on this basis as well as chemical imbalance from lack of essential nutrients.

Glutathione is one of the most effective methods for enhancing liver and brain detoxification. In general, this has to be given intravenously, although I will talk later about a product that aids in absorption by mouth using a means called liposomal encapsulation. I have actually seen patients who have had gray hair turn back to its natural color and pigmented age spots become lighter following detoxification. Lipofuscin is found in these pigmented spots and contains iron. Iron is one of the first heavy metals removed with EDTA chelation, which will be discussed later. Iron increases oxidation in the body, just like rust on steel. You do not want too much iron.

The skin is the largest organ for excretion of toxins. Many rashes and skin conditions may be a manifestation that the body is trying to eliminate toxicity and may become worse during detoxification. Psoriasis has been shown to improve following systemic detoxification.

Water is an important nutritional aspect of health. Good hydration at the cellular level allows optimal chemical functioning. Water is a means to rid the body of toxins through the kidneys. Good water is not widely available, and many filtration systems lack a true beneficial result. Chlorine and fluoride in water are killers. As physicians, we now see more thyroid dysfunction than fifty years ago. The periodic chemistry table shows that chlorine, fluorine, and bromine are all in the same line as iodine. These other halogen elements may compete with iodine and affect thyroid function.

Not only are we exposed to these substances in drinking water that is not filtered properly, but they can also be absorbed through the skin during long, hot showers. Another gray area has to do with pharmaceuticals used by patients that go into our sewage. Water treatment plants may not filter out all these chemicals which can be ingested or absorbed during a shower or bath. Too much iron in water is not good.

Two quarts of water a day should be a reasonable minimal goal. One way to achieve this is to drink 20-30 oz in the morning upon arising. Ingesting more than two quarts of water daily only improves the filtration through the kidneys and excretion of toxins from our system. It would be quite rare to overdo the intake of water. Bottled water may contain dioxins from the plastic containers. Amines are another toxic water contaminant that damage DNA by a process called methylation. This affects genetic expression, which will be discussed later.

While coaching my son's Little League baseball team in the middle of a hot summer, I always encouraged the intake of water. I look at professional athletes who may be having an "off day" as a reflection of some nutritional aspect or mild dehydration affecting their overall performance. I know when I told the boys on the baseball team to "tank up on water" intake was still inadequate since they did not relate to a specific quantity. A very good marker for sufficient fluid intake is the frequency of visits to the bathroom. I certainly note on travel days when it is difficult to find a restroom and I decrease my water intake I just feel more "draggy." I told the baseball team to drink water until they had to go the bathroom every thirty minutes as a sign they were adequately hydrated. Chronic dehydration is a major element in premature aging.

The ideal world would have a whole house water filtration system that not only treats the drinking water, but also that coming from the shower head. The real world would at least have some sort of filtration system for the drinking water and very short, cool showers. I have even become more aware of this from a wellness standpoint for my puppies. Although they drink out of a puddle of water when we are out for a walk and they are thirsty, I feel much better when for the most part they are drinking filtered water from home.

The best natural source I have encountered is water directly from the lakes in the Canadian wilderness or from a spring in the Flint Hills of Kansas. I do not need to use filters with water from these areas. This water may contain many important trace elements currently missing in our processed food.

Perhaps some benefit from natural water sources is ozonization, which increases the oxygen content in the water. The cost of an ozone system at home would be out of the price range for many people. Formation of a hexagonal structure of the water molecules can occur after water passes over a magnetic field. This may allow improved absorption leading to better hydration inside the cell. I am not convinced that ionizers and alkalinizers actually add any benefit to water preparation. Diet is probably the most important element in trying to maintain an alkaline environment.

An interesting aspect of water and natural medicine is related to cold water therapy. Sebastian Kneipp, among others, utilized this treatment over one hundred years ago. Father Kneipp discovered the healing power of the cold gush or pour, and also used cold compresses. Cool or cold water was poured over the entire patient or a body part several times a day. Think about diving into a cold pool and how this seems to take your breath away. What happens is that blood contained in the skin surface is shunted internally. This shunting of blood has been shown to boost the immune system and increase lymphatic flow. There may also be some stimulation as far as hormone secretion.

As an example, try taking a regular shower, and when finished, turn the water to cold and stand in this for thirty to sixty seconds. An indication that there is improved lymphatic flow and shunting of surface blood to internal organs is the resultant increase in urination in the subsequent hour. Comfortable? Remember, you decide where to be in your real world. This aspect certainly is not expensive.

Vitamins and supplements are another component of nutrition. As pointed out in my dissertation, many billions of dollars a year are spent on these items. Basically, taking high doses of vitamins and supplements while continuing with a high-glycemic, fast-food diet is a complete waste of money. The fact that we have to fortify processed food with vitamins is a travesty of the industrialized world. In addition, chemically manufactured vitamins may actually be a mirror image of the natural molecule. These are called isomers. As such, they may not fit precisely into receptor sites on the cell and therefore are recognized as foreign to the body and not utilized properly. Natural sources are best.

With a proper diet and food preparation, handfuls of vitamins and supplements are not necessary and may not need to be taken on a daily basis. However, with the widespread interest in these nutraceuticals, I fear the pharmaceutical industry will soon lobby for control over these items. After all, there is money to be made in an industry. The quality of the resultant product may not be efficient or favorable to optimal health. In addition, television commercials will begin to push "magic bullets." Pyridoxine (vitamin B6) is an example of a current vitamin being reviewed for availability by prescription only.

Taking certain vitamins or supplements in high doses may also alter the chemical balance in the body. Vitamins are defined as micronutrients which are substances required in small amounts to facilitate function at the cellular level. Review of nutritional textbooks will explain the interactions between various micronutrients. High doses of a specific one may work against the fine chemical balance in the body. For instance, concomitant vitamin A intake may decrease vitamin D levels. One source can be a high concentration of vitamin A that is found in fish oil preparations. Surely the body may compensate at times for this, but vitamins/supplements still present some type of exogenous substance to the body. In addition, many vitamins are synthetically manufactured and may be recognized differently by the body than natural sources as explained above.

There is quite a balance between different trace minerals. Absorption of calcium is improved by simultaneous ingestion of magnesium and zinc. Zinc, at the same time, may compete with copper and selenium utilization. These trace minerals are cofactors involved with many enzyme systems. Taking too much of one could upset the balance. Relatively small doses of many nutrients working together is the key rather than large amounts of certain supplements.

Soy products provide another example of balance. The active chemical component in soy is genistein. At a low dose this may have an antiestrogen effect, whereas at a higher dose it simulates estrogen. Depending on the processing of soy, the amount of genistein available can vary in products. As pointed out in my dissertation, there may be a genetic difference in the assimilation of soy in the body. In addition, ingesting soy in certain amounts at different ages can also lead to a variable effect. Men do not do as well with high amounts of soy products. Estrogen is a man killer.

Intestinal health and gut flora, as well as a deficiency in digestive enzymes that occurs as we get older, may also affect the digestion and assimilation of soy as well as other nutrients. Look at this as far as the absorption of fat-soluble substances and minerals. For example, calcium requires acid for optimal absorption. The purple pill commonly taken for acid reflux problems affects assimilation of many supplements. Protein digestion can use enzymes from vegetable sources as well as the pancreas, such as papain from papaya and bromelain from pineapple. Bromelain has excellent anti-inflammatory properties and is used in anti-aging programs.

The word *probiotics* means the good bacteria that make up the intestinal flora. I think of this in terms of "the good guys." These good bacteria balance and stimulate normal immunity. There is an extensive lymphatic system in the gut that makes up a significant portion of the immune system. In other words, we need to balance our system and learn to exist with other living organisms in the world. Concomitant probiotics need to be considered, when antibiotics that disrupt the normal gut flora are given. This is more than the *Lactobacillus* in yogurt, which is the right idea, just not the right product and not enough of "the good guys."

MRSA, the so-called "flesh-eating bacteria," is commonly found but does not attack everyone like a wild tiger waiting for a kill. Why would God make the world and then leave us to coexist trying to wipe out all the bacteria? Yes, there are some that cause disease, but when our system is out of balance, natural resistance is lowered. Certainly, there is a place for antibiotics, but an intact immune system continues to be essential in fighting an infection.

Another example is colitis diarrhea from *C. dificil* bacteria (clostridium colitis). This can occur following antibiotic treatment for an infection in the face of an overall lowered resistance. Probiotics should be considered in patients treated for MRSA, as well as other infections.

When taking probiotics, these little guys need to be fed, and that is referred to as prebiotics. Intestinal flora will thrive on a ripe banana or raw vegetables. These should be taken at the same time that any probiotics are taken. "The good guys" do not do well with fast food. Routine probiotic use can be helpful but is even more important after someone has been subjected to antibiotics.

Colonoscopy screening for colon cancer is currently promoted in cancer prevention. During these exams, many patients will be found to harbor small polyps. I always wondered if this could be the response of the inner lining of the colon to whatever irritant may be in the waste material contained in the bowel. Currently, many patients are subjected to repeated colonoscopies to burn and obliterate these polyps since they can be precancerous.

I looked at improving bowel health and changing the environment where these polyps grow. Using probiotics, along with milk thistle and dandelion root for liver detoxification, I found many patients would be free of polyps on subsequent scope exams. Now, frequent repeat colonoscopies were not necessary, even though I was making a living with this procedure.

One of the most commonly used drugs is the purple pill for acid reflux or GERD. When there is not enough acid or digestive enzymes, the body reacts by keeping food in the stomach and not letting it pass on to the intestine. Delayed emptying from the stomach aggravates acid reflux. Although it makes the patient feel better, the purple pill cuts back on acid production and further interferes with proper digestion. Our stomachs were made to function with acid. One of the drugs used to help the stomach empty better is metaclopramide. There is a current class-action lawsuit pending because of side effects from this medication.

Garlic and ginger are spices frequently used in third world countries and recommended by the local physicians for acid peptic disorders. H. pylori is a bacteria that has been implicated in stomach ulcers, GERD, and possibly stomach cancer. The two above mentioned spices have antibacterial, antiviral, and antiparasitic properties. Here is a natural medicine tip. I have found that fresh garlic alone can wipe out residual H. pylori in patients who have a resistant form that does not respond to the usual antibiotic regimen given in this country.

Ginger root can be prepared as a tea. It is a natural prokinetic that improves emptying of the stomach and transit of material through the intestine. Using a combination of ginger root, a small amount of additional acid, such as betaine hydrochloride and supplemental digestive enzymes, I have seen many patients resolve their acid reflux symptoms. Probiotics also play a part in proper digestion and improving transit through the intestinal tract.

There have been many studies and a lot written about vitamin C, a natural chelator as well as antioxidant. It generates hydrogen peroxide in spaces outside the cell which may be how it affects cancer cells. Our white blood cells (leukocytes) do the same when attacking bacteria, viruses, or parasites. The limiting factor with vitamin C use relates to the amount that can be absorbed when taken by mouth. This allows only so high of blood levels before the body begins to excrete ascorbic acid in the urine. Large amounts taken by mouth may also be irritating to the stomach. The reason for giving vitamin C intravenously in certain conditions is to achieve higher blood levels than those obtained from oral intake.

Liposomal encapsulation is a recently available new technology. Liposomes are phospholipids, or a healthy type of fat that is incorporated into our cell membranes. With a poor diet, healthy phospholipids are replaced by oxidized fat which results in a weaker structure. This process affects every cell in the body and leads to the degenerative changes in tissues seen with aging. These include sagging or wrinkled skin and weakening of connective tissue, such as ligaments and tendons.

Liposomal encapsulation is based on a process where attraction of individual phospholipid molecules forms globules. When this is performed in a certain solution containing, for example, vitamin C, the phospholipids form around and encapsulate the vitamin C. After ingestion, these phospholipids are absorbed directly from an empty stomach, transported to the liver where they enter the liver cells, and then release whatever chemical they contain. Supposedly, higher blood and intracellular levels of vitamin C are obtained comparable to an intravenous dose of ascorbic acid. The phospholipids do not taste the best, but can be mixed with juice or another liquid to be made more palatable. Besides their utility as a delivery agent, ingestion of liposomes may provide repair of cell membranes. Saggy skin improves without plastic surgery.

I performed some personal experimentation using liposomal encapsulated EDTA. EDTA stands for *ethylenediaminetetraacetic acid* and is used for chelation. Without going into the details of chelation or arguing its beneficial effects, I found that this is quite similar to using EDTA intravenously. EDTA by itself is not absorbed well orally (only 5%). However, with liposomal encapsulation there appears to be about 80% absorption. I checked a twenty-four-hour urine collection after intravenous infusion and also after oral chelation using the liposomal encapsulated form. There were similar results of heavy metals removed with both methods.

Glutathione is another substance that cannot be given by mouth and previously was effective only by intravenous administration. The body manufactures glutathione from precursors. As glutathione is used up, it needs to be replenished. Liposomal encapsulation provides another more practical alternative as a method in delivering glutathione for detoxification.

The advantage of liposomal encapsulation allows chelation or detoxification to be performed in the home setting while maintaining a normal daily routine. Again, talking about a real world versus an ideal world, the use of liposomal encapsulation with certain substances may be beneficial and avoids having to go into a doctor's office or clinic setting once a week for an intravenous infusion. The one to four hours the IV would take may not be practical for many people. This provides an example of how preventive measures can be made to fit a real world.

The bottom line is that the human body assimilates foodstuffs and micronutrients and can provide a better balance than that provided artificially by trying to ingest and manipulate certain amounts. Consider alkalinized water to try to achieve a less acid system. Despite alkalinization of ingested water, the body will still tend to provide an acid-base balance relative to its overall chemical status. This is basically what is meant by the holistic approach—that is, allowing the body to act as a whole machine with self repair and control of the individual parts.

Chemical balance is the key to prolonging health and longevity. It allows optimum gene expression in cells so that they may function in the manner which was intended. This chemical balance will also allow what Donna refers to as her "freedom day," where she can trash her system a little bit with fast food. If the majority of the time the body is in good chemical balance, it will compensate and recover well. However, regular daily insults allow the system to be overwhelmed. Thus, the body produces symptoms of disease, and we see the degenerative conditions that arise with aging. It is amazing how long some people like alcoholics survive despite significant self-abuse. The body has a remarkable ability to reverse changes and heal itself if the proper groundwork is done. It continues to fight back until it finally wears out. Changes seen with premature aging can be slowed and possibly reversed to some extent.

An example of proper gene expression is the p53 gene, which inhibits malignant transformation of cells. There are many environmental insults which may turn off the protective properties of the p53 gene and allow cancer cells to develop. Another gene that has been studied is the so-called sr gene for longevity. Resveratrol is a supplement that is being promoted as far as stimulating this particular gene. I am not convinced that one agent is able to promote gene expression *without* an underlying receptive environment. The bottom line is a chemical balance in the entire body to allow proper gene expression for cancer and disease prevention along with promotion of longevity. The goal is to establish an environment where genes express themselves as they did in our 20's and 30's.

Another modality currently available in many European countries, referred to as "live cell therapy," uses injectable nucleic acids. Nucleic acids make up our DNA. A dietary source of nucleic acids is chlorella, rich in proteins, vitamins and minerals, and growth factors. Remember that chlorella also serves as a natural chelator and detoxifier. Folic acid is important in supporting DNA. Brewers yeast is an excellent source of primordial nucleic acids which can be used as building blocks for repair of genes.

One thing covered extensively in the dissertation was the complexity of the hormone axis. Let us discuss some aspects. Thyroid dysfunction seems to be increasing. I pointed out the chlorine and fluoride in the water to which we are exposed. One of the common preservatives in bread contains bromide. This can be another current factor that possibly interferes with iodine utilization by the thyroid gland. I also look at the dental x-rays we have all received in the past without a shield placed over the thyroid gland for protection. Although each time represents a small amount of x-ray exposure, repeated doses over many years may have something to do with a hypoactive thyroid. These are simply observations to try to explain the increasing frequency of thyroid problems.

Consumption of coffee reportedly decreases the incidence of some cancers. This may be due to antioxidants (polyphenols) in the coffee bean. Green tea also contains polyphenols. Some promote caffeine as the helpful chemical in these drinks.

However, caffeine also works as a whip to the adrenal glands to put out catecholamines (adrenaline) and cortisol. Many popular street drugs and some medications do the same. High cortisol levels are definitely an adverse factor involved in aging with opposite effects to those of growth hormone. I am not promoting exogenous administration of growth hormone as the "fountain of youth" since in most instances, certain patterns of exercise, nutritional aspects, and a good sleep cycle will naturally stimulate sufficient amounts of growth hormone for prolonging health and longevity. Then we get back to the real world and the ideal world: Am I willing to give up my daily Starbucks? What is the balance that I am willing to accept?

HRT (hormone replacement therapy) in females has followed a swing in the pendulum during my career. The most comprehensive evaluation of HRT is the WHI (World Health Initiative) study which shows that the benefit of hormones in women far outweighs no hormone replacement. These include cardiovascular health, improved bone density, less diabetes, and prevention of dementia. A recent study also showed a decreased incidence of colon cancer in elderly women receiving HRT. This probably reflects boosting the immune system. However, there were also some confusing results.

The increase in strokes that was seen in one arm of this study occurred in females who were more than ten years postmenopausal and had not received any hormones prior to the start of replacement therapy. Tissue changes that occur in this time period from lack of hormone stimulation may play a part. It takes healthy tissue to allow a response to estrogen. It is important to maintain continuous chemical balance.

In addition, hormones used in this study were not bioidentical but consisted of synthetic progesterone and an estrogen derivative from a pregnant mare urine. The increase in breast cancer seen in one portion of the study is a gray area when trying to make firm conclusions. It is important to use bioidentical hormones with careful monitoring of overall health. Women also need some testosterone, and this can be compounded with an estrogen cream. Donna's cancerous nodules seemed to respond better when she used progesterone.

As far as male hormone replacement, it is interesting to note that in age-related groups of men today, compared to the 1950s, the testosterone levels in the 1950s group were 35% higher. This either means that we are not as much "men" today as in the past, or is a reflection of chemical exposure in our current environment to substances that mimic estrogen (xenoestrogens), as well as other toxins. Testosterone can be metabolized to estrogen in a process known as aromatization. This occurs with increasing body fat, so obesity encourages much of the naturally produced testosterone to be converted to estrogen. The result is feminine-type symptoms, such as a further increase in body fat around the hips and waist. A vicious cycle has started.

Another aspect that needs to be considered is the fact that the organ with the most testosterone receptors in the body is not "that little guy between our legs" but the heart. Heart health in men is closely related to testosterone levels.

Many male patients with adult-onset diabetes are also found to have low testosterone levels. Boosting testosterone does not cure the diabetes, but improved sugar metabolism may allow simplifying the medications used in management. Some trace elements, such as chromium, are also helpful.

Testosterone replacement is not expensive and costs about $25 per month. As far as the prostate cancer scare with testosterone, I refer you to Abraham Morgentaler's work in my dissertation. He actually found an increased incidence of prostate cancer in testosterone-deficient men. The important aspect is maintaining an even physiologic level with appropriate monitoring. Improved immune function may also play a part. There is no quick fix, and HRT should be viewed as a process. There is safety and benefit in hormone optimization.

Congestive heart failure (poor pumping ability) is one of the more common conditions leading to hospitalization of patients. There may be a slow accumulation of toxins causing a chemical imbalance that affects the function of heart muscle. Hormone deficiency can play a part. Besides considering the importance of testosterone in heart disease, growth hormone has been shown to improve the contractile ability of heart muscle. It may be more rational to consider hormone replacement with or without other drugs as part of the treatment. The effect of calcium as far as muscle contraction will be mentioned in chelation.

Exercise has certainly been shown to benefit good health. Results of different patterns of exercise are reflected in body habitus. Compare a long-distance runner to a sprinter. The long-distance runner generates lactic acid through anaerobic activity. This type of exercise tends to use fat as an energy source. Short bursts of high-intensity output with sprinting will stimulate growth hormone and will increase lean muscle mass.

Overall, an interval, high-intensity pattern can be used with any type of exercise program, including resistance training. This should be considered when looking at personal goals. Many long-distance runners have worn-out joints and show premature aging when they hit sixty years of age. Too much exercise may generate excessive free radicals that could overwhelm the antioxidant stores in the body. Benefits from high-intensity exercise can be achieved in a matter of fifteen to twenty minutes total exercise time per day. All exercise stimulates endorphins, which chemically feed into the hormone axis. Even low-intensity exercise, such as walking, increases lymphatic flow by muscles acting as a pump, squeezing lymph fluid and blood back to the heart. We were made to be active.

All of the above are vital components to improve health, but the conventional third-party health-care system has many weaknesses that inhibit wellness programs. Generally, part of a complete longevity workup on a patient includes an extensive panel of blood to look at the metabolic and hormone status. One component is a vitamin D level. Currently, it is difficult to jump through enough hoops for the insurance companies to approve paying for a vitamin D level.

Why are these tests important? There are several silent markers that, if abnormal, can be addressed before symptoms arise. Practicing in the Midwest, I have had a lot of patients, such as farmers and ranchers, with extensive sun exposure over the years. Some of these appeared to be patients for life as they returned time and again with precancerous skin changes or skin cancers. As part of a wellness program, I began to draw vitamin D levels and many times found blood levels that were quite low despite the apparent amount of sunlight that these patients received. Boosting vitamin D levels definitely improved the status of their skin, with resultant decreased skin breakdown and lowered incidence of skin cancer. This emphasizes the importance of vitamin D in skin healing and repair.

Do we hide from the sun that is provided for us? There is a proper balance. Ravaging the skin is not good but energy from the sun is part of the natural world. Ultraviolet exposure itself promotes vitamin D synthesis in the skin. There has to be some other benefit since depression has been shown to be higher in patients deprived of certain levels of sunlight for an extended period of time. This is related to melatonin secretion—another hormone. Also, the chemical structure of vitamin D is made up of a steroid ring similar to other hormones. Can you begin to see the complexity?

Other benefits from vitamin D on cardiovascular health and cancer prevention have been shown. This may be the result of the ability of vitamin D to decrease inflammation, such as an inhibition of the oxidation of fats, which form buildup in arteries.

Vitamin D is not expensive. Consider what the system is paying for treatment of skin cancers. I now see less skin cancers in patients with high-vitamin D blood levels. I have seen no evidence of vitamin D toxicity when giving up to 10,000 units per day and I try to boost levels to the 75 ng/ml-80 ng/ml. range. Look at the application of PABA as a sunscreen. There goes another chemical to be absorbed. Fernblock is a natural product that concentrates in the skin to protect from harmful effects of ultraviolet rays. We were made to be outdoors.

Insurance programs do not permit a bone mineral density in middle-aged men as a screening test. Low bone density is a silent aspect of health. Obviously, the importance is to identify the patient who is on a path to develop osteoporosis. Low bone density also represents a symptom of a chemical or hormone imbalance.

A bone mineral density test is permitted after a hip is broken. Men have a mortality rate three to four times higher than that of women when a hip fracture occurs in an osteoporotic bone. By the time the patient arrives at that point, they have lost a lot of ground, and it is almost impossible to reverse the changes. Treating bone mineral density early with significant amounts of vitamin D, possible hormone replacement therapy (testosterone in men), and appropriate combinations of mineral supplements (more than just calcium) that will be adequately absorbed is another potential aspect of a wellness program that benefits the whole system. Although it is difficult to justify to the insurance company a bone mineral density test on middle-aged men as part of a preventive health program, there is no problem paying to repair a fractured hip.

To take this a step further, blood clots are frequently seen as a complication in patients with hip fractures, presumably from immobility. I would suggest this occurrence also implies an underlying chemical imbalance that increases the coagulation properties of the blood. Increased clotting problems are also seen in smokers even in the face of normal blood tests.

Scanning the carotid arteries in the neck with ultrasound is an inexpensive and noninvasive means to evaluate the lining of the blood vessel. Eighty percent of strokes are caused by buildup in this location. Since hardening of the arteries is a systemic condition, this scan also reflects what may be occurring in other blood vessels in the body. Thickening of the inner lining (intimal thickening) is very good marker of aging. Again, in my experience I have found that it is very difficult to justify this test to the insurance companies unless the patient has already had a stroke or is having current symptoms. The horse is out of the barn.

Many people are scared that the recently passed health-care plan might ration care. The above examples show that it has been rationed for many years. I suspect that thirty years ago a group of men in suits and ties saw the money involved in health care. To share this wealth, a "health-care industry" was developed. Profits became a priority over patient care. I used to be a doctor. Now, I am a "health-care provider" for big business. Professionals become employees. Decision making is taken out of my hands.

Concerning the extensive metabolic and hormone panel that I draw as part of a wellness exam, patients have brought me the billing statement showing that their insurance companies have been charged approximately $3000 for this lab work. When copayments and non-allowable tests are factored in, many patients wind up paying $500-$600 of the bill. I am currently using a lab where this same panel can be obtained for about $600 as a cash only price. In addition, I do not have to pay one of my employees to make phone calls and fill out forms trying to jump through appropriate hoops with third-party payers. Furthermore, there is no paperwork or registration required at the hospital to draw the blood. As far as the patient is concerned, the part that they pay is the same. As far as my office is concerned, there is less employee time required. As far as the system, $2500 that previously disappeared into some black hole is now not available to support the health-care industry. I do not see an incentive from the industry standpoint to decrease this cost.

As stated earlier, there are alternative treatment modalities that are not approved by third-party payers. EDTA chelation has benefited many patients. Some of the benefit may be due to drawing heavy metals out of the body. We all have extensive exposure to these since the Industrial Revolution. As mentioned previously, high fructose corn syrup may slowly add to body stores of mercury and progressive development of a variety of subtle symptoms.

Multiple sclerosis (MS) is an elusive disease that fits in the category of an autoimmune disorder. This may be secondary to an exaggerated immune system response to a viral illness. There is a recent report showing an accumulation of iron in the tiny blood vessels in the brain in patients with MS. Some patients have shown an improvement in symptoms after chelation and detoxification using glutathione. Iron is one of the first heavy metals to be removed by EDTA chelation. Interesting! How about the detox?

I really do not want to get into the complex pathophysiology of the chelation treatments, but the cardiovascular effects are really more than just pulling calcium out of plaque buildup inside arteries. For example, too much calcium inside a cell may affect its function. In heart muscles, this can alter the ability for contraction, as well as increase oxygen demand, of the cell. A common heart and blood pressure medication is called a "calcium channel blocker." These affect the so-called "calcium pump" in muscle cells to achieve results. Chelation may balance calcium levels inside and outside the cell and accomplish the same thing as these drugs.

Chelation increases the secretion of parathormone, which is involved with calcium balance and bone growth. As such, it may also play a significant role in treating osteoporosis. Chelation to stimulate improved bone density is overlooked along with providing adequate vitamin D. I am not talking about those four hundred units of vitamin D, which is the amount usually provided with a calcium supplement, but more in the range of 5000 to 10,000 units per day. Chelation treatments are not approved by Medicare or third-party payers. Commonly prescribed for treatment of osteoporosis, bisphosphonates are covered. These are expensive drugs. Comparatively, vitamin D is cheap. There may be effective alternatives to treat osteoporosis. The fact that this is a frequently seen condition suggests a significant portion of our population has a metabolic and/or hormone imbalance.

Let me relate another observation. During my father's treatment for cancer, a bone scan showed spread of tumor to the pelvic bones. This was discovered when Dad began to have groin pain and thought he had pulled a muscle. Tumor weakens bone and there was concern he would fracture the pelvis while standing or walking since this is a major weight-bearing part of the skeletal structure. A pelvic fracture would have left him bedridden.

My father had significant underlying osteoporosis involving the vertebral (spine) bones and ribs. After treating the cancerous spot with radiation treatments, it was recommended that he receive a bisphosphonate by IV to strengthen the pelvis and prevent a fracture. Although immediately prior to this treatment a bone scan had shown tumor only in the pelvic bone, within two months a repeat scan showed spread of the tumor throughout the ribs and spine. Apparently, as the body tried to build up bone in the pelvis that was eroded by tumor, it also worked to restore bone in the most severe osteoporotic areas. Unfortunately, cancer cells were incorporated in the repair process. My father continued to teach me lessons until his death.

I am not faulting the doctors for what went on, although my father had significant bone pain and a difficult final month of his life. The thought process to attempt to strengthen bone and prevent a fracture was good. An established quality clinical pathway was followed. The point is to try to learn from this encounter. There is not a simple answer, but this example emphasizes the importance of observation to improve judgment in the care of subsequent patients. Good judgment comes from experience. Experience comes from making errors or having adverse results. Blindly following guidelines promoted by the health-care industry without individual consideration is one weakness of the current system. Physicians need to be able to use their experience and not be forced to follow established clinical pathways out of fear that they will be punished for stepping outside the box. Non-physicians can follow a cookbook. Judgement requires more. For instance, current clinical pathways for diabetes do not say anything about checking testosterone levels. The definition of insanity is doing the same thing over and over, expecting different results.

Another unapproved beneficial treatment is prolotherapy. This stands for "proliferative" therapy and consists of injection of an inexpensive combination of substances, which stimulate growth factors in tendons, soft tissue, and joints. Ozone can be added to the prolotherapy solution (called prolozone), when injected into large spaces such as joints. This adds an antiviral, antibacterial, antifungal, and antiparasitic benefit to the treatment. The ozone releases additional oxygen and provides a free oxygen molecule, serving as a scavenger which attaches to many substances that should not be in the body and promotes their elimination. Prolotherapy serves to strengthen supporting structures of the joint, such as the ligaments, and may even promote cartilage growth.

My personal experience with the use of prolotherapy involves chronic tendonitis (tennis elbow) and a lax ligament around one knee from an old injury. Since ozone cannot be injected into a ligament (there is no space for the ozone gas), I added a small amount of hydrogen peroxide to the prolotherapy solution. This resulted in intense inflammation and increased pain for about a week, with subsequent resolution of the tennis elbow pain I had for more than a year. In addition, the ligament around the knee tightened. I have been impressed by these personal results as well as those in many of my patients.

Prolotherapy is not approved by Medicare or third-party payers, but the use of cortisone for injections is permitted. If there is an inflammatory process taking place and causing damage in a joint, cortisone injections may settle down the pain, but the destructive elements of the underlying inflammatory pathway continue, and rebuilding does not occur. The result is eventual joint destruction to the point where replacement is required—a further example of an expensive treatment used and a preventive modality ignored. But the healthcare industry was developed to generate income.

Oxidation is the process by which sugar is burned for energy in our bodies. Oxidation also generates free radicals, which are harmful and need to be cleared out of our systems using antioxidants. We have covered some aspects of antioxidants in the section on vitamins and supplements. As mentioned previously, oxidation of fat is bad for us, leading to weakening of cell membranes and buildup inside blood vessels.

Oxidative therapy focuses on the use of hydrogen peroxide which breaks down to form water and oxygen. The foaming that is seen with peroxide represents the release of oxygen in this reaction. As discussed previously, vitamin C and white blood cells use hydrogen peroxide in normal body chemistry. It is a natural substance found in our systems. As such, it cannot be patented, which lessens interest from the industry standpoint.

Intravenous hydrogen peroxide has been used since 1920 in attempts to provide more oxygen for tissues to promote healing. Charles Farr in Oklahoma City began using this in 1984 for treatment of a long list of various conditions, and it is now utilized in more than fifty countries. Why have you not heard of the availability? Insurance companies will not pay for medical services or care, which they do not classify as "usual and customary." Usual and customary means that most physicians provide the same service or treatment. The average physician is not educated about oxidative therapy. I know I did not hear about this in medical school. Therefore, coverage for this service is denied by insurance. Are there benefits? No doctor is going to spend his time to look at this if he has no way to be reimbursed.

I was also told in medical school that chiropractors were quacks. Patients have been sent to me because of swelling in one leg or a cold or discolored extremity. After I ruled out a serious circulation problem, I found that many of these patients resolved their problem after a visit to the chiropractor. Structure somehow must play a part that interferes with lymphatic flow and leads to swelling. Nerve endings affected by a structural problem might lead to a cool or discolored limb because these nerve endings go to tiny blood vessels, which then dilate or constrict causing these signs.

When my son was in sixth grade, he woke up one morning with a swollen knee. He did not remember any injury or event that might have caused this. The orthopedic doctor recommended crutches to relieve weight bearing. Cory was a good athlete, and after two weeks he was in my face to find some way to make him better. He next underwent an arthroscopy (looking into the joint with a scope) and had fluid drawn off his knee. Nothing abnormal was found. He was told to continue crutches and take ibuprofen. Two more weeks went by. I was going to kill him or he was going to kill me. We then went to see a rheumatoid specialist. The doctor came into the room and told us he had good news. This was not rheumatoid arthritis. I asked him about the diagnosis. He told me it was "idiopathic monoarticular arthritis," which means "His knee is swollen, and we don't know why." His recommendations: continue crutches and take ibuprofen.

At this point Cory was almost in tears. He wanted back into sports and to be a normal thirteen-year-old boy. I took him to the chiropractor who examined my son and said, "Cory, you must've taken a pretty good lick on the football field. One side of your pelvis is locked up." Corey underwent an adjustment, and within two days, the swelling of the knee, which had been present for eight weeks, was gone. Apparently this was related to structure. I learned something and soon developed a good relationship with many chiropractors. This is only one example of similar results I have seen over the years.

CAT scans and expensive imaging techniques are replacing a careful history and physical exam in the evaluation of patients. I was taught that if you listen to a patient 85% of the time they will give you the diagnosis. The system reimburses for procedures, not physician time and judgment. Simple treatment that requires lifestyle changes is not acceptable to many patients. These are not comfortable and take time to see results. Short-term Band-Aids with instant relief are preferred. Also, think high tech. Some of my patients request a CAT scan as if it were the diagnostic machine seen on Star Trek. The x-ray exposure from a full chest, abdominal, and pelvic CAT scan is equivalent to five hundred chest x-rays and eight years of normal background irradiation. Can this cause DNA damage? The threshold to affect or break genes may be lower depending on underlying chemical balance.

CAT scans routinely used to diagnose appendicitis in young patients can deliver a dangerous dose of radiation. Physician judgment may not be perfect with the preoperative diagnosis of appendicitis confirmed at operation in 95% of patients using clinical judgment alone. However, CAT scans are not perfect and can also miss appendicitis in addition to adding x-ray exposure and expense to the evaluation. Again, what balance are we willing to accept?

One of the most important elements of Donna's recovery has to do with spirituality. As mentioned in the dissertation, this is certainly an aspect that is difficult to quantify or identify quality. However, spirituality involves personal responsibility and the capacity to change in dealing with life's stresses. This personal responsibility is seen in many patients, who take supplements, since they also tend to change other aspects of their lifestyle.

My grandmother used to say if you start the day by opening your eyes, it is already a good day. She also told me to begin with "Good morning, God." If it was "Good God, it's morning" an attitude adjustment was needed.

Patients comment that my life as a surgeon must be stressful. To me, it is no more stressful than what occurs on a daily basis for most people. What is important is to do your best and tackle life one moment at a time. If the present is not handled properly, everything that follows will contribute additional stress. It is essential not to create our own difficulties. My brother once told me, "If you enjoy what you do, then you never work another day in your life." Unfortunately, surveys have shown that 70% of Americans do not like their job.

What is difficult for me to accept when dealing with cancer is the statement, "There is nothing further we can do." How about addressing the patient's fears? How about communicating with the patient and family regarding what to expect and potential comfort measures? How about giving the patient a hug or holding their hand? These measures cannot be evaluated in the lab or with sophisticated imaging techniques, but I am convinced they play a part in health and well-being.

I know this is not a complete synopsis on healthy living. There are many other detailed sources available. I look at the road to better health as a journey—one step at a time. There are no magic bullets. It is difficult to do everything at once. We are not changing oil in a car. In dealing with patients, I attempt to reach certain goals and then change the game plan as overall health changes and a new level is achieved.

I want this book to begin to help direct patients in their search for prolonging health and longevity. The comments are my current opinion and can change as I continue to review more literature and gain more experience with observations.

I hope you are inspired by Donna's story. I hope you find the scientific analysis interesting. I hope this arouses your curiosity about the function of "the human machine."

SECTION II

Donna Elizabeth Storrer
Bibliography

Donna was born in Wheeling, West Virginia, in 1947. After graduating from McGuffey Joint Junior/Senior High School, she worked in the Air Force as a military supply clerk for two years, ten months, and sixteen days. There she met her husband, Jerry, and they moved to Kansas in 1968. Donna attended college for one and a half years and then worked outside the home for eleven years. The next twenty-two years were spent homeschooling four children. They currently live in a remodeled rural schoolhouse, Harmony Hill School. Their bedroom is on the stage of the old gymnasium. She works outside the home as head cook in the food service at Logan Avenue Elementary School. She and Jerry have enjoyed forty-three years of married life and also have five grandchildren. They enjoy summers in their cabin in the mountains near Rocky Mountain National Park.

Living Well with Stage III Cancer

(Despite the Medical Experts)

Donna E. Storrer

Contents

This book is dedicated to my husband, Jerry, for all his support and love; to Dr. Joe for all his support and open-minded care; and to all the people who brought forth my name in prayer before the Lord.

Preface

I did not start out to write a book about my cancer journey, so much as to vent my feelings of fear, anger, betrayal, injustice and confusion. I started out with the conventional—standard—American College of Surgeons, NCI, AMA, and FDA recommendations for my cancer treatment program. It was not long before the Lord helped me to realize that much money was being made off of my cancer and that much harm was being done to my body. The Lord showed me that if I continued on with the standard medical treatment for my cancer, even more damage was going to be done to my body and mind. I picked up all the booklets and pamphlets put out by the NCI and the American College of Surgeons on cancer treatment. One of the pamphlets titled "Questionable Methods of Cancer Treatment," by the American College of Surgeons, stated on page three that "Fear and desperation drive many people to try methods of cancer management that are promoted to the public despite lack of real evidence that they are safe and effective." *Fear* and *desperation* are exactly what drove me to try the standard method of cancer management promoted by the medical community, despite its horrible track records of mutilation, maiming, and debilitation.

Some may argue that the mutilating surgery that I went through gave me a better chance to try an alternative route. Perhaps the mastectomy may have helped in taking the tumor load off initially, but the side effect of having my lymph nodes routinely torn out was a serious consequence—of ignorance personally and medically—that I will have to deal with the rest of my life, and the surgery may have helped spread the cancer as more tumors appeared within a couple of months of the mastectomy.

Many cancer patients survive traditional treatments just because of their "strong will to live," or their belief (placebo) that mutilating, burning, and poisoning will rid their bodies of cancer. (Anne and David Frahm, who wrote the book, *A Cancer Battle Plan*, felt that her life was saved due to standard treatments, but David immediately started her on juicing therapy after standard treatments sent her home to die. The Lord had shown him the need to build up her immune system, which had been thoroughly destroyed by all of the standard cancer treatments.)

In the past fifteen years, I have personally witnessed the death of loved ones who were persuaded to undergo traditional treatment for their cancers; they were told by the experts that they got it all, only to find out in a very short time span that the cancer was back again—bigger and faster growing than ever! Even though I was not told that they got it all, I was told that statistically I only had about a year if I did not have six months of aggressive chemo followed by radiation. The Lord—the Great Physician—said differently; for it has now been fifteen fantastic, full, fun and sometimes frustrating years living well with a Stage III cancer diagnosis (the credit goes to the Lord's biological immunotherapy program).

The American College of Surgeons claims that "Use of these (alternative) approaches can divert people from effective treatment and cause physical, emotional, and financial harm." (Does anyone in their right mind believe that no physical, emotional, and financial harm is done with the standard "approved" methods of cancer treatment?)

The American College of Surgeons "urges consumers, health professionals, educators, journalists, legislators, and law enforcement officials to become knowledgeable about questionable methods of cancer management and take action to curb their use." I urge everyone to become knowledgeable about *all* methods of cancer management and to take action to curb the attempts to take away the people's right to choose their own health-care management. Sadly, many people choose traditional treatments simply because their insurance companies will not pay for anything not sanctioned by the American College of Surgeons or the FDA—even though an alternative therapy may be less expensive and may allow a more productive life due to a treatment that gives quality of life. We are all created as unique individuals with unique and individual health needs.

With all the pollutants and chemicals bombarding us daily in our air, food, and water supplies, and with a medical community pushing drugs (and their many side effects to compromise our health even more), it is more important than ever that people take a more active role in their own health-care management if they want better health because neither our government nor our medical-pharmaceutical community will put our health before their own interests.

There are many fine and wonderful people involved in medical and health care, but human greed has corrupted many organizations that were founded on the concept of helping to better mankind. It is up to each individual to educate, research, and pray about the kind of medical care they want and or need.

Chapter 1

In the Drama of Life, God is The Director Behind the Scenes

December 20, 2008

Fifteen years ago today (December 20, 1993), we were sitting at the supper table when the phone rang.

"Good evening," I answered.

"Is this Donna?" asked the voice on the other end. "This is Dr. Joe."

"Yes, it is, Dr. Joe," I answered somewhat nervously.

"Donna, I got the results back on today's biopsy, and the results aren't good," he said softly and compassionately.

"Cancer?" I asked, as tears filled my eyes. I was looking at my husband, Jerry, and three of our four children sitting around the table. They were looking and listening to every word.

"I'm afraid so. I would like to see you and your husband on the twenty-second to discuss what you want to do. Just call the office for the time schedule."

"All right, Dr. Joe," I mechanically answered, trying to keep my emotions under some form of control. "Thank you for taking the time to call. We will see you on the twenty-second."

Jerry came over to me, and we just held each other. We still had three children in home school. Our oldest son had moved out three months earlier to discover the world of reality for himself. We still wanted to own a piece of Colorado. We had no time for cancer. There were too many things that we still wanted to do.

We were not shocked at the news, but disappointed. It was disappointing to have our fears confirmed. The left breast itself had been preparing us for nearly seventeen years when the first lumps appeared. Six to eight months before the diagnosis, an eyeball exam showed obvious problems.

My home church pastor said that he did not believe in accidents. I did not either, but we don't always listen to our "little voice inside."

Books had been brought into our lives in 1976, regarding cancer and the cancer industry, but we had just put them in our personal library for future reading, some day.

Jerry and I had been too busy trying to save our eight-year-old marriage to really be concerned about cancer. We had been classic examples of pure selfishness and materialism.

I had suffered with chronic yeast infections for years, possibly because I had been on birth control pills nearly eight years before I got pregnant in 1975 with our first child, Ryan. I had been selfishly content without children when I suddenly decided that I wasn't being fair to Jerry if he wanted a child. My doctor had said that it might take a couple of years before I could become pregnant after being on birth control pills for so many years. At the age of twenty-eight, I did not feel that I could delay pregnancy much longer if Jerry wanted a baby. We had gotten into a bad habit of double communication (not expressing our true feelings but saying what we thought the other wanted to hear).

When I asked Jerry if he would like to have a baby, he thought that it was not fair to deny me a baby just because he had no desire to be a father. So, he assured me, "It sounds okay to me."

Two weeks later, I had the worst case of flu that I had ever experienced. About the time I decided to go to the doctor, it was suddenly over. As long as I had been on the birth control pills, I had been very regular with my periods, but again, I was told by my doctor that I probably be off schedule for a few months. However, I knew by my tight-fitting clothes three to four months later that I was pregnant.

The pregnancy was normal as was the delivery, except for my reaction to the standard drug relaxant given to me when I reached a certain dilation size. I went into another world on a high trip and left reality behind. Naturally, the Lamaze classes for a drug-free delivery were of no value since I was not able to relate to the idea of labor or delivery. My reaction had been similar in the past when I had been given pain medication for smashed fingers (ten years before Ryan's birth), and when I had been given Darvon for wisdom teeth extractions (eight years before Ryan's birth). I had told the obstetricians of my reactions, but either the nursing staff ignored the warning, or the doctors felt it was of no importance. These were the only times that I had ever had any medications other than aspirin.

About six weeks after Ryan's birth, the selfishness and immaturity of our marriage "hit the rocks." Even though I found myself in a love-hate relationship with Jerry, I did not want our baby to grow up in a split home. I had discovered the miracle of life that God gives when a child is born, and I also discovered that I did believe there was a God in charge of the universe. I found myself praying, "Dear God, if you will give me a marriage with love, I will give you my life." That was a prayer bargain that God took me up on, even though there are folks who do not believe that anyone can bargain with God. Perhaps it depends on the bargain being made.

Our marriage was slowly but surely getting stronger by the time our second child, Michelle, was born in 1977. After my horrible hospital experience of adverse drug reactions during Ryan's birth, I chose to deliver Michelle in a birthing clinic. Delivery was drug free and normal until time to get the placenta out. The placenta would not release, so I was transported by ambulance to an osteopathic hospital, where I underwent quite an ordeal. I had to have three pints of blood before the placenta could be torn out piece by piece. Due to my lungs starting to collapse, I could not be put under anesthesia. I was given a local injection to try to hold down the pain as much as possible. When a brusque Dr. Came into the room and looked at me, he suddenly yelled to a nurse, "Get stocking on her right away!"

I asked—in what I thought was a normal voice—"Don't you like hairy legs?"

He bent his ear down to my lips and said, "I'm sorry, I couldn't hear. Could you repeat what you said?"

So, I said again, "Don't you like hairy legs?"

He laughed, put his hand on my hand and said, "Honey, your hairy legs are beautiful. It's the blue color that I don't like! The stockings will warm your legs." He went on to add in a very soft voice, "You are in the basement right now, and I'm not sure we are going to be able to pull you out."

I remember ignorantly praying to God, "I guess I'm ready to meet you if I die, but I don't think it's fair to bring a little girl into this world without a mommy to help her."

God, in His mercy and grace, probably shook His head in sadness at my stubborn ignorance of His ways. I had been reading the Bible faithfully since I had made the bargain with God about a marriage with love. I knew of His Son, Jesus Christ, but had never acknowledged my need of a Savior for my sins. I had become frustrated as I tried to live by The Ten Commandments. It seemed as if I was breaking some of them every day. I just wasn't able to be good enough to live by God's laws. I certainly recognized everyone else's sins, and their need to be forgiven by Jesus, but not my own need of Him. To my foolish way of thinking, I was as good, if not better, than most.

Needless to say, God knew I was not ready to meet Him, yet, so He blessed the doctor's valiant attempt to save my life. The good doctor told Jerry and I that I would probably not have a period for a year or more, and that I would probably never be able to have any more children. Since Jerry and I had the perfect family of a boy and a girl, that news was not heartbreaking for us.

I had breastfed Ryan for only eight weeks before putting him on formula so I could go back to work, and so I could appease the pediatrician who had a fit over Ryan's loss of a pound of his birth weight.

"What are you trying to do, starve the baby to death?" She demanded.

Jerry and I were stunned, as Ryan had been a very happy, contented baby, and he had even slept four to six hours straight during the night. Common sense should have told us that Ryan was doing great, but we ignorantly listened to the so-called expert on babies!

Well, I was determined that I would have plenty of milk for Michelle, so I started pumping my beasts to insure a good milk supply for her. By the time I got home from the hospital, I had enough milk for twins. Michelle was a good nurser, but she could not begin to drink all the milk I was producing, so I pumped to get relief. I did not realize at the time that pumping was the wrong thing to do. For the first time in my life, I had cleavage (age thirty), but I was in absolute pain and agony. My armpits were so lumpy that I walked around with my arms outstretched. My breasts were as hard as bricks.

My family doctor told me to quit pumping and let the milk supply meet Michelle's demand—they would soon match. After more than two weeks of continual pain, I asked the doctor to help me dry up as I could no longer tolerate any more pain. I put Michelle on formula and felt like a total failure as a good mother and a first-class wimp!

I started my period within a couple of months after Michelle's birth. I continued having lumpy breasts and armpits, but with the arrival of the irregular periods, I would get relief from the pains, and the lumps would go down. I went to a couple of doctors about the lumps, but they felt that the mammary glands were the problem—no need to concern myself with thoughts of cancer as cancerous lumps would not rise and fall as my lumps were doing! So, why bother reading the books we had about cancer?

In the meantime, Jerry and I were still working on our marriage. I was having a difficult time forgetting the hurts of the past years, even with dealing with life going on. One day it all came to me as a gentle breeze would. I was kneeling at the bedside trying to pray to God, but the past was burdening me to the point of weeping. A little voice inside me seemed to be saying, "Donna, you recognize others' need of a Savior, yet even though you daily break the commandments, you have not accepted the fact that you need saved from your sins, too. 'No man cometh to the Father, but by Me.'" I humbly asked Jesus to forgive my sins and to become the Lord of my life. I received a peace that passed all understanding.

Of course, the trials of life continued. About the time Ryan was six and one-half years old and Michelle was four and one-half years old, the lumps were quite active, and at times, sharp, shooting pains would stab through my chest. One night I went into the children's bedrooms and cried, because I just knew that I probably had cancer and might not get to raise them.

Since I had Jesus as my Savior, I felt no fear for my life. I feared what would become of my wonderful family.

Chapter 2

Pray First

Did I get busy and read to start taking action against cancer? No, I did not! I had a far greater fear of my traditional cancer treatments due to watching my grandfather and other family members die slowly and miserably with the various cancers they had. I refused to openly acknowledge my cancer fears, but I did pray, "Lord, please speak to me clearly as to when I need to get serious about cancer."

In 1983, I became pregnancy with our third child, Jeremiah. The lumps and the sharp, shooting pains in my breasts and underarms disappeared. I agreed to another hospital birth, but in a birthing room only and with no drugs. The pregnancy and delivery were great, even at the age of thirty-six! We attended church, as usual, the evening that Jeremiah decided to make his entrance into this world. The labor pains started in the afternoon, but I was not about to rush to the hospital to just lie around all night. I did not say anything to Jerry, but during the service I took hold of his hand. Each time a labor pain hit me, I just squeezed Jerry's hand. When the service ended, our pastor came back to see what was wrong with Jerry. We told him that we were heading directly to the hospital. He said to Jerry, "I noticed some pretty painful expressions on your face, but when I looked at Donna, she was sitting with a very calm countenance, so I didn't know what was going on." The delivery was just as easy as possible. I was in the hospital a little over an hour before Jeremiah safely arrived. It was a fantastic experience—no drugs, no complications, no freezing delivery, no retained placenta, and no extended pains.

Jeremiah was a very strong nurser and extremely demanding—every two hours or less. After two weeks of breast feeding Jeremiah, the doctor and I both knew that I would have to have to supplement him as he seemed to be constantly hungry. So, after nursing him on both breasts for thirty minutes or better, I offered him formula. To my utter chagrin, he drank an entire eight ounce bottle of formula in fifteen minutes. He then went to sleep for five straight hours! When he awoke, and I offered him the breast instead of the bottle, we had a royal battle of the wills. Poor Jerry was about to lose his mind over hearing both of us cry. By the third day, Jeremiah won, as I developed 'milk fever' and had to go on antibiotics. It was then that I decided that just because God made women able to bear children and produce milk to feed them, did *not* mean that all women could or would do either. If she can, great. If she cannot, then praise God that she lives in a country that has the scientific knowledge to make healthy formulas for a healthy baby. I told Jerry and the Lord that for something so normal and natural, I hadn't found it to be so easy.

The lumpy breasts did not return until a few weeks after our fourth child, Deborah, was born in 1984. I had a tubal ligation the day after her birth. I was turning thirty-eight years old within four months. The pregnancy had been normal until the seventh and one-half month. We started getting extremely fast heartbeats. I had a weekly sonogram until she was born. The caring Dr. Did not want to deliver her in a birthing for fear of complications. He wanted better light and more room to maneuver around. I wanted a warm room and Jerry free to come and go. We compromised with my wearing knee socks and the door to the delivery room remaining open so the range of motion wouldn't be so cold. Jerry was free to come and go, as his nausea allowed him.

I had gone into the hospital too soon, so my labor was ten hours long. I was attached to a heart monitor and Deb's heart rate was so fast at times that the dial would go off the paper and a loud beeper would go off. I was at seven centimeters when my Dr. Came in with another man. When I discovered that the other man was not a doctor, but a nurse, I freaked out! My modesty was offended! No one had asked me how I felt about having a male nurse. The seven centimeters dilation dropped back to five centimeters (that is a strong indicator of how much the mind can control the body). I started crying and would not talk to Jerry or anyone about my problem with a male nurse. A wise head nurse soon noticed that I became stressed every time I saw the male nurse, so she sent him on a lengthy errand. My dilation then took off, and Deb was safely delivered.

For three months after Deb was born, we took weekly trips to Wichita (eighty-one miles away) to see a heart specialist. He said that Deb had an extra nerve causing the problem. Since her heart was starting to enlarge from the hard work of beating so fast, he put her on heart medication to slow down the rate. She slept most of the time. She would awaken four times in a twenty-four-hour span for feeding. She would nurse off me then drink about two ounces of formula after nursing. Within a few weeks, my milk production dried up. The lumpy armpits and breasts came back after the return of my period. I was not concerned that I might have cancer any more. I figured the lumps had to do with the hormones put into my system from female babies, but the hormones did not get into my system from male babies. I had nothing scientific to back up that belief, nor could I ever remember reading any such thing. I just put the lumps and sudden sharp pains in the Lord's care. I did not plan on forking over hard-earned dollars for more doctors to tell me that it was mammary glands acting up. After all, I had dealt with the lumps and pains for five busy years before Jeremiah's birth, so I figured, I could do it again.

I did deal with the continually rising and falling lumps and pains for another busy nine years. I was tired all the time, but I figured that home schooling four active children could keep anyone tired. I had been having hot flashes off and on since age thirty-five, therefore I felt that a lot of my body's fatigue and hormone problems were menopausal.

There was no history of breast cancer in my family, but plenty of other cancers abounded, since I came from a family of smokers. I had never read anything to indicate that cancers could be transferred in blood transfusions, yet cancer cells *do* get into the bloodstream. I was far from obese, but certainly could have afforded to lose a few pounds in the hips. In general, I did not feel endangered. Being tired constantly, yet able to function and care for my family just seemed to be a normal thing. We had an acre of ground to be mowed, trees to be trimmed, a large garden to care for, four very active children and their playmate friends to watch after, church and homeschooling activities, and all the other responsibilities involved in caring for a family. It was just normal to be so tired.

We were also involved in patriotic activities, involving writing letters to our congressmen about various issues affecting our country. We were having a hard time trying to understand how our government was always making deals with other countries that helped those countries, while those same deals hurt our countrymen. It seemed to us that our government was not looking out for the welfare of its own people.

Chapter 3

Without Christ, We're Not Ready to Die; With Christ, We have Every Reason to Live

On December 22, 1993, we had a $70 consultation with Dr. Joe. He was the surgeon that did my left breast biopsy. The nipple had pulled into the breast and was secreting a smelly liquid, so there had been no guesswork involved as to where to do the biopsy. We did not discuss a lumpectomy at all; just a mastectomy. Dr. Joe said that he would do a right-breast biopsy before doing the left, modified radical mastectomy. He would send the biopsy to the lab immediately, and if the rest was cancers, he would remove both breasts.

Jerry made it clear that cancer on location would be the only reason for the loss of either breast. He saw no reason for unnecessary mutilation. Even though my breasts had been lumpy and hard for several years, Jerry knew they were a part of my feeling good about myself. If Jerry had been a "breast man," he certainly would not have married a size 32AA gal!

On December 23, 1991, an eight-and-one-half-centimeter malignant tumor was removed with the left breast. The thickened tissue in the right breast was benign. My body had reacted differently to the two different biopsies. The left breast had become swollen, red, and angry-looking, plus it hemorrhaged. The right breast felt as if nothing had ever happened to it. I do not know if the antibiotic that I had been put on before surgery (due to a bladder infection showing up in the urinalysis) was responsible for the physical reaction differences in the two biopsies or not. When the left breast tissue was examined by the pathologist, it was found to not only have the eight-

and-one-half-centimeter tumor under the nipple, but the tumor was completely surrounded with all kinds of benign lumps and tumors possible in a breast. It was no wonder that I was hard and lumpy!

Even though the right breast was hard and lumpy too, no cancer was found. However, it did occur to me that if the surgeon had done the left biopsy in the same location as he did the right breast, it was likely that no cancer would have been found in it either, since the tumor had been under the nipple, not out in the outer quadrants. The Lord had given us clear-cut signs with the retracted nipple, leakage, and odor.

During the mastectomy surgery, Dr. Joe removed fourteen lymph nodes that were found negative of cancer cells. I was never told that the lymph nodes would be jerked out as a standard procedure. If I had known how integral the lymph nodes are to the immune system, I would not have allowed any such procedure, but I was not an informed person—my own fault for ignoring the cancer books sitting on my personal library shelves.

After the first biopsy, I had been given Vicodin for pain. After taking just one tablet, I spent several hours low to the floor, nauseated and dizzy. For the three days that I was in the hospital, I felt fine, but did have two nasty reactions. Apparently, the valium given to me before surgery to relax me caused a bad case of hives. I was given an injection to treat the hives. As soon as the nurse left the room, Jerry's mom went to say something to me when she noticed I was having difficulty breathing and holding up my head. Mom immediately ran after the nurse. The nurse rushed back in, looked at me, and said, "What's wrong with you?"

"I don't know," I said, "Don't feel so good . . . feel sick . . . dizzy."

The nurse reached into a pocket of her uniform jacket and brought forth another needle for another injection. I just lay in the chair too weak to object or ask questions. In a few minutes, I could lift my head. Within ten minutes, I was back to normal. I never did find out what two injections were, specifically. I thought about what might have happened if Mom had not been there.

I did fine on the 325 milligrams of oxycodone HCL 5 m for pain after the mastectomy.

It was the first Christmas that our family had not had a large gathering or been at a large gathering. It was a scary time for them—I have regretted my foolish fear and panic that motivated me to rush into surgery. No one was pushing me. I could have done some research for a couple of days or weeks to learn what options I might have had. Instead, I panicked. I wanted that treacherous breast removed immediately. I did not seek the Lord's direction, guidance, or perfect will. The only thought I had for my family was: "How are they going to manage without me."

On December 28, I had the drainage tubes and the right biopsy staples removed. I was weak, but not in any pain or physical discomfort. My head was still in a whirl, and I could not keep tuned in to any particular thought except, "What next?"

The mastectomy staples were removed on January 4, 1994. Dr. Joe expressed concern about the lumpy masses in the right breast, so he ordered bone and liver scans to be done on me. I did not like the liquids that I had to drink, but the technician that operated the bone scan equipment was a delightful character. His name was similar to a favorite cookie enjoyed by most children. He asked questions to get me thinking about other things besides my cancer. He shared things going on in his own life. He had positive feelings about life in general, even though he had just undergone surgery and was moving about with extreme care. He wasn't stiffly professional, but radiated warmth and caring as did Dr. Joe.

Of course, my body reacted to the nuclear medicine that I had been given to drink for the scan. I spent the next six days near a toilet as the diarrhea kept me moving quickly. The only other time that I remembered having such severe diarrhea was when I picked up a bug in my digestive tract (giardiasis, caused by drinking contaminated water). We had put our pop cans in a beaver stream for cooling purposes. Even though we wiped the cans off before drinking from them, it wasn't clean enough for my system (that bug was with me for several months).

Chapter 4

The Right Kind of Fear
Prompts Us to Do Right

On January 18, 1994, I had a $166 consultation with Dr. C, the local chemotherapy oncologist. He barely looked at my face and my body not at all. He spent most of the forty-five minutes reading my surgery and pathology reports that had been in his office for over a week. Dr. C pushed for six months of aggressive adjuvant therapy (Adriamycin-based or Mitoxontrane-based Systemic Chemotherapy). He also pushed for local radiotherapy to the operative field—left upper chest—because the deep margins of my section were not clear of tumor. Dr. C then proceeded to push for an oophorectomy (the removal of the ovaries to stop estrogen production). Since estrogen feeds breast cancer, he felt that he could control the amount of estrogen in my body better with hormone replacement therapy (HRT) for the rest of my life, whereas, my ovaries natural estrogen could not be controlled. Admittedly, my ovaries functioned irregularly, but they did function. I had the philosophy, "If it isn't broken, don't try to fix it."

I explained my fear of chemotherapy due to my body's prior reactions to ordinary drugs. He believed that the adverse reactions to the various medical drugs that I had taken before were just perceived as drug sensitivities on my part. Dr. C felt that we needed to give the chemo a try and then go from there if it did not work. I disagreed emphatically. Jerry was getting the feeling that the doctor was not listening or did not care. Jerry backed me completely on no chemo at this time, even though I was classified Stage III cancer. We all three agreed on getting a second opinion and starting me on Tamoxifen (ten milligrams, twice daily). I had heard and read pretty good reports on it from the news media and had not heard of any bad side effects. The Dr. Did say that it would throw me into full-blown menopause, but there would be no vaginal dryness or osteoporosis. Dr. C indicated that I had very high risk of local and systemic recurrence due to my margins not being clear of tumor.

I took my first Tamoxifen tablet that night at bedtime. During the night, I was awakened with horrible stomach cramps, nausea, and barely made it to the toilet before vomiting. The next morning, I tried the dosage again. In a couple of hours, I was sick again. I believed that the drug was good for me, so I cut the dosage in half. It worked, and I was satisfied that it would battle my breast cancer.

On February 4, 1994 (the day before my forty-seventh birthday), I had my second opinion with Dr. D in Wichita. Prior to my $194 consultation with him, he had requested a whole life medical history on myself and any drugs taken by me. After examining me, Dr. D expressed that I was only taking one half of the prescribed Tamoxifen dosage. The mastectomy was well healed. Since I had a difficult tolerating any type of meds whether oral or IV in the past, with significant reactions, this to some degree, had an effect on his overall recommendations for my care.

The left chest wall showed no evidence of any gross tumor, but small lumps on the staple sites were noticeable to me. Dr. D felt it would be literally impossible to get me through six months of adjuvant chemo. However, he did want me to really try to go full dose on the Tamoxifen. Each time I tried, the results were as before. I was not able to make any headway and was disappointed, because I believed the Tamoxifen would help me fight the breast cancer.

Dr. D had insisted that I see a radiation oncologist also. He made an appointment for me to see one that was in the same cancer treatment building as he was located in. Jerry and I discussed the eighty-five mile trip to Wichita every day for six to eight weeks, versus a sixty-mile trip to Topeka every day for the same time frame. We opted for Topeka since we knew the daily trip would take its toll on me even if I had not had cancer. Jerry had made that daily trek for three months when he was assigned to Forbes Air Force Base after his return from Vietnam in 1969, and it had taken quite a toll on his energy level then.

Since we did not have the money for an apartment or motel for me to stay in while undergoing the radiation treatments, that option was out. Even if we had had the finances, I am not sure that I could have handled being away from my family for more than a couple of days.

On February 16, 1994, I had a $289 consultation with Dr. J in Topeka. I was delighted to finally get a female doctor at last—it was a short-lived delight. Her first words: "It's too bad you had the breast removed first. I would have been better to radiate the tumor in the breast, then have it surgically removed. Now some damage to the heart and lungs could occur with the radiation treatments."

Jerry and I were stunned as it immediately reflected poorly on our lack of knowledge and the other doctors that we had been dealing with. We had been relying on the doctors to know the best and latest breakthroughs in cancer treatments, instead of relying on ourselves to research all cancer treatments before doing anything. We justified this belief with the high prices charged for our consultations, surgeries, tests, and medications.

Dr. J did a thorough examination (pelvic, rectal, and breast) as well as questioning my health background. I was feeling good, but I told her (as I had Dr. D) that my arm bones and muscles hurt all the time. I had noticed that when I tried increasing the Tamoxifen, the pain increased in my arm and axillary area. With the smaller dose of drug, the pain was more manageable. Her answer was about the same as Dr. D's. "It is probably due to the mastectomy surgery and some nerve damage. It should pass in time. Try to increase the Tamoxifen."

Dr. J discussed radiation treatments with us. She told us the good and the bad effects, and we discussed the differences between cobalt and brachytherapy. She had me start "porting" that same day after Jerry and I agreed that the brachytherapy might be the best way to go as it was just surface application. Cobalt would have clipped my heart and lungs, even though the Dr. D did not feel that the damage would clinically significant. Since my heart and lungs were in excellent working order, I told her that we did not want to do anything to hurt them. I had already experienced (in 1990) an episode of walking pneumonia that had taken me nearly five months to get over, and I was not anxious to experience lung problems again. It had taken three different antibiotics (with the third one being repeated) before I was able to function normally again in being able to talk to people without continually hacking in their face or ear. It may not have been clinically significant to the medical world, but it certainly was life altering to me in my communication with others, even if it did not hospitalize me.

Jerry and I were at Dr. J's for three and one-half hours for questions, exams, and porting (being set up with x-rays and lead plates to protect areas from exposure to the penetrating rays). Dr. J was thoroughly professional and slightly brusque. She said that there was no evidence of local recurrence. I pointed out a tiny lump that had arisen not long after the drainage tubes were removed. The lump was located above the drainage tube scar.

She answered my statement with, "Patients with breast cancer think every little pimple is a cancer tumor." (In March 1995, this "pimple" proved to be more cancer.)

I went back to see Dr. Joe on February 17, 1994. He was happy that I was going to have radiation treatments because he too felt that I would have recurring cancer without further treatment than surgery. He told me about one of his patients who had taken vitamin C and beta-carotene in large doses while undergoing radiation for breast cancer. He had been surprised by her lack of side effects with the radiation. She had no seeping cracks or dry cracks. It made sense to me to avoid any pain or discomfort that I could, so I started taking vitamin C (1,500 mg) and beta-carotene (25,000 IU) that very day. Dr. J, as well as the ACS booklets, was quite thorough in explaining the nasty side effects of chemo and radiation treatments while undergoing them. They don't put out much information about the long-term side effects *after* the treatments are over with. I could not help but wonder how anyone could survive at all after surgeries, six months of poisonous chemo, and six to eight weeks of burning radiation. I concluded that the human body could take a tremendous amount of punishment and torture if there was enough will to live through it.

I asked Dr. Joe about my hurting arm. He felt that it was related to nerve damage during the mastectomy. He, too, felt that the pain and discomfort would pass, eventually. None of the doctors had recommended painkillers to combat the pain, so I did not have to add side effects piled on top of side effects. Except for Dr. C, they acknowledged my adverse reactions to drugs as being a genuine physical threat—not just a mental perception on my part.

I was back in Topeka on February 18, to finish porting before beginning my radiation treatments on the twenty-first. While talking to the technician, I learned that he was setting me up for cobalt.

"There's been a mistake, because I'm to get brachytherapy—not cobalt," I told him not so calmly. He beeped Dr. J and within a couple of minutes, she came hurrying in. He motioned toward me.

"What's the problem, Donna? I thought we discussed everything." She brusquely eyed me.

"You said cobalt might clip my heart and lungs," I shakily answered back.

"Yes, but it should not be clinically significant," she replied.

"You also said that I might experience chronic lymphedema of my arm," I stated more shakily.

"Well, you'll just have to learn to live with it. Now just trust me—okay?" She patted my arm and walked out.

"Dear Lord, what am I going to do now?" I whispered in prayer as tears filled my eyes.

The technicians continued to tattoo my chest area. They marked my upper chest with blue and black markers that I was not to wash off. After they finished the porting, they took two Polaroid pictures of their handiwork. I was dizzy when I was told that I could get up and dress (after lying as still as possible for about an hour and one-half in an awkward position). So I just sat there and glanced over to the counter where the pictures had been placed. I saw a body that looked like a diagramed chart of choice cuts of meat! The next thought was a body at the morgue, ready for an autopsy dissection! As soon as the thoughts went through my mind, I became panic stricken. I had been praying for guidance and knew at that moment that I could not and would not go through the radiation treatments. I did not know what I was going to do, but radiation was clearly out of the question for me. It is said that "a picture is worth a thousand words," and those Polaroid pictures spoke volumes to me. I knew that the Lord was eliminating this treatment for me just as He had eliminated chemo for me. I was thankful for the clear-cut message, but I still went home in a mental turmoil.

Chapter 5

For a Good Night's Rest, Rest in the Lord

I was angry with my body for having cancer. I was angry at my family for wanting me to do something. I was angry at the medical profession, the ACS, and the NCI (National Cancer Institute) for having made very little progress in the past fifty years of cancer research. It seemed to me that the billions of dollars poured into someone's pockets as it was drained out of cancer patients' through surgery, chemo, radiation, and tests.

On February 19, 1994, a friend called us to tell us to turn on our radio to a certain station. We did so and heard a woman's voice saying, "I had surgery for breast cancer, and my doctor put me on Tamoxifen and recommended radiation therapy."

A male voice answered, "Tamoxifen has been linked with uterine and cervical cancer, and I sure would pray about the radiation therapy. I would recommend using progest cream in place of the Tamoxifen, as it balances out a woman's hormone levels naturally." He went on to tell her who made the product and where she could order it.

I got on the phone after hearing their call-in number, as I had just finished reading a book given to me by a friend (*A Cancer Battle Plan*, by Anne and David Frahm). After going through all the standard treatments, plus bone marrow transplant, Anne used supplements and dietary changes to restore her destroyed immune system. Her diet was loaded with nutrients. The ACS and the NCI booklets had diets loaded with calories to offset the weight losses due to the body's attempts to rid itself of the poisons of their harsh treatments. Those organizations made it clear that diet could not cure cancer, but now they are touting the antioxidants, because grassroots pressure is forcing the issue.

I asked the doctor on the call-in program what he would recommend for a supplement program for me after I explained where I was with my breast cancer. His recommendations were the following:

> One-half teaspoon progest cream every other day
> Two teaspoons barley green, three times daily
> Slowly increase vitamin C to ten grams daily
> Vitamin E, 400 IU daily
> Beta-carotene, 25,000 IU daily

I hung up the phone with a feeling of excitement, instead of dread.

A friend, who heads our home schooler's group, called that evening. I told her about the radio program. She laughed and said that she, as well as her parents, went to that doctor personally. Her father had been going blind with diabetes and had been persuaded to try chelation therapy (a synthetic amino acid called ethylenediaminetetraacetic—EDTA—is administered by means of a slow intravenous drip. Once in the bloodstream, this chelating agent grasps free-floating ions of heavy toxic metals, forming a chemical bond with them, then passing through the kidneys and expelling from the body.) His eyesight slowly improved. Her mother had colon cancer, but after going into a coma during her second chemo session, her mother chose chelation and supplements. My friend herself had severe allergies which were brought under control with supplements. It just happened that her mother had a good supply of progest cream and green barley on hand, as they bought it at a discount for ordering in large quantities.

Jerry and I drove to their home out in the country and bought a jar of the cream and a jar of the barley green. I started my program of these natural supplements and quit the Tamoxifen that night.

Within two days, it dawned on me that my left arm was no longer hurting. I was no longer propping the arm up to relieve some of the pain. We decided then to read the pharmaceutical fact sheet on Tamoxifen and Nolvadex. Imagine our chagrin and anger as we read the following:

1. It was contraindicated (inadvisable for medical treatment) in patients with known hypersensitivity to the drug. Could this apply to a person with hypersensitivity to most drugs? Wouldn't it be expected that the doctor or doctors pushing it at thousands of women each year—for the past twenty years—would observe their patient carefully for any side effects?
2. Hypercalcemia has been reported in some breast cancer patients with bone metastasis within a few weeks of starting treatment.
3. Twenty-five percent (25%) of patients may experience hot flashes and nausea and/or vomiting.
4. Increased bone and tumor pain and local disease flare have occurred. Patients with increased bone and/or musculoskeletal pain (3-6 percent) may require additional analgesics.
5. Visual disturbance including corneal changes, cataracts and retinopathy have been reported in patients using Tamoxifen.
6. A conventional carcinogenesis study in rats (doses of 5, 20 and 35 mg/kg/day for up to two years) revealed hepatocellular carcinoma at all doses.

I decided to write Dr. J, trying to explain why I would not undergo radiation. I delivered the letter to the van driver who drove from Topeka to Emporia daily, to pick up cancer patients for radiation treatment. While waiting at the pick-up location, I visited with others who were waiting also. One poor fellow was being treated for mouth cancer. He could no longer eat because the radiation burned his mouth and caused big, ulcerated areas. He said that he would rather be dead than go on with the treatments, but the tears of his distraught and overwrought wife forced him to continue on with the radiation. A woman came into the room using a walker. She said she was now seeing doctors to see if they could do anything for the paralysis occurring from the radiation to her pelvis for cervical cancer the year before. Her story brought back the memory of a dear fifty-nine-year-old neighbor friend of ours who had been treated with cobalt for uterine cancer. Within two years, she was in a wheelchair due to the paralysis caused by the radiation, but the doctors told her that the radiation saved her life. She felt that she was now a burden on her family and would rather have taken her chances with the cancer that had not been bothering her (it was discovered when she had her pelvic exam), than to lose her independence. She wasn't interested in quantify of life, just quality of life. A lifelong friend of the family had his pelvis radiated for treatment of prostate cancer, and found himself walking with a cane within a few short months.

I also wrote a letter to Dr. Joe, similar to Dr. J's. I had told both that I would be glad to discuss it in person if either cared to have any more to do with me. Dr. J called Dr. Joe, and she agreed not to contact me at that time. He would refer me back to her if possible.

For the first time in several months, I was now sleeping peacefully through the night. I was asking the Lord to show me each step to take for a quality journey. I wasn't asking the Lord to extend my life. I was too much of a wimp to endure pain, agony, or suffering.

Dr. Joe called me about two weeks after receiving my letter. He made arrangements for us to talk and to examine me. He said that he believed in medicine, miracles, vitamins, and prayers. He was not a cancer specialist, therefore he was limited in cancer advice for me. When I had last seen him on February 17, he had suggested that I read *The Breast Book*, by Dr. Susan Love and *Love, Medicine and Miracles*, by Dr. Bernie Siegle (while undergoing radiation treatments). Before we hung up, he asked me think and pray about the oncologist's recommendations before making a final decision. I told Dr. Joe that I would talk with the Lord, as I trusted Him completely with my best interests.

Chapter 6

Our Problems Can Be Opportunities to Discover God's Solutions

I wised up and started reading about breast cancer. I read all there literature that I could get from the ACS and the NCI. I picked up one pamphlet entitled, "Unproven Methods of Cancer Treatment." This turned out to be the ACS "blacklist" of alternative treatments.

I had noticed in the ACS and NCI pamphlets and booklets that new, experimental treatments like "biological immunotherapy" were into clinical trials. The pamphlet, "What Are Clinical Trials All About," stated on page 18:

> "combination therapy was the use of two or more modes of treatment—surgery, radiotherapy, chemotherapy, immunotherapy—in combination, alternately or together, to achieve optimum results against cancer."

It stated on Page 19:

> "Immunotherapy—a form of biological therapy. An experimental method of treating cancer, using substances which stimulate the body's immune defense system."

I called the ACS about getting into a clinical trial on the biological immunotherapy. On March 1, 1994, I was told that even though I was diagnosed as Stage III cancer, I was not a Stage IIIb! Those are people with cancer who have gone through the standard big three treatments with little success. Since I had gone through surgery (mutilation) and not chemo (poisoning) or radiation (burning), I was not eligible!

"You mean because I don't have one foot in the grave, already, that I'm not eligible?" I loudly exclaimed to the ACS female voice on the other end of the phone line.

"Well, we don't see it that way. People with cancer tend to get overemotional," she calmly replied.

The irony of her statement hit me, and I started laughing at such reasoning—which just confirmed her statement. I told her that I would do it a different way then, that I did not need the ACS telling me that I had to be on "death's door" before I could try an alternate route!

I finally listened to the still small voice of the Lord and decided to check out the treatments blacklisted by the ACS. I went right down the "Unproven Methods of Cancer Treatment" list. Some of the books that tell about these "unproven methods" are:

> *Options: The Alternative Cancer Therapy Book*, by Richard Walters
> *World without Cancer*, by G. Edward Griffin
> *Cancer Therapy: The Independent Consumer's Guide to Non-Toxic Treatment and Prevention*, by Ralph W. Moss
> *A Cancer Battle Plan*, by Anne and David Frahm
> *The Immune System—How It Works*, by NCI
> *Amazing Medicines The Drug Companies Don't Want You To Discover!* by University Research Publishers.
> *Laetrile Case Histories: The Richardson Cancer Clinic Experience*, by John A. Richardson
> *My Triumph over Cancer*, by Beata Bishop
> *Prescription for Nutritional Healing*, by James F. and Phyllis Balch
> *Spontaneous Healing*, by Andrew Weil

A book I read for enjoyment, but found very uplifting was *Stick a Geranium in Your Hat and Be Happy*, by Barbara Johnson. It had nothing to do with cancer, but had everything to do with attitude in the midst of great stress and trials. Her advice and shared experiences were extremely encouraging to me.

As I was reading the various books on cancer, I noticed a common thread in them—nutrition to build up the immune system. Since I had very little control and limited finances on procuring totally natural grains, fruits, vegetables, etc., I changed my diet to a more natural diet, as much as possible, with supplementation.

It took Jerry and I several months to make the changes. We added supplements of vitamins, minerals, and herbs to make up for the dietary deficiencies of our particular environment and circumstances. If an herb prevented tumors, prohibited the growth of tumors, fought tumors or in any way was anti-tumor, we tried it out.

Since I wanted my liver to remain strong and carry off the destroyed cancer cells, I used herbs like dandelion, alfalfa, chaparral, garlic, milk thistle, pau D'arco, and red clover. The budget determined how much and how often I could obtain these products. Monthly specials determined what supplements I would use that particular month.

Our insurance company—Aetna—would only pay for "mutilation," "burning," and "poisoning" as it only approved what the ACS or FDA approved. Even though my therapy program was dependent on our limited finances, the Lord stretched those dollars, guided me in my selection, and blessed their use to superb health in my body.

My not being able to enter a clinical trial was another blessing from the Lord. Only the researchers know who is getting what. They compare the results of those who did not get the new item to those who did. Of course, the placebo effect (faith or hope) is taken into consideration, but more as an irritant that people get better by believing they are getting something that will help them if they are not getting it.

The ACS, the NCI, and the public would probably be shocked at how many people won over cancer simply due to their faith and hope (placebo) that the torture they were undergoing in conventional cancer treatments would win out if they just hang in there long enough. They also might be shocked at how many died because their faith could not get them through the mutilations, poisonings, and burnings.

It is my belief that if the public knew just how many people died of the conventional treatments' toll on the body, the ACS and the NCI would be out of business. But, when a cancer patient dies of heart failure, lung collapse, or any other organ failure due to the harsh cancer treatments, the death certificate more than likely does not read "cause of death organ failure due to chemo and radiation treatments."

The Lord saw to it that I got exactly what I was supposed to get to do the job that He saw fit to be done.

Chapter 7

God Supplies All Our Needs— One Day at a Time

After examining me on March 16, 1994, Dr. Joe asked, "Are you going to do the radiation treatment, Donna?"

"No," I emphatically stated. "As I explained in my letters to you and Dr. J, I would be going against what God is showing me to do."

I proceeded to show him several books that I had read, including the two that he had recommended that I read. I also told him what supplements I was now taking.

"How have you been feeling, and have you had any side effects?" Dr. Joe inquired. "Tell me why you are taking each supplement."

"Other than breaking out with a good case of poison ivy, which I haven't been around for two or three years, I feel fantastic," I replied.

I handed him a list of my supplements, and I showed him a pocket book card file that I was carrying. It listed each item and what that item was good for in helping my immune system. My memory was not the best so the pocket file was carried in my purse to share the information wherever and to whoever was interested in my biological immunotherapy program.

When I asked Dr. Joe if he would consent to document and semisupervise my progress, he agreed to do so. He was not of the same denomination as I, but we both agreed that there is a mighty God in control of our universe. He agreed to try to work with me.

Chapter 8

Even If You Have Nothing Else to Give, You Can Give Encouragement

In April, 1994, I joined a small cancer support group of five people. The leader of our small group was Patty. She was diagnosed with breast cancer at forty-four years of age. She had undergone a modified radical mastectomy, lymph node removal, chemo for six months, and radiation for six weeks. Patty did not remember much of her first year after her diagnosis. Her treatment and her job were all she had energy for. Her family took care of themselves and the home. Patty attended the Nazarene Church. By the time I met her, she was back to being involved in many things; she operated well under a lot pressure.

Katherine was a caring, giving, Catholic lady, whose husband had also been diagnosed with prostate cancer a few years before she was diagnosed with breast cancer. She was sixty-six years old when diagnosed. She too went through the standard cut, poison, and burn therapies. She said that she had experienced extreme tiredness and one hospitalization stay due to her lymph node removal. A nurse took her blood pressure on the arm that had the lymph nodes removed during her mastectomy. Instant lymphedema was the result. If most women were told of the lifelong consequences having their lymph nodes jerked out, they would tell the doctors to forget removing their lymph nodes as more harm is done to the woman than any benefit from knowing if cancer is in the lymph nodes. The recommendations seem to be the same whether one had cancer in the lymph nodes or not. Even though Katherine's husband had undergone cancer treatments too, he did not care to talk about their cancers to her or anyone else.

Phyllis was our Baptist socialite who was a bubbly person; she kept very busy to keep from worrying or fretting herself sick. Her husband did not like her to be in a support group, as he felt that she was highly suggestible. Phyllis was fifty-five years of age when she was diagnosed with breast cancer. She had gone the same traditional route as the others and seemed to have several long-term side effects, but she was on several different medications so it was impossible to tell what was causing what.

Laurie had been battling breast cancer since 1989. She was thirty-seven years old when she was first diagnosed. She and her fifth husband were already having problems in their marriage, so it did not take him long to flee the scene. (I do not say that in any condemning way as it takes utter devotion to help someone going through traditional treatments, and even some alternative therapies can be quite stressful.). Laurie had been through the standard treatments each year for four years straight. She had also undergone an oophorectomy, then a hysterectomy in her cancer battle. When I met Laurie, she had just finished another round of chemo at the Cancer Treatment Center of America. Her previous treatment programs had been here in Emporia and St. Francis Hospital in Topeka. She attended a Christian church and had just recently accepted Jesus as her Savior. She admitted that she wished she had started her treatments in Tulsa at the Cancer Treatment Center of America, because they did try to treat the whole person—mind, body, and spirit.

Richard was a military man, diagnosed with rectal cancer. He was in his thirties, and he and his wife were expecting their third child at the time that I met them. He went through surgery at Fort Riley, Kansas, but had to go to San Antonio, Texas, for chemo and radiation. He underwent several surgeries doe to various infections with the installation and maintenance of his "Hickman box." That is a chamber installed in the chest area—under the skin—to enable easier access for a lot of intravenous injections, thereby helping to avoid collapsed veins. Richard was not able to come to the group meetings often, because he was so tired and ill most of the time. He and his family moved out of town before we had the opportunity to really get to know him.

Nancy was another Catholic lady who joined our group about a year and a half after I joined. She was a retired teacher and a very well read, caring individual. She was diagnosed with breast cancer at seventy-two years of age. She had a history of dealing with cancer as her two husbands had died of cancer. Nancy also had quite the medical history for herself. She had cataracts, a heart pacemaker that was on the recall list, and Parkinson's disease. She had had a mastectomy on the cancerous breast and was put on Tamoxifen therapy. A couple of months later, her doctors and she decided that the other breast should also undergo a mastectomy, just in case her cancer might recur. Surgery would not be as convenient if her Parkinson's disease advanced. About two and a half months after the second mastectomy, she underwent a complete hysterectomy for uterine cancer. Nancy "took quite a licking, but just kept on ticking," with a very upbeat personality to carry her through.

The cancer support group became good friends and we stayed in contact even after events forced our group to stop meeting. It was surprising how good a person felt just being able to talk to others who had been or were going through similar trials and fears. It was a good place to vent good and bad feeling, to be with and talk to others who knew the same fears, the same ego-shattering mutilations, nausea, stomach cramps, and vomiting.

We did not all experience the same treatments, and in my case, they just confirmed the gladness in my heart in not going through chemo and radiation.

Chapter 9

Feeling Tense about the Future?
Remember That God is Always Present

On May 16, 1994, Dr. Joe expressed concern over several lumps on the mastectomy staple scars, but he was especially concerned over the largest lump above the drainage tube scar. He found lumps at the base of my neck, and an angry-looking, raised mole on the back of my neck. He ordered a blood analysis, as he was concerned about the quantity of various supplements that I had been taking. Dr. Joe marked my chart with the positions of the mole and lumps. He measured the largest at two centimeters (the width of my thumb nail).

The blood work showed no signs of trouble in the bloodstream. The liver, thyroid, and protein checks were fine. I was feeling so physically fine that I bounced out of bed in the mornings—even before the alarm went off. I did not awaken with aches and pains, nor did I drag myself out of bed (as I had done for many years previously).

By June, my exam revealed the lump to be a bit smaller, as well as the mole, but the neck lumps were still present in the same form.

I decided to go with my cancer support friend, Laurie, to the Cancer Treatment Center of America in Tulsa, Oklahoma. We left on June 21 for an exciting yet frustrating event. The center concentrated on the whole person—body, soul and spirit—but unfortunately, still relied heavily on the big three money makers (surgery, chemo, and radiation).

I attended nutrition classes taught by Dr. Patrick Quillin, author of *Beating Cancer with Nutrition*. I attended prayer sessions with folks from different denominations, but we all had the belief that God had the final say over our afflictions.

The people at the center seemed to be very caring, and the patients were all in various stages of treatment and disease progression. There seemed to be a desire to get everyone involved in as many classes as possible and to encourage them to talk about their feelings.

Their cafeteria was fabulous! It offered a wide variety of natural and wholesome foods on one side and the standard American diet on the other side. The center felt that it was important that patients eat heartily, even if the patient chose an imbalanced diet. It was necessary to keep the patients from wasting away due to the nasty side effects of chemo and radiation treatments. Fruits and juices were available as snacks for the patients whenever they desired them.

Other than become homesick by the third day, I enjoyed the trip with Laurie for educational purposes. I did not enjoy seeing Laurie become ill after her chemo treatments. Since she was too ill to attend the classes, I took notes for her. She was also too ill to eat any food at all. This distressed and disturbed me, as I knew that Laurie needed nourishment to help strengthen her from the cancer, as well as the standard, harsh treatments.

Even though the center treated patients with supplements, nutritional diets, shark cartilage, prayer, meditation, visualization, etc., it still pushed the big three moneymakers. In order for Laurie's yearly treatments (costing over $100,000) to be paid by her insurance carrier, Blue Cross and Blue Shield, her standard treatments had to be ACS-approved. After three years of Emporia- and Topeka-standard treatments, Laurie was into her eighteenth month with Tulsa's program. She was usually so sick during and after her treatments that she had very little strength to prepare any kind of meal for herself or to even take the supplements sent home with her. The cost of the supplements from the hospital center was just like any medications given to patients in a hospital—*exorbitant*! But Laurie had to get them through the hospital so that her insurance would pay for them as she could barely make expenses meet (since she could only work part time due to her treatments and the resulting sickness).

When Dr. Joe examined me in July, the neck lumps were gone, the mole was almost gone, and the chest lump was a little smaller than in June. Dr. Joe felt confident enough not to see me for two months, and to tell me to keep doing what I was doing, as we were both able to see positive results going on with my body.

My biological immunotherapy program was as follows:

Two tablets multiple vitamin and minerals, with iron
One tablet multiple vitamin and minerals, without iron
Six tablets (1500 mg each) vitamin C—a power antioxidant
Three tablets (750 mg) bioflavonoids—synergistic with vitamin C
One tablet (125 mg) DMG—improves cellular oxygenation
One tablet calcium (1,000 mg) and magnesium (500 mg)—essential
     for normal cell division and function
Two tablets Echinacea (380 mg)—lymph system stimulant
Two tablets chlorella (350 mg)—detoxifies the body
Three tablets potassium (99 mg)—normal cell division and function
One tablet acidophilus—aids digestion
Two tablets garlic, with lecithin (500 mg each)—enhances immune
     system
Two tablets Bromelain (500 mg)—aids digestion, plus helps
     control inflammation and swelling
Two tablets zinc (25 mg)—acts as a "spark plug" to activate the
     enzymes that digest cancer cells
One tablet chromium picolinate (200 mcg)—helps bring protein
     to where it is needed
Two tablets vitamin E (400 IU, mixed tocopherols)—aids in
     normal hormonal production and immune function
Two tablets beta-carotene (25,000 IU)—powerful antioxidant that
     destroys free radicals
Four tablets selenium (50 mcg)—powerful free radical fighter
     and it is synergistic with vitamin E (good partners)
One tablet CoQ10 (50 mg)—improves cellular oxygenation
One tablets SOD/3 (2,000 McCord Friderich units)—destroys
     free radicals
Six tablets alfalfa (500 mg)—good fiber, natural laxative and
     natural diuretic
Progest Cream (1/4 t. daily)—applied to soft parts of the skin for
     balancing hormonal levels
Water—(one-half gallon to full gallon, daily)—basic solvent for
     all products of digestion—essential for removing wastes—
     regulates body temperature

Chapter 10

God Can Use Life's Setbacks to Move Us Ahead

In our budget, we set aside $25 weekly for motor gas expenses. Whatever did not get used for gas went into our vacation fund. Jerry and I had been blessed to take at least a one-week vacation every year since Ryan's birth. Sometimes it was back east to Pennsylvania, West Virginia, Ohio, and Indiana. Other times it might be Colorado, Wyoming, western Kansas, Oklahoma, Arkansas, Tennessee, or North Carolina. We had friends and family scattered throughout the United States, so there was no lack in places to go. We had even been blessed with a variety of vehicles to take us on our trips.

We started out with a Ford Mustang, then a Pinto station wagon for our growing family. Next, was a VW van. Jerry and his dad customized a Ford Econo van into a camper for us. Dad liked the job they did so well, that he bought his own Ford Econo van for his and Mom's trips. As the years progressed and our family continued growing, the Lord opened the door for us to get a 1971 Winnebago motor home that we used on a regular basis for the next nine years (1984 to 1993).

The Winnebago took the six of us—sometimes more—over twenty-five thousand miles in comfort to see and enjoy many great sights. However, since the Winnebago had finally reached the age where it needed major repairs before each trip, we had to sell it. With the cost of the biological immunotherapy program that I had adopted, we did not feel that we could take 8 mpg trips any longer, plus the children were all capable of roughing it a little better than when they were a lot younger—actually it was because I could handle trips better now that the children were older. With the sale of the motor home, we got a tent camper as part of the deal. It was old, but it was roomy. Since we had sold our customized camper van years before, we borrowed Jerry's folks' van (they rarely took theirs out of the garage due to Dad's health problems) to pull our tent camper. Dad's van had drawers, cabinets, closet, and storage seats that converted into a three-quarter bed.

Our first trip with Dad's van and our tent camper was in June 1994. My sister, from Oklahoma, went with us to see our parents and other family members. Jerry's youngest sister, her two small children, and our oldest daughter were traveling with us, but in a separate vehicle. Michelle's job was to help look after Brenda's children so there would be as few distractions as possible.

Our first stopping place was in Ohio at Jerry's other sister's home. After a couple of days, we left the two sisters to visit for a few more days while we went on to West Virginia and Pennsylvania.

My sister, Ginger, and my husband were both having trouble with joint pains. The two of them discussed how disgusted they were feeling that even with the probability of more cancer in my body (the lumps on my chest), my energy and vitality amazed them. Ginger questioned me about the supplements, the quantities, and the prices. She and Jerry decided that they had best get started on a program toward arthritis problems.

Our visit with our parents and with our brother, George, and his wonderful family was with mixed feelings for Ginger and me. The weather was nearly one hundred degrees with high humidity. All of us were quickly sapped of any energy during the day. Our beloved parents' lifestyle of smoking indoors, drinking alcoholic beverages, and continual bickering about everything made us uncomfortable. We stayed at George's home in the beautiful countryside of Pennsylvania; we would drive each evening to our parents' house for a few hours visiting time. Our parents were about thirty to forty minutes from George, even though they lived in West Virginia.

One dark night, on our way back to George's, I made a derogatory remark about Jerry's fast driving on narrow roads. Tempers were short, and I found myself in the driver's seat. I turned into the wrong driveway; it had deep culverts on each side. In trying to back out, I got into a cross-wise mess, but Jerry was determined not to help out, so I temperamentally said I would "walk to George's." Of course, Jerry and I were guilty of making Ginger and the kids very uncomfortable with our mean words to each other and our very immature behavior. It was pitch-black outside, so one of the kids handed me a flashlight. Ginger said she would walk with me. Jerry and the kids drove on to George's house.

"You know that you and Jerry are being guilty of misplaced aggression right now, don't you?" Ginger asked. "You are both really upset with Mom and Dad's lifestyle, and you can't understand why they won't change it for even our brief visit. Like me, you love them and hate to see them so miserable. That's why I'm not staying with them—why I'm sleeping on that hard bed in the van—because I can't handle their drinking and fighting. It hurts too much to see them hurting themselves."

By the time we walked the dark road to George's, I was much calmer. It helped to talk to Ginger, because I knew from her former life as an alcoholic, she was hurting for them even more than I was. She had overcome alcohol by letting her Savior, Jesus Christ, become the Lord of her life.

Jerry met us at George's driveway, as he also felt bad about our raunchy behavior. Ginger went on to bed, as Jerry and I hugged each other and apologized to each other. We were relieved to be heading back to Jerry's sister's home in Ohio the next day.

The rest of the trip back to Kansas was hot but pleasant. We shifted the kids around at various rest stops, which gave them variety—which, in turn, kept our sanity.

A few weeks after we were back from the trip east, we received a call from George's wife. Her mother had just been diagnosed with breast cancer and was being prepared for surgery. Her mother had a history of heart problems, but had a strong constitution in spite of her heart. George's mother-in-law was persuaded to start taking some supplements, but the oncologist did not encourage much besides chemo and radiation—even with heart problems! George's mother-in-law went steadily downhill as she tried to build up a body being bombarded with poisoning and burning.

At the end of July 1994, we decided to take two weeks and go camping gain in Estes Park, Colorado. Ryan had not been able to get away from his job to go with us on our two previous trips, so he determined that he was going to meet us in Colorado this trip. We, again, took the folks' 1976 Econo van and our tent camper. We left our '86 Aerostar at home for Ryan to drive to Colorado to meet us at a designated campground that all the kids had enjoyed in years past. Since Jerry and I planned on looking for real estate to buy (a habit that we did not seem to be able to get away from, we agreed to a more costly campground in Estes, instead of a campground in Rocky Mountain National Park (RMNP) that Jerry and I liked better. The kids preferred swimming pools, miniature golf, and shopping to hiking beautiful scenery.

I had pretty much been doing anything that I wanted to do physically such as: building a railroad tie and gravel walkway; planting and digging up flower gardens; mowing an acre of ground with a push mower, and going swimming with the kids. After a very bad sunburn from a hot July day at the swimming pool, I had several oversized freckles left on my skin when the peeling was done. I also had some knots rise on my back. They did not hurt; just itched occasionally.

Since the sun is so much more intense at a higher altitude, I declined swimming with the kids. Jerry went along to supervise the horseplay, since Deb did not know how to swim yet. Jerry tossed balls back and forth to the kids for hours. He was amazed at how much shoulder movement he could now do without pain stopping him. He previously had sharp, shooting pains in his shoulders whenever he played catch and pitch. After a few throws, he would have to quit because of the pain. He realized the pain-free throwing meant improvement in his health and that the Lord had blessed the use of the vitamins, minerals and herbs for better health to Jerry's body—which was also a temple of the Lord's.

Jerry and I spent several hours looking at properties, but every year the prices jumped by several thousand dollars, and we were not able to catch up to the prices with our savings account—which was actually getting less as we spent money for the biological immunotherapy program. We decided to quit looking at properties and go on a hike to Twin Owls. It was a shock when we saw smog over Estes valley. It was not a lot of smog compared to what we had seen over Denver and Boulder, but it rather surprised us as we had always thought of the Estes Park—Rocky Mountain area as pure mountain air. We realized that we too contributed to the pollution problems by being there, but staying away was not an option for us. (We had been working with an

Estes Park realtor since August 1991, but we had worked with other realtors trying to buy a campground for several years before that.)

Since Ryan had not been with us on our July 1993 trip to the Loveland—Estes Park area, we took him to the Cedar Springs area that a Loveland realtor had shown us. It was two and one-half miles of switchbacks on a public forest access road. Ryan was a daredevil, but he did not care for the road at all. We told him how much it had improved in a year's time, because in 1992, there were no guard rails. He could not believe that anyone would want to live in such a secluded area. He did admit, however, to it being beautiful once he arrived at the top of the switchbacks. He had also enjoyed seeing the rock climbers on one of the sheer walls seen from the switchbacks. (We learned that this wall was called Combat Rock.)

Our 1986 Aerostar had no problems with altitude adjustment, but the 1976 Econo van ran very roughly and died several times in Estes Park, so we did not dare try it up the switchbacks. (Once Jerry changed carburetors, it did fine in the higher altitudes.)

We were all sad that Ryan only got to spend a week with us as he had to go back to his job and his nice girlfriend, Lisa. It was hard to accept the fact that our family was growing away. Cancer was just one of the many trials ahead in living life as each new day presented itself.

It was also with more sadness than I had ever felt when we packed up the camper and van and headed back to Emporia. I felt that now my cancer and the cost of the treatment program would mean that we would never realize our dream of living in the mountains. I very selfishly cried for many miles of traveling as I said good-bye to a lost dream. I felt bitter, cheated, abused, and misused by the Lord, so I inwardly ranted and raved at Him. I had already ranted and raved at Jerry on our Twin Owls hike about his not making enough money to get out to the Estes area; about his not wanting me to quit homeschooling the kids; about his not wanting me to get a part-time job and homeschool part time; and his irritating patience.

I finally exhausted my raging thoughts and was quietly sitting with my head against the backrest when a still, small voice inside me seemed to say, "Donna, Donna, don't you know that I only want what is best for you? If I let you move out here, it will take both of you working full-time jobs just to make ends meet. The children that I have given you will have to go to the government schools, as there would be no time to school them. There will be no time to enjoy the beauty that I have created, because you will be working constantly to just survive. I have come that you might have life more abundantly."

I humbly gave my dream to the Lord, with a peace that passed all understanding. I could not begin to understand how He could love such a selfish person like me, but I knew beyond a doubt that He did love me.

Chapter 11

Seeing God's Work in Our Life
Puts a New Song in Our Heart

The mole that had been on my back of my neck was history—just a memory—by my September 1994 exam. The chest lump was still reducing, while the six smaller lumps along the mastectomy scar seemed to do nothing. They just remained the same. Dr. Joe felt that we could move the examinations to three-month intervals.

On December 5, 1994, I had a complete blood count, a linear profile chest x-rays, and a right mammogram. On December 12, I discussed the test results with Dr. Joe. All the tests had come back fine, except for the recommendation that another mammogram be done in six months. The mammogram had shown small masses, but I was irritated by the fact that it had not been compared to the mammogram taken a year ago. Both Dr. Joe and I knew from the breast itself, that the breast was no longer hard and lumpy. It was soft and smooth to the touch. I came to the conclusion also that I was not having any more mammograms, as it had been a proven fact since 1946 that x-rays caused cell mutations.

Dr. Joe wanted me to consider having a biopsy on the largest lump, as it had remained the same size as it was in September. We thought that the immune system might have encased it. We decided to give it another three months for the lump to do something or not, as well as give me plenty of time to pray about its removal and the removal of all the small lumps along the mastectomy site.

I was not comfortable about disturbing all those lumps. I was not comfortable about making my immune system concentrate on healing surgical wounds in my body instead of concentrating full force on destroying tumors (benign or malignant).

On March 8, 1995, I met with a very alarmed doctor. My chest lumps were noticeably larger. I tried to explain what I thought I had done wrong and that I corrected my mistake (the lumps were actually smaller again from when I started the correction in my program). I had started taking DHEA supplements twice every other day for thirty-four days. As soon as I noticed a definite increase in lumps and size, I quit taking it on January 17, but not enough time had elapsed before my appointment with Dr. Joe.

Dr. Joe got pretty insistent on surgically removing all the lumps. He was such a caring doctor that I could not get agitated at him. He was truly trying to save me from a cancer takeover, if at all possible. He suggested another try at radiation, or an oophorectomy or trying the Tamoxifen, again. He argued for cleaning up all the lumps, for a major biopsy along the scar. As much as I valued the advice of this wonderful physician, I valued the Great Physician's leading the most. I had received a peace in my heart about a small biopsy on the largest lump. Dr. Joe asked me to please go home and pray more about the major biopsy and removal of all the lumps.

After losing two or three nights of sound sleep because of no peace, I finally called Dr. Joe and told him that I would only go for the originally planned biopsy. I only wanted him to take half of the lump, but he gave me two sensible reasons for removal of the entire lump. Too small of a sample of the tumor might not be able to be examined properly, which would be a waste of time and money on the biopsy. Second, a tumor area does not heal well when part of it is left behind.

On March 31, 1995, I had the 1.1 cm lump removed. (Remember that the tumor had been measured at two cm when we first measured it.) The incision was approximately one and one-half inches long. I refused to be sedated so Dr. Joe did local injections. I would not care to go through it every month, but it was amusing and interesting to hear all the verbal interactions. Dr. Joe did have to remind me to quit laughing, as he needed me to not move, but his lively medical crew were thoroughly enjoyable, so all had to cooperate in the matter of my not moving.

The lump was verified as cancer, but I was not upset at the news, because we had watched it reduce in size before its surgical removal.

The Lord had been blessing the new food choices of whole grains, fresh fruits, and vegetables, the supplements and the large amount of water daily.

On April 7, Dr. Joe removed the stitches. He had not used staples this time, because of all the lumps on the staples sites of the mastectomy scar. The biopsy area looked great and was healing nicely. Dr. Joe wanted to see me again in a month to get a baseline on the remaining lumps.

Chapter 12

God's Love is Persistent but Never Pushy

When I met with Dr. Joe again on May 9, the biopsy site was fine, but the lumps were still a source of concern to him. The measurements showed them to be a little larger than last month. I explained to Dr. Joe that my emotions seemed to play a very big part in the ups and downs of the lumps. He asked me what was going on to distress me. I started with my deeply depressed father-in-law, who was to have surgery in a few days. I knew he would lose his mind again with the drugs that would be given to him for pain and everything else that would arise. Secondly, I was disturbed at the rumors flying around town regarding Dr. Joe's marital breakup and the possibility of his leaving town. He assured me that he was staying put.

My third emotional upheaval was over our beloved son and his fiancé who were bouncing back and forth on whether they were going to get married or not. His fiancé was carrying his baby, our first grandchild, and we did not know if we would be the baby's grandparents indeed or not. We did not want the kids to get married if they did not love each other, and we were hurt that their upbringing was betrayed by their deliberate sexual temptations that they had put before themselves. However, we were proud of the kids in that the taking of the baby's life by way of abortion was never a consideration for either of them. They both accepted the responsibility of deciding what was best for the baby.

Fourthly, I was concerned about my own mother who was scheduled for prolapsed bladder surgery, and she was not very good about telling her kids all the facts as she felt they all have enough of their own worries without adding hers to theirs. The lack of information usually just caused us more doubts about the routineness of her health problems. My mother definitely was not a whiner or complainer to her children.

The final thing bugging my emotions was that Jerry and I agreed to help Brenda set up a twenty-fifth anniversary celebration for their sister and her hubby (who were coming to visit from Ohio). We knew this would be our only chance to help them make their twenty-fifth anniversary very special. Brenda did most of the planning so Jerry and I just ended up doing the setting up of the layout. I was concerned how we were going to manage the surprise. They had cleverly managed to help give Jerry and I—as well as his brother and wife—surprise twenty-fifth anniversary celebrations at the same time that we had believed we were helping set up a celebration for the folks' fiftieth anniversary. After we left from helping to decorate the church gym for the fiftieth, our children and their aunts and church folks turned around and added all the touches needed for two twenty-fifth anniversary celebrations at the same time and place.

Dr. Joe kindly reminded me to practice "thinking on things that were good, pure, and lovely" as God's word instructs us to do. He suggested that I practice relaxation techniques such as deep-breathing exercises. (I have found the deep-breathing exercises to not only help reduce mental stress, but to actually relieve many physical ailments like back and shoulder pain, indigestion and tightness of the chest with cold symptoms.)

I agreed to see Dr. Joe in three to four months or sooner if anything came up that I felt needed his attention or advice. I told him that I was considering trying to locate a bloodroot powder salve to put on one of my chest tumor lumps. I read a portion of Dr. Andrew Weil's book, *Spontaneous Healing*, regarding this specific herb and its effect on dogs with tumors. Dr. Joe said to let him know if I found the formula.

Chapter 13

Each New Day Gives Us
New Reasons to Sing God's Praise

In June 1995, Jerry, the kids, and I took a trip to New Mexico for nine days. From the very start, it was a nerve-racking trip for me.

Ten miles out on a highway running beside swirling floodwaters, the 1976 Econo van started shaking horribly. When Jerry stopped and then started it again, it was fine. (It did that to us almost daily, and it could start shortly after we began the day's travel or five hours later.)

We lost the driver's windshield wiper during a rainstorm—naturally. By the time we stopped that night in Las Vegas, New Mexico, Jeremiah was running a fever because he had caught his older brother's cold. We had planned to spend the night at Storrey Lake, but it was cold and very windy. We chose a motel instead, as we did not want Jeremiah to become chilled.

Day two was when we lost our antifreeze at a rest stop before reaching our destination at Soccoro, New Mexico. For some reason, we decided to drive up to the Magdalena Mountains once we reached Soccoro. Over two-thirds of the way to Magdalena, the fuel filter decided to act up so we barely made it to the small town of Magdalena. As it was, there were no businesses open for mechanical problems because it was a Sunday.

On the third day, we developed a hole in the oil pressure sending unit as we were traveling to the Very Large Array (VLA)—huge satellite dishes. Needless to say, we never got to see them. The good news was that I had been complaining about smelling gasoline since we left home, but no one else smelled it. When a mechanic at Magdalena was checking out the oil problem, he discovered a gas leak. My nose was vindicated, and there was a perverse pleasure in my attitude.

We spent a large part of day four sitting at a service station getting our gas and oil leaks taken care of. I had caught our sons' colds, plus started a full-flowing menstrual period, so we headed back home after the van repairs were made. Needless to say, I was not handling this stressful trip at all well as we spent the rest of the day looking for a campground that was not mosquito infested. We finally found one before sunset on top of a hill with a cooling breeze. Unfortunately, the breeze stopped, and the mosquitoes found us.

We had been fighting the heat every night after the first cold, windy night when we stayed in a motel. Sleeping inside the closed van (due to the mosquitoes) was not at all comfortable.

Day five proved as frustrating as the other days with smog in Albuquerque, higher-priced real estate in Las Vegas than what we had found in Soccoro and a high-priced campground with freezing pool water and cold showers. However, we had a great night's sleep in the pines, even though it was another warm night. However, we were able to open the van doors for ventilation, because there were no mosquitoes.

After a great night's sleep, we decided to head back to Santa Fe and Los Alamos. We all had a good time in Los Alamos, but it was sad to think about the atomic bomb being developed there. It was sad to think that such an instrument had to be used, but force is sometimes necessary to stop evil. When mankind begins to believe that they are gods, they must be stopped, and sad to say that innocent ones will be hurt in the stopping process. We thought it rather interesting but not amusing, that the government was still the largest employer in Los Alamos and that the per capita income was around $50,000. It also seemed strange to see all the security and barbed wire enclosures still in full force. It seemed to us that a lot of secret or mysterious happenings still abounded behind closed government doors.

Our camping at a Los Alamos city park was comfortable even though we had to keep opening and closing the van door between rain showers until it was cool enough to sleep under a light blanket with only the roof vent open.

We went hiking in Bandelier Monument State Park on day seven of our trip, after checking out more real estate prices in Los Alamos.

New Mexico property prices made Colorado prices seem reasonable. When we left Bandelier, we headed for Santa Rosa. We had our daily problem with the van shaking, but other than terribly strong winds, it was a day of beautiful desert scenery.

After a cool night's sleep in Santa Rosa, we went on to Liberal, Kansas, to the airplane museum. We enjoyed our tour and then headed for the Dodge City Campground. We had stopped there before and knew it to be reasonable, clean, and spacious. The winds were still going strong, but we enjoyed a nice evening stroll.

We had experienced a long spell of the van shimmying again before reaching Dodge City, so we were anxious to get on home and find the problem.

The five-hour drive home on day nine saw the van starts shaking first thing on the road, but otherwise the trip was pleasant. Jerry made the brakes top priority after arriving home, as he had discovered they were locking up and causing the van to shimmy.

After arriving home, unpacking, and reflecting on the nine-day trip, I realized that even with all the problems that we encountered, God always had a blessing right alongside the problem.

The roads were always clear of traffic when the van started vibrating. There was no traffic on the highway when we lost our windshield wiper in the rainstorm, or when smoke was pouring out of the van due to the broken oil sending unit. The mountain road was easy to coast down to get to a town for parts. The rest stop had plenty of water to clean up and fill up the radiator after we lost the antifreeze. The people who we met were friendly and helpful. The scenery was fantastic. We had enough money to get parts and repairs. We had safe places to camp each night, and the 1,900 miles we traveled were scenically spectacular!

I started looking at my cancer in the same way—a problem with many blessings from the Lord. The cancer forced me to take charge of my own health and body. Through cancer, the Lord showed me how to say no to things with which I was uncomfortable. I was learning to prioritize my life, to do what I could—decently and in order. For the first time, I was no longer a respecter of persons just because they had degrees, position, or monies. I had foolishly equated those items with knowledge, wisdom, and expertise—especially in the medical profession. The Lord gave me a discerning spirit on therapies to toss out and therapies to consider. If the therapies did harm, forget them.

If the therapies did not harm, try them. The Lord had shown me that doctors did not have all the right answers, but I—like millions of others—had made gods out of them (which might account for the many doctors who think they *are* a god).

With the Lord's blessing upon the dietary changes and supplements, my body felt better than it had felt in nearly twenty years. I awakened fresh and ready for the day. There were no aches, pains, or stiffness unless I had done a lot of hard physical labor to earn them.

I was slowly learning how to lean more securely on the Lord. Being a person that never liked being out of control, I had a tendency to borrow trouble constantly. I tended to worry about problems that were totally beyond my ability to do anything about. But the Lord was showing me "one day at a time is sufficient for today's trouble."

Chapter 14

You Can Be Confident About the Future
If You Walk with God in the Present

Between May 1995 and September 1995, life went on with blessings, trials, and the rise and fall of the chest lumps.

Our son and his fiancé decided that they truly loved each other and wanted to be married, but not because of their expected child. They set a July 1 wedding date at our church. We told our pastor that we would not be offended if he refused a public ceremony for them, but our pastor felt that if he could in any way encourage a young couple to turn their lives over to the Lord and to make right choices, he would do so regardless of what public opinions were. We were amazed at the support and love shown to these children who had strayed from their moral upbringing, yet it should not have surprised us, for that is how our loving, caring Lord is with us. He does not put a stamp of approval on our wrong choices, but He shows us love despite of our sins and wrongdoings. He shows us there are consequences to all our choices and even though He forgives His children when they ask for forgiveness, wrong choices have a price tag. The Lord's Word says, "Be sure your sin will find you out," and "You shall reap what you sow."

On September 7, 1995, a dearly loved friend suddenly died of an aneurysm. He and his wife were vacationing in Colorado when the Lord called him home. I could picture him greeting many others in heaven who we had known here on earth. My sadness at his earthly departure turned to happiness for him and his grand, heavenly reunion. I started looking more and more forward to my heavenly reunion too. I could envision him talking to patriots, like George Washington, Abe Lincoln, Booker T. Washington, Chang Kai-shek, George Washington Carver, Congressman Lawrence McDonald, and other Christian patriots, who we and he had come to love and admire through our studies together in Christian and conservative publications and organizations.

Our friend's death made me realize that even though I feared the thought of my cancer taking me from my earthly family, I was ready to see my Savior, Jesus, as well as friends and family who were already serving Him in heaven. Our friend's death was not a long, lingering, pain-racked existence. He was not in a nursing home or hospital in excruciating pain, or in a drugged state of nonexistence to his surroundings or family.

I thought about how many friends or family members had died just since my cancer diagnosis, and how many more would depart from this earth before I might be called home. It gave me peace and contentment to know Jesus as my Savior and to have no fear of my soul's future.

When I expressed no fear of dying, the oncologists, acquaintances, and even some friends and family members, asked me if I had a death wish. They could not comprehend that my body was a temple of the Holy Spirit and therefore it was my desire to care for it to the best of my limited ability. Using toxic chemicals or burning it were not options in caring for *this* temple.

Chapter 15

Self-indulgence Leads to Self-Destruction

On September 11, 1995, Dr. Joe scheduled me for another chest x-ray and blood chemistry profile. The results were good—as previously—and my energy level remained high. I did whatever I liked in the physical realm.

However, I had mental irritations to deal with. I loved the gentle, intelligent, and thoughtful ladies in the cancer support group that I attended, but I would get so irritated when they got excited over their new prosthesis or hat and wig to cover their bald heads. I had experienced the same irritation when I went to the Cancer Treatment Center with Laurie. They had classes for head coverings to help the side effects of chemo. They had staff on hand to help one find the right prosthesis (from plain falsies to flesh-colored breasts with nipples on them—they were stuck to the chest wall with adhesive strips).

I just did not feel that women were doing right in hiding the effects of current cancer treatments. I felt that if we women would all go braless, we would be making a loud statement that said, "If you do not want to be mutilated like this, then start demanding that other treatments be considered by the medical establishment and by the ACS, the NCI, and the FDA. Start *demanding* that the billion-dollar cancer industry of cutting, poisoning, and burning get a smaller portion of the money pie. Start demanding that more research dollars go to natural alternatives and that the FDA stop the chemicals from being added to our food and water supplies. Start demanding that the FDA stop the growth hormones being used in the meat and dairy industries, because those hormones could easily affect estrogen levels that feed breast cancer." I could not understand if the FDA was established to protect our food supply for us or for the food industries' profits.

In October 1995, we took a geography field trip/vacation to the West and southwest United States. Our first night found us enjoying the generous hospitality of Jerry's brother, Bill, and his wife, Irene. They lived in western Kansas, and we always tried to stop at their home whenever possible. They are wonderful people. (We have been blessed with nine great sisters- and brothers-in-law.) Irene told us about a friend of hers who had gone through the big three cancer treatments several years ago. Breast cancer had struck her friend again, and the friend chose to go through the nightmare all over.

I could not decide if she and others like her were some of the most courageous people in their desperation to beat cancer, or if they were the most foolish people to allow such torture to their immune systems. Again, I could not comprehend why dietary changes to more natural foods were not stressed by the AMA, the ACS, and the NCI.

Common sense seemed to me to suggest that cancer gets ahold of the body from a weakened immune system, so the immune system should be strengthened—not weakened—through poisoning and burning. There was a bit of consolation that medical journals were now telling doctors not to rip out the lymph nodes anymore. It had been discovered—it took nearly fifty years—that a person did better in fighting cancer if their immune system was left intact. In the case of breast cancer, it was more harmful to the woman to deal with the side effects of ripped out lymph nodes (edema is the common problem and having blood pressure taken on an arm that has had the nodes removed can cause hospitalization). I could only hope that the doctors themselves had the time to read the medical journal reports. I was terribly remiss in not researching the latest cancer technologies and from all indications, I was in the company of millions. I would have to live the rest of my life with the consequences of my ignorance.

I could not understand why we deliberately chose to stay ignorant of our body and the importance of our organs (beyond reproduction). Why did women allow doctors to routinely cut out their ovaries to stop estrogen production just so they can then be put on the latest hormone replacement therapy (HRT)? HRTs have been linked closely to cervical and uterine cancers. I had read that over six hundred thousand hysterectomies were done yearly that were not necessary, but they were quick and easy incomes for hospitals and doctors. When I read that, I was skeptical, but after reading how many mastectomies were done routinely—even after lumpectomies were proven to be as efficient but less mutilating—then I realized sadly that much of the medical establishment was not looking out after the best interest of the patients—many of whom could get by with lumpectomies. We, the general public, can take our share of the blame too. Many doctors have bowed to our expectations with our desires for quick fixes—not long-term solutions. Too many women get fed up with PMS, monthly periods, birth control that takes self-control, unplanned pregnancies, irregular cycles, hot flashes, and many other inconveniences related to the female reproductive system. Too many men get fed up with all of the above-mentioned facts of life also, not to mention their inconveniences of self-control, commitments, family support, midlife changes, etc.

Since the general public wants quick fixes, the pharmaceutical companies are only too happy to oblige. With our medical schools and medical publications being financed by pharmaceutical companies, the medical establishment naturally pushes (by way of written or called-in prescriptions) the drug of the month, which may or may not solve the ailment. More often than not, another drug will be prescribed to counter the side effects of the previously prescribed one (especially in older adults whose metabolism has slowed down and cannot rid the body of the drug as quickly as a faster metabolism used to be able to do). The original problem gets lost under the newer side effects of the next prescribed drug. It becomes a vicious cycle.

The dangerous drug Tamoxifen is soon going to be touted across the news media as some kind of boon to women to combat PMS or possible prevention of breast cancer. Will they be told of the risk of cervical or uterine cancer, blood clots, eye problems, bone and/or muscle pains, or any of the other very real side effects? What about the side effects with tubal ligations—severe cramps and huge blood clots? Whether it is the pharmaceutical company, the pharmacist, the doctor, or the patient's responsibility to know what to look for in immediate as well as long-term side effects is split four ways as far as I am concerned. People have got to get rid of the notion that they are not responsible for their well-being—that it is someone else's responsibility.

Doctors have taken a big toll in lawsuits. A few of the lawsuits were probably well justified. The majority were not. Because of our sue-happy mentality and the lack of common sense in the courtroom today, doctors now order thousands of dollars worth of tests to make sure they cover everything possible so thoroughly that no judge or jury could accuse them of negligence. Should the doctor take the path of common sense and nondrug treatment, the patient would more than likely go to another doctor anyway. Many doctors have learned for survival's sake to give the general public what it wants—temporary quick fixes.

In comparing the quality of lives with those who survived traditional therapies and those who survived alternative therapies in cancer treatments, the quality seemed superior in the alternative therapies. The biggest complaint seemed to be adjusting to a more natural foods diet.

In one of the ACS pamphlets, it was stated that those of us who used alternative or "unproven" therapies were desperate and wasting our valuable time and money. Those of us choosing alternative therapies claimed that desperation was the only reason that anyone would allow their body to be burned, poisoned, or mutilated deliberately.

Since most insurance companies will not pay for alternative therapies, our costs vary with our affordability. Traditional treatments for Laurie averaged over $100,000 for each year of treatment using the big three treatments (see chapter 9). Laurie died in December 1994, after five years of mutilations, burnings, and poisonings. She had undergone two different mastectomies, an oophorectomy, a hysterectomy, a neck surgery, and finally a shoulder carving (all accompanied by the poisoning and burning). After all this standard treatment, Laurie had no quality of life. Laurie's death was excruciating pain, hallucinations from morphine and other pain killers, tranquilizers, and finally starvation.

According to *Time* magazine, 147, no. 14 (1996): 60, "The American Cancer Society estimates that in 1996, 317,000 Americans will be told they have prostate cancer, more than the 184,000 new cases of breast cancer and nearly a quarter of all non-skin cancers expected this year. That figure represents a staggering increase over last year's 244,000 new prostate cases and the fewer than 85,000 recorded as recently as 1985. The American Cancer Society predicts that deaths from prostate cancer in the U.S. will reach 41,400 this year, a number fast approaching the annual breast cancer toll of 44,300."

Every time I read these types of statistics, I cannot help but put dollar amounts like 184,000 times $100,000 equals $18,400,000,000 to the cancer industry! The only incentive to cure cancer is from those who have it or those who have a loved one who has it—not from those making a good living from cancer.

The doctors and/or researchers who find an inexpensive cure or effective treatment for cancer are quickly squelched by the billion-dollar cancer industry and organizations that were set up to watch out for the interests of the people, but seem to have found it more lucrative or powerful to aid the industry. Insurance companies such as AEtna will not pay for treatments that are not FDA approved! As long as I went through the standard big three therapies, the insurance company paid the majority of the $17,000 bill for the three months it took me to start listening to the Lord and researching other alternatives. However, AEtna balked at paying for any alternative treatments of vitamins, minerals, and herbs (approximately $2,500 a year for my program).

The Lord had blessed me with a doctor who accepted the insurance payments as full payment for his services. I have heard that this wonderful doctor has done the same for other individuals also. His acceptance of the insurance payments as payment in full allowed me to continue on with my biological immunotherapy program. I looked at my particular program as saving the insurance a bundle of money, so I could not understand why they were not doing anything to encourage alternative treatments. After all, it has cost Laurie's insurance company over half a million dollars for her standard treatments over five years. At the rate that I was going with my biological immunotherapy program, it would only cost the insurance company $100,000 over forty years! It sure seemed like a wiser, more cost-efficient program for insurance companies to encourage rather than discourage. I realize that they just turn around and raise everyone's premiums, but in the long run, it could save them from going out of business due to the duped people turning to nationalized health care.

As long as people can be convinced that the cancer industry is making progress in the fight against cancer, the true statistics will be covered up. When anyone bothers to mention that prostate and breast cancers are more prominent now than ever, it is always pointed out that new screening technologies help in early detection. I am beginning to get the idea that early detection may actually translate into an earlier death due to the treatments to which the body is subjected. A lot of women will not die of breast cancer, but of uterine and cervical cancer much later in life due to earlier treatment practices of their breast cancer. A huge percentage of men die *with* prostate cancer, but not *of* prostate cancer. How many more men are dying years earlier from having gone through treatments because of early detection? I do not know the answers to the statistics, but I think the questions and observations are valid.

I know my advice to anyone contemplating any kind of cancer treatment would be to educate one's self. We all have our prejudices in everything. There are good treatments and bad treatments—good doctors and bad doctors—good people and bad people. Check them out.

Chapter 16

To Change Your Outlook,
Remember Who's Looking Out for You

Even with the extra monies going for my biological immunotherapy program, we still managed to save $600 for our yearly vacation. We had two weeks time allotted for this trip, but due to the small sum saved, we expected to be back home within a week due to us running out of money. So we decided to cure our homesickness for Rocky Mountain National Park and the surrounding area.

After leaving Jerry's brother and wife, we went straight to RMNP where it cost us $5 for a week's pass. Since it was after the main tourist season and most of the water facilities were shut down, camping was free. We had packed a nice supply of food to go along with our camp stove and equipment, thereby making meals very economical and convenient. We camped in a great spot for watching herds of elk nearby. The bull elk in mock battles was a sigh to thoroughly enjoy. Hundreds of cars lined up alongside the roadway just to watch the elk and to hear the bulls bugle. We could not have picked better time or location to see such a display. The weather forecasters had been calling for snowstorms and generally bad weather (before we left home), so we had been a little skeptical about the vacation timing. We had originally scheduled our vacation for September, but the company bosses had extended the annual two-week plant shutdown (for repairs and overhauls) for an additional two to three weeks. Since Jerry had two weeks' vacation time coming that had to be used by October 19, 1995, or lost with pay, we had decided to take our chances against the weather reports for the RMNP area.

While we were hiking the RMNP campgrounds and trails, a ranger delivered the message to us that we needed to call home. We did so, and learned that our son and daughter-in-law were the proud parents of our first grandchild! Mother and baby girl were doing fine, while Daddy and Auntie were arguing over who was calling who first. It was an exciting time for everyone.

After the sun went down, the four of us would shut ourselves up in the van, wrapped in coats and blankets, and play simple games like "triominoes." By dark, we were curled up nestled deep into our sleeping bags. After all the exercise during the sunny days, sleep was never a problem, and the cold nights did not bother us.

For three gorgeous days, we hiked around the park. The blizzard was delayed so our days were sunny and warm. We continued being fascinated by all the elk and the hundreds of sightseers. The biggest surprise to us, however, was the nesting snakes! Over the past several years, we had been in RMNP at least a half a dozen times on vacations, and could not remember having ever seen even one snake in all the miles we had been blessed to hike. But this trip was a different story. We found them all over the trail to Cub Lake. Deb and I had stepped off the trail to avoid a couple of snakes lying on the trail. The grass was fairly tall where we were standing, so when two more snakes headed between our legs, it did not take but a second or less for Deb and I to be back on the open trail! Jerry and Jeremiah just stood quietly watching the snakes as they moved across their shoes. Deb and I found it fascinating *from a distance*.

We could not be around the Estes Park area without looking for some property to call our own. It had become an obsessive ritual over the years and even though we really did not expect to find anything—in our poor price range—that could be called a decent building site, the looking always takes to us to interesting places. The realtor that we had worked with the most over the years sent us to soaring heights to see several building lots. Her map showed the road going all the way around the area that she sent us to. We went up and around, and up and around, and more up and around! The cliff-top houses and mansions built on these sites were spectacular and insane. The lots at our price range had to be dynamited to get a spot level enough to put a small or tall house on it.

We loved the eagle's view, but since God had not put wings on us or our vehicles, we could only shake our heads in the negative.

The road ran out on us on our way back down the mountain (at least the map had indicated that it went back down on the other side). We could not back up or out of the mess we had driven ourselves into. I threatened to "string up" one realtor who knew we had an old 1976 Econo van—not a four-wheel drive vehicle like she drove. True enough, it *had* been a road of sort many years ago, but now it was strewn with rocks, small boulders, and deep washouts.

I pushed and shoved and heaved the rocks that I could, while Jerry—with great driving skill—humped, bumped, dipped, and climbed the washouts. With fervent prayer, the Lord helped us get down the used-to-be-road. I *did* inform our realtor that she should get an up-to-date map of the area, as well as take the trip herself before she sent any more trusting, unsuspecting souls into the area.

The one buildable lot at the base of that particular road was $35,000, which was far beyond our ability to pay. We told our Estes Park realtor that we were going to go back to an area that a Loveland realtor had shown us in July 1993, and that we had again visited in August 1994, when our oldest son had driven our Aerostar out to Colorado to join us on our vacation. The prices had been reasonable when we first saw it, but the two and one-half miles of switchbacks were not quite what we had in mind at that time. We knew that it was a beautiful area but figured that prices had probably skyrocketed there too. Even though we were no longer looking for a house big enough for a family of six, we were thinking about a small vacation cabin that could be used as a getaway or retreat ministry that could slowly be built over a few years' time, as our financial resources allowed us. The Loveland realtor had shown us a small A-frame for $15,000, but we either were not listening to the Lord's quiet voice at that time or the timing was not right, then. In the meantime, our Estes Park realtor gave us the name of a realtor living in that particular area, whom she had just sold a lot to, and we headed back for a third visit (in three years).

The Lord's timing was exact, as we had just made the decision that morning to head for warmer parts as the snow had finally arrived. We had awakened to a gorgeous winter wonderland in RMNP. There was no wind yet, so the snow was delightful to watch the deer and elk pawing it to get to the grasses beneath.

The realtor was not home, but we had a nice visit with his lovely wife and children. It was getting colder and windy, we told her that we were going to drive around and mark down any lots for sale that we might be interested in, and that we would contact her husband after we got back home. Well, her husband caught up with us while we were in a discussion over two small parcels. He was as homely and nice, as his wife had been pretty and nice. He asked us a few questions and then told us to follow him. He took us to two parcels that he had just been contacted about selling. We looked at our dream lots that were in our price range! They totaled nearly four acres of very buildable sites, with lovely views of the Rocky Mountains, tree-covered slopes, open fields, and breathing space between neighbors. The paperwork was done by our Estes Park realtor, as she was determined to get something out of us for all the time she had invested in us over the years.

We were happy that the Lord opened the door to our dream of owning a little piece of the Rockies finally, but we did not understand His timing. The land was covenanted, with a $75 yearly road fees. (It later proved to be a big mistake in not having the realtor put this in writing. We did not have any extra monies for building, as my immunotherapy for cancer took the extras, but we knew the Lord would put a cabin there if He wanted it so.)

Chapter 17

Gratitude to God Leads to Grow in Godliness

Since we were now nearing the end of our first week of our geography field trip/vacation, and we had spent only a fraction of our small vacation fund, we decided to travel south for a day or two. Jerry and the kids enjoyed the sights of Denver, Colorado Springs, Pueblo, Santa Fe, and Albuquerque—I am not much for big cities, so I did a lot of stewing over Jerry's looking and driving at the same time.

We enjoyed stopping at God's Painted Desert and His Petrified Forest. It was disgusting to read the evolutionary garbage put on the various information signs the state and federal governments. We found the evolution information to be as repugnant as atheists find creation information, but we believers in an Almighty God have not done our jobs of "occupy until I return," and Satan has had a field day with our forced tax dollars being used to spread his deceit in trying to oust God out of anything relating to government. Separation or church and state simply meant that the governments were not allowed to make any law for or against religion. Satan has deceived many into acceptance of government laws against religion specifically, Christianity. This nation had become great under the establishment of Biblical principles to guide it, and we should not forget God's goodness to our nation. But, as we forget God, as we toss out His standards, and as we turn to our own devices, we will experience the lack of His blessings. It is beyond our comprehension how anyone can look at the magnificent national parks and wonders of the world, and deny the God who created them! It should not surprise or shock us about government edicts, because God's word says: "For we wrestle not against flesh and blood, but against the rulers of the darkness of this world, against spiritual wickedness in high places." (Ephesians 6:12) Only spiritual wickedness could make such decrees as these:

1. A corporation is considered a person with legal protection, yet a baby in the womb is not a person.
2. A federal employee's life is worth the death penalty, automatically, to anyone who takes that life, but a nonfederal employee's life is not worthy of an automatic death penalty to anyone taking that life.
3. Evolution will be taught as fact, but creation will not be mentioned.
4. Our men and women will be sent to wars in other nations, but not allowed to win those wars—just a few battles.
5. The government will pay large corporations huge subsidies to hire non-Americans, thereby taking jobs away from its own citizens.
6. The official language of the American people will be questioned as a main language or not.

Even with the knowledge that our government was not equal, fair, non-discriminating, or looking out for the best interests of its citizens, we still thanked the Lord for the freedom that we still had to travel the United States and see His glorious wonders!

We were blessed to be able to stay overnight at some lovely rest areas that had good lighting for safety and plenty of warm water for washing up. We were surprised at all the travelers and tourists in the southwest in October. When we reached the Grand Canyon National Park, it was to find long lines waiting to get into Mather Campground. Through the Lord's management, we got the only site open in the campground, and we were able to keep it for three days! The weather was superb. We stood with open mouths at the sight of thousands of foreign visitors (from Japan, China, Taiwan, France, England, Germany, Switzerland, etc.). It seemed as if we were visiting another country ourselves.

The brochure prices of the hotels on the rim and the mule rides were staggering (I did not hesitate to tell the lord that I would love to take a mule ride to Phantom Ranch and stay at a hotel on the rim someday, if He ever saw fit for us to have the money to do so.)

However, it did not hinder our pleasure in hiking down Bright Angel Trail for a few miles—we had to force ourselves to turn back so that we would be sure to have enough time walking back *up* the trail.

The walk back up Bright Angel Trail reminded me of the trail of human sin. We find it so easy to go down into sin (the beautiful canyon), but a lot tougher and harder to get back out of that sin (canyon).

Our 1976 Econo van was doing great on this trip. It ran rough in the higher altitudes, but otherwise trucked right on down the road. Jerry did find a broken spring in the left rear wheel brake, but it did not cause us any problem.

We left Grand Canyon on the eleventh day of our trip and traveled through lovely Flagstaff, stretched out Phoenix and Tucson, where we stayed overnight. We saw the sights of Demming, Las Cruces, and Alamogordo, New Mexico, on day twelve. We had a ball climbing and running over the White Sands National Monument and were ready to settle down for the night at Oliver Lee State Park. The night sky was so clear that we were able to study the Milky Way Galaxy through our binoculars. The moon was so bright that it was absolutely gorgeous outside, with a warm, gentle breeze during the night.

On our thirteenth day, we took the scenic route to Cloudcroft-Artesia and saw more of God's handiwork. We were doing well on our vacation fund, so we went to the Carlsbad Caverns for more study of God's marvelous creation. The hours we spent in the caverns were exciting and wondrous. We truly appreciated the God-given ability that man has used in making it easier for us to appreciate God's creation—the vehicles in which to travel, the gas to propel the vehicle, the power and ingenuity to get electricity to out-of-the-way spots for our better enjoyment of His majestic wonders.

When we left the caverns and headed for Texas, the van started making a terrible engine rattle, but it kept going on down the road with us to see the sights of Palo Duro Canyon. I had been in the canyon over thirty years ago. It had taken a couple of hours by horseback, and it was thrilling. Now the canyon had roads, campgrounds, hiking and horseback trails for everybody's pleasure. The thrill was not the same for me, but I knew that I would have to keep in mind that: (1) Driving a vehicle compared to riding a horse was no fair comparison for me; (2) No canyon could compare to the awesome Grand Canyon, in which we had just been a couple of days ago; (3) The weather was cold and extremely windy at Palo Duro, so we did not have the pleasure of hiking the area for any enjoyment. We did not care to try to swallow at the sand, dirt and dust fiercely blowing about.

Due to the cold, blowing wind, our stay at Palo Duro was short. We headed to Liberal, Kansas, where we stayed the night in a motel range of motion with southwest décor, green plants, spacious sleeping, dining and bathroom arrangements. We got some nice ideas for a little cabin on the acreage that the Lord had allowed us to find and buy on this trip.

On the fifteenth and final day of this blessed trip, we visited Cheney State Park and saw about 150 miles of new territory in Kansas that we had wanted to see before, but had never taken the time.

The Lord stretched our $600 over 3,500 miles, many scenic wonders, clean motels, lovely and safe rest areas, wonderful state and national parks, good food, and two weeks of a fantastic geography field trip/vacation. But that is how the Lord does things in our lives. Just as the Lord stretches our finances, He stretches our faith and trust in Him—one mile at a time, one dollar at a time, and one day at a time.

Considering how many times we have provoked the Lord with our lack of faith, His mercy shows His *love*.

Chapter 18

Sorrow Looks Back, Worry Looks Around, but Faith Looks Up

In November 1995, we had a Thanksgiving Day dinner as usual for our families. We had been blessed to have these dinners since 1977 (except twice). This was our second big family dinner since the cancer diagnosis nearly two years before. The Lord just continued confirming that even with active cancer in my body, life still went on with many blessings to accompany the trials.

Also in November, dear friends had their adoption party for the second adopted child. It was a gala festivity and another reminder of God's strengthening process of His children. Their first child was diagnosed with leukemia two weeks before my diagnosis of breast cancer.

Again, I learned how marvelous the human body was created. It can take unbelievable abuse from itself, others, and the medical world. The parents did not have the freedom to choose a therapy for their child. As soon as the youngster was diagnosed, he became the doctor's child to be treated therapeutically as the medical profession saw fit. The parents were only allowed to pick one of the hospitals named by the doctor.

The parents had to stand by and watch their child swell into non-recognition, vomit constantly, lose his hair, get physically violent due to the painful side effects of the chemo, and go through surgery for the Hickman box for the many injections of chemo and counteracting agents. No such thing as a balanced diet was recommended, as the parents were instructed to let him gorge on whatever he liked so he would not waste away. Many cancer patients die from malnutrition or "wasting away." His favorite foods were hotdogs and lunch meat. All I could think about was that poor little body trying to fight cancer, trying to fight the side effects of the chemo, and ingesting more carcinogens (nitrates and nitrites).

I, foolishly, tried to tell my friend about the link between hotdogs and childhood leukemia. Naturally, she was offended, as she was already under tremendous stress, watching what her child was going through, the continual eighty-five-mile trips to the hospital in Wichita, the horrendous medical bills received daily in the mailbox, and continual guilt that they could be responsible for their child getting cancer, because they had catered to his picky eating habits. She did not need a thoughtless friend, like me, to feed her guilt, so she felt compelled to tell others to stay clear of my information when I tried to share some suggestions with them.

At first, I was terribly hurt, but after praying for all of us, the Lord helped me to understand what was going on after she had expressed her displeasure with me. I had active cancer too, but I was the picture of perfect health, experiencing very little pain or discomfort. Her son was being tortured with the traditional cancer treatments that he was forced to receive.

I made comments that I would go to Mexico to get alternative treatments, if necessary. She had felt that I was condemning them as not being good parents for not taking their child to Mexico. I clarified that mistaken belief very quickly. They were much stronger parents in this situation that I ever could have been. They took an active part in their son's care and treatment. They watched the doctors and nurses to make sure that every proper precaution was carried out. Through their watchfulness, many infections caused by carelessness, were avoided. They were devoted parents, who were strong enough to go through the treatments every step of the way with their son. They made me realize how blessed I was that God allowed cancer to strike me and not one of my children, for I am a weak person even with the Lord's help.

On December 15, 1995, I had my regular appointment with Dr. Joe. We talked about the bloodroot powder that I had received from an herb company, but I had not been able to get the formula to know the right proportion to use as a paste over the tumor/lumps. He was not comfortable about its use, as bloodroot is caustic. I was not real gung-ho about using it yet, as I was not sure I could handle the drawing out of the tumor or any accompanying pain. I easily agreed to hold off using it until I felt it was absolutely necessary. Dr. Joe did suggest that I try to find someone who practiced alternative medicine, if I felt the need.

"In the field of medical science, we have attained about 20 percent knowledge," Dr. Joe explained, "I am learning about this as you learn too."

We agreed to another visit in three or four months or sooner if I felt it necessary, as I now had several new lumps under my left armpit, but no discomfort or pain.

I had called Dr. Andrew Weil (who wrote the bestseller book, *Spontaneous Healing*), but was unable to get him. I wrote twice to try to find the bloodroot formula, since I had read about it in his book. After a few weeks had gone by, I called again. This time, I had reached his kind, courteous, secretary. Dr. Weil had not been able to get in contact with the aged gentleman who had sent the bloodroot salve sample to him. I was disappointed, but I just figured that it wasn't in the Lord's plan for me at this time. It had taken quite a number of phone calls to various herb companies to locate bloodroot powder in the first place, so I decided to freeze it just in case I needed it for an emergency alternative therapy, someday.

Even though I did not get what I wanted from Dr. Weil, it in no way took away any good that I had obtained from reading his book. He just confirmed what I had been observing for a while that the mind is a powerful tool given to us by the Lord to use in ways to honor and glorify Him and to use for the care of His temple. I am committed to try to do no harm to this temple that His Holy Spirit indwells within. It does not mean that I will not make mistakes, after all, I do get very impatient.

The Lord cares for me and loves me even if He allows unpleasant things to come into my life. He loves the world so much that He gave His only begotten Son, that whosoever believes in Him shall not perish, but have everlasting life (John 3:16).

Chapter 19

The Power That Drives Us Comes from the Spirit inside Us

Near the end of December 1995, the new lumps, as well as the old ones, seemed to have strong activity going on. They were going up and down. The original larger lumps on the mastectomy scar were turning brown and feeling crusty. I was thankful they were on the underside of my skin where I could monitor them daily—no guesswork involved.

I had been on progest cream since February 1994, so I decided to take a three-month break and see what would happen. I had a period on January 17, 1996, and then the next one was thirty-six days later. I had averaged twenty-four-day cycles from February 1994, until January 1996, each period lasting five to seven days. On February 22, 1996, the period lasted twenty-four days! I had no cramps or loss of energy, just the discomfort of wearing pads for so long.

Jerry's father was getting the runaround on his health problems, as he had been for many frustrating years. The family tried various doctors in Emporia, Topeka, Halstead, and Kansas City. It was always more drugs and tranquilizers. He had been diagnosed over the years with heart problems and Alzheimer's (neither of which could be proven—just alluded to). Then, because he had tremors, a shuffling gait, and slumped shoulders, he was diagnosed with Parkinson's disease. We could not get any doctors to believe that long-term laxative use could be causing some of his dementia, as well as some of the tranquilizers that he had gotten addicted to over the years.

The doctors had just patted us on our concerned heads and basically said to leave the doctoring to them. It is with shame that we listened to them for so long. We could not help but realize that much of Dad's medical problems were a direct result of misprescribed medication, piled on top of overmedication.

According to Sidney Wolfe's book, *Worst Pills/Best Pills*, several medication used long term and prescribed regularly for older people can cause Parkinson's disease—Elavil, Prozac, Haldol, Thorazine, BuSpar, etc. "Each year there are approximately 61,000 older adults with drug-induced Parkinsonism . . . . 70% of doctors treating Medicare patients flunked an exam concerning their knowledge of prescribing to older adults. Between 40% and 50% of drugs prescribed for older adults outside the hospital were overused."

One hundred nineteen (119) of the 364 most commonly prescribed drugs for older adults—one out of every three drugs—should not, according to published studies and/or Public Citizen's Health Research Group and its medical consultants, be used by older adults because safer alternative drugs are available." (see chapter 3, p. 55, for the 119 drugs which they say "Do Not Use" and their safer alternatives.)

When we checked every prescription given to Dad by several doctors in several cities, we found most to be a "Do Not Use" drug, as well as the higher-priced drug prescribed for the particular diagnosis of the moment. It put us on guard for all future medications prescribed for any of us to be checked for side effects, as well as price.

We decided that maybe we might try an alternative clinic location about an hour's drive from Emporia. It had been mentioned in the book, *The Cancer Solution*, by Robert Willner. We thought since our homeschooling friend's parents had done so well on chelation therapy in Kansas City, maybe we should give it a try for Dad. The family also wanted me to give the clinic a try as they were concerned about my ongoing period and my new lumps that started at the beginning of my arm pit.

We started our new adventure on March 12, 1996. As stated before in one of the previous chapters, chelating agents are used to bind with heavy toxic metals, such as cadmium, lead, and mercury (standard toxic metal put in our mouths routinely for fillings and approved by the very agencies supposed to be protecting the general public), and to excrete them from the body. It has been used effectively to treat arteriosclerosis for more than forty years in the United States. EDTA (ethylene diamine tetraacetic acid), a synthetic amino acid, is the chelating agent administered intravenous to treat ailments. It is slowly released into the bloodstream over several hours. It attracts lead, strontium, and most divalent metals. It has not been found to be toxic when used correctly.

We felt that it would not hurt Dad, but the chelation might actually remove some of the toxic material out of Dad that might be there. Dad had been an electrician, a plumber, and a carpenter throughout his life, and those trades certainly had some hazardous materials involved in them.

My own treatment at the clinic consisted of hydrogen peroxide in the veins, once a week for four weeks, then vitamin C intravenously (started at twenty grams because I was already taking twenty grams orally each day). Since I was still on the extended period, I was told that I would be given a shot of progesterone if I was still flowing by my next appointment the following week. I decided that I would go back on my own progest cream program, from which I had taken a three-month break. My period stopped after four days of the cream being applied directly on my chest tumors.

Dad and I both had complete physicals, including blood and urine samples before we started any treatments. His blood work came back very poor. Mine was marvelous, except for low sodium and iron. With the extended menstrual flow, I was not surprised at being low in iron.

The consultations ($165), tests ($240), enzymes ($46), four hydrogen peroxide treatments ($320) for a total of $771 in six weeks, were mostly out of pocket expenses for us. However, Medicare did pay some of Dad's, and AEtna paid 80 percent of the first four treatments for me. They balked at the next six, and when I called them and questioned them, I was told that AEtna would not pay for over-the-counter remedies. I asked them, "Where can I get over-the-counter injections?" They chose to ignore my valid question and denied any further payments. I reminded them that they paid $5,500 for my consultation and radiation porting. They, again, pointed out to me that the FDA-approved form on cancer treatment! Big government was looking out for my welfare!

It is too bad that the framers of the constitution did not see fit to put medical freedom alongside freedom of speech, press, and religion. I am sure that there would not be any more quacks in the alternative field of medicine than there are in the traditional field. Just as in other walks in life, we must be on guard, use some common sense, learn about our particular body as much as possible, and be willing to take on more responsibility for our actions. Just swallowing mainstream medicine that is being pushed by the media, as well as the medical establishment, is not going to solve our health problems. The message the media puts out on upset stomachs is, "It's okay to pig out or eat foods that your body clearly shows you that it does not handle well and probably is not good for your health. Just take Mylanta, Pepcid AC, Maalox, Zantac, or Tagamet, etc., because you do not want to show self-control or self-denial just for your health's sake."

With the hydrogen peroxide and vitamin C treatments, my tumors seemed to flatten out, but otherwise, tumor life continued up and down. We did not see much, if any, improvement in Dad's condition, either. He still had trouble with tremors and his shuffling gain. He would now freeze suddenly, and we would have to talk him into moving. He had gotten more mentally flaky with each week.

Over the Easter break 1996, friends volunteered to look after Jeremiah and Deb while Jerry and I took a quick trip to our lots near Drake, Colorado. It was the first time since 1980 that Jerry and I had been away from the kids. We surveyed and measured our lot boundaries, but without much success. It involved a lot of up and down hillsides, over tall brush, around some trees and then driving steel posts for markers. The sunshine was intense with about two inches of snow on the ground. Our top parts were nice and toasty, but our feet were wet and cold by evening of the first day of our arrival.

We decided to go into Estes Park to a motel since we knew that tourist season had not officially opened yet. Therefore, prices would be reasonable. We enjoyed our hot showers, a quiet dinner in front of the TV, and just each other, without the thousands of interruptions common in our household.

The second day was perfect all day long, with gorgeous weather and a dry ground. It was grand exercise in a mountain setting, and we were able to meet some of our neighbors who were in the process of building a chalet-style home. Imagine our delight when we discovered that they were homeschoolers also! We were looking forward to getting to know each other better over the upcoming summer months.

We had no idea what we were getting ourselves into, with the covenants and an association, but the Lord knew the future and the land was His—even when I had the tendency to forget who was in charge.

Chapter 20

If You're Filled with Pride, You Won't Have Room for Wisdom

By my May 8, 1996 appointment with Dr. Joe, my lumps were still noticeable with the eye, but they felt and looked much flatter. He asked what I was doing, so I told him about the alternative clinic. He asked several questions about the treatment that I had chosen and about the cost of the program. He seemed relieved as well as happy that I was trying it. He wanted progress reports if I continued in the program. He was still very much concerned that the lumps were still in clear existence, even after five hydrogen peroxide injections and three vitamin C injections of twenty, thirty, and forty grams. Dr. Joe, again, suggested (in a kind, subtle manner) removal of the ovaries, because of the new lumps in my armpit.

In the meantime, Dad was getting feebler and more cantankerous. It had been discovered at the alternative clinic that he had rectal polyps, so Dr. Joe was asked by Mom to do a colonoscopy and surgical removal of the three polyps. The polyps were benign. Dad seemed to heal quickly, but his mind got stuck on bowel movements and urination. If someone brought up "plumbing" for any reason, Dad wanted a plumber to work on his internal pipes! If someone changed oil in a car, he wanted to be lubricated too. We tried to see the humor in all of this, but knowing that Dad was mentally leaving us was hard to take. He couldn't seem to get any interest in anything but himself. He was infantile in his behavior toward Mom and his active, older grandchildren. He acted as if he thought they were bad people who were out to get him. That was not the Dad we loved and respected. Of course, he was always stubborn—that was a family trait—but there was no reasoning with him now. He would get physically violent with those trying to help him, and with his adrenaline pumping him up in his anger, he was as strong as any mule.

Dad was aggressive toward me when I was driving their car back from the alternative clinic (Mom usually drove the seventy-four miles going to the clinic). One week, as I was driving us back home, Dad suddenly jerked the gear shift from drive to second gear. Our speed was about 75 mph. It naturally shook me up, and I yelled at him. He said that he hadn't meant to touch the shifter, and that he was just reaching to adjust the air conditioner control. I shakily told him not to let his hand move toward the shift column again and reminded him that he was to stay buckled up.

Another week, he managed to upset me to the point that my leg started shaking badly. I was learning to quickly call upon the Lord to calm and strengthen me and to quiet Dad's mind. The Lord would graciously answer my prayers, and we would continue on toward home. I had to remind Dad about the shift column only one other time, and he remembered with remorse what he had done. When I asked him why my driving upset him so, he said it wasn't my driving. (Later, we learned that he blamed us for the loss of his driving ability and skill.)

A large percentage of parents probably go through periods of wanting to run away from home, children, and responsibilities as much as children want to run away at times in their lives. We all fight the pain of disappointments, and I definitely admit to wanting to be a runaway parent at times as well as a runaway daughter and/ or daughter-in-law.

Even with the Lord to lean upon, life can be tough. I knew the Lord was working on me to think of things that were good, lovely and pure. I knew the Lord wanted to see more gratefulness in my attitude. Our eldest son was a good provider for his family. He loved us all and missed us when he was on the road. Our eldest daughter scheduled her days around my treatments so she could look after Deb and Jeremiah for me. Even though she had moved out on her own (so her lifestyle choices would not be an irritant to my health), she tried to help us when she could do so even when it was inconvenient.

In my heart, I knew that the Lord had blessed us with fine children who would, one day, let their Savior Jesus, also be their Lord. I would just get so impatient with them as well as myself. Because I am a person who likes to be in control, it was difficult for me "to let go and let God" take charge of the children that He had loaned to me for a short time.

Our daughter-in-law continued being a blessing to us in her care of our granddaughter. We never lost one night's sleep worrying about the kind of care that Ashley was getting. She and Ryan were both proud parents and were trying to be good parents to their precious child.

What a delight our granddaughter was to us in her pure innocence and discovery of the world about her! She loved everyone, accepted everyone, but her favorite was Aunt Deb. Our daughter-in-law had to hide Deb's photo as Ashley would see it and cry to see Deb.

Life went on with its ups and downs, its joys and sorrows, its tears and laughter. The Lord's variety made life very interesting—never dull.

We had planned on stopping the alternative injections after a total of ten treatments, unless the Lord worked a miracle by letting us see a definite improvement in Dad or myself. Since there were no changes, we had our last injections on May 21, 1996. Dad had continued to decline, and Mom felt that they would be bankrupt before much longer, since Dad insisted on seeing the doctors at each visit for his obsessions with his malfunctioning body. The doctors were too costly and unproductive in diagnosis and treatment (for out-of-pocket expenses).

My energy, stamina, and vitality remained good, but some of the tumors were now into the muscle tissue, instead of just attached to the skin. It was interesting watching how tall they could rise after each treatment, then how flat they were before the next treatment. They seemed to be in a consistent crisis mode for a couple of days for calming (just as with my menstrual cycle).

On May 28, 1996, I added shark cartilage supplements to my biological immunotherapy program. I took nine tablets of 740 mg each in daily, divided doses. I set a three-month trial period, as I felt that to be sufficient.

Chapter 21

Others May Prove Untrue,
but Jesus Never Fails

The summer of 1996 involved several trips to Colorado to get a small cabin/house built, so on June 7, we were packed and ready to leave town shortly after Jerry got off work. A realtor friend had left a message on our answering machine, while the kids and I finished mowing our acre of ground. It seemed that she had a young couple—with three children—who wanted a country home in the city such as we had. Even though we did not have our house on the market, over the years we had let it be known that it was always for sale at the right price. Since selling our house was the last thing on our minds, Jerry and I made a quick decision to let it be in the Lord's hands as to whether this was the right time or not to sell out. We dropped the keys off at the realtors and headed west for a nine-day vacation to the Colorado lots in the Lord's Rockies.

We planned on getting a septic tank installed first, so we could properly dispose of our port-a-potty waste—without having to travel up and down the switchbacks daily. However, all the county red tape squelched that plan. Newton's third law of motion states: "For every action, there is an equal and opposite reaction." Murphy's law states: "For every action, there is a reaction." Donna's law states: "For every action, there are at least ten reactions!"

We managed to get our thirty-inch perk holes dug with a helpful neighbor's post hole digger. I only managed to get one of the holes dug due to the rocks. Poor Jerry had to do the other three holes. We had to keep in mind, as we fought the rocks, that it was our dream to have our own piece of the Rockies! Our next step was having an eight-foot septic, but it filled with water. Our neighbors said that it was just springtime water—not a spring.

Our week was filled with many blessings to offset the continual red tape frustrations. We were able to meet the lovely families of the two gentlemen whom we met over the short Easter weekend. They kept us supplied with good drinking water and great fellowship. Deb enjoyed playing with their daughters, while Jeremiah enjoyed teasing and tormenting all of them—the girls kept coming back for more.

Deb and Jeremiah also made friends with more neighborhood children, which in turn encouraged us to meet the parents of their new friends. Another older and delightful couple took us under their tutorship. They did not live year round in their beautiful little cabin in the mountains, but they did get to spend several months in their cabin each year. He would usually get a part-time job while they stayed in their cabin to help stretch their retirement dollars further. He asked us if we had ever gone rock rappelling and if we were interested in him showing us how to do it. We did not turn down his offer at all.

The rock rappelling was terrifying, initially taking that first step over the edge. I found it to be much like dealing with my breast cancer. The initial first step in making a decision of which choice of treatment to undergo, was just as terrifying as stepping backward over the cliff face. But, just as in rock rappelling, I had to use a guiding hand and a brake release hand at the proper times. My cancer therapy program was guided by the Lord through prayer and release of one therapy step to move on to the next therapy step.

We met one of the current board of directors, and he told us to use his phone any time we needed to. He had big equipment available for our hire, so we used him and his partner for all our dirt work. They were very helpful to us and not just because they wanted our money. They sent several people our way to help us to get our cabin built as quickly, efficiently, and as economically as possible.

We met folks that built gorgeous log homes, but unfortunately not in our price range (we thought at that time). Then, we met a carpenter/contractor who had the philosophy in life, "I try to keep in mind that the guy I'm mad at today will probably be pulling me out of the ditch tomorrow." We came to terms on time and price, and he agreed to put in a basement and to put up our cabin shell for us.

One of the county inspectors visited with us about getting started on the paperwork trail. He let Jerry accompany him through an inspection on a new hole under construction.

We also met an ex-airplane pilot (who had lived in a small trailer for three years while building his cabin). The county laws allowed him one year in the trailer—the same as the covenants—while building a home. The association board of directors (abod) took him to court. Since he was violating the county rule too, and since the parcel owners pay yearly taxes, we really did not understand why the association felt the need to spend road dues on legal fees. The pilot lost in court, but he was only responsible for his own legal fees—not the abod's legal fees taking him to court. We assumed that the abod found it easier to sue him with road dues than to get the county to enforce their rules. We should have taken warning of the abod's wayward management of road dues as it was our belief from reading the covenants that the yearly dues of $75 was specifically for road maintenance.

Before leaving our town, we had received a letter from the abod stating that funds for the roads were low due to a lost court case and the abod wanted the parcel owners to pay their road dues immediately if they had not already done so. We had been disturbed at the letter, as we had not been told by the realtors or informed as a parcel owner that a lawsuit was in action. The way we read the covenants was that each parcel owner had a right to sue in his own behalf if anyone was in violation of the covenants, but nowhere could we find in the covenants that we could be forced to pay for other parcel owners' lawsuits.

The abod lost the court case, due to a mistake made in the filings of one and two. The abod, therefore, had no jurisdiction over filings one and two, and not only lost the court case, but also lost the revenue from those two filings (two hundred lots). The majority of those parcel owners were happy to no longer have anything to do with a petty, vindictive board of directors, nor were they displeased to no longer pay road dues for public, federal, and county roads that the abod insisted the parcel owners had to maintain. It was true that the county did not plan on taking over the maintenance of the public roads over which it claimed jurisdiction, but the abod had always found it easier to get road dues from the parcel owners than to argue or petition the county.

When questioned later about who voted for the lawsuit, the abod insisted that the parcel owners (the association members) voted for it. We found out by reading the court report for ourselves, as well as the abod's letter to the parcel owners, that the sued parcel owner had brought in a used double-wide mobile home, after receiving permission from board members. The covenants did not allow for the used portion, so someone brought it to the abod's attention. We also discovered that the abod's lawyer warned them there was a problem with the filing records. However, the abod used the same voting method that had been wrongfully used for many years. They just collected a quorum of twenty votes, and thirteen of those votes then represented the majority vote of all the parcel owners. They refused to back off from the lawsuit as they hoped the judge would just overlook the filing error and concentrate on the covenant violation. Justice did prevail for filings one and two, and the judge freed them from the covenants and the abod. It was good news for one and two, but the remaining filings were expected to make up the lost revenue!

The legal bill for this piece of mismanagement was nearly $18,000 out of the road dues. The covenants read that the owner of each tract should, during the period of ownership, automatically be a voting member. However, past boards had arranged things so that only those parcel owners present and in good standing could vote (but of course, all parcel owners, present or not, would pay what those present and in good standing voted for).

How easy it is to lose track of one's responsibility, role, or function when dealing with unaccountable funds! Just as the association was voted in originally to see to the care of the roads, the American Cancer Society was set up to find ways to defeat cancer. It was to examine all research fairly—not just concentrate on entrenched, expensive medical procedures already in use with a very poor record. An inexpensive therapy (compared to the big three) was not acceptable regardless if it worked on some cancer patients—it was just a spontaneous remission. It amazed me at the gullibility of the American public in its continued giving to an organization interested far more in protecting its own interest than the interest of the people it was formed to help.

Jerry and I did not feel that there was anything we could do to enlighten the public about the ACS and the NCI, but we certainly felt that we could shed some light on abod's errors.

We could not point at a specific individual in the abod who was deliberately doing wrong. At this particular time, we felt that the abod was just financially ignorant—not misappropriating road funds feloniously, but in error. After all, some of the present board members had reached a neighborly hand out to us in helping us to get started right in building.

So Jerry and I wrote a letter to the abod, expressing our concerns and our *no* vote on increasing road dues. We signed our letter and gave it to a neighbor friend to read at the annual summer picnic/business meeting that we were not able to attend. We did not know at this time that there were bylaws set up for the association allowing proxy votes, but we had felt that as out-of-state parcel owners, our signed proxy letter with its two *no* votes would be acceptable. A couple of the board members were good neighbors, and we had already expressed our concerns, personally, to them.

It was with great disappointment and sadness that we learned our proxy letter and votes were not allowed to be read nor counted. Even their own bylaws permitted proxies, but *ours* were not acceptable!

It was the beginning of enlightenment of how entrenchment can lead to despotism even in a small road maintenance association. When good people did nothing, then wrong would prevail.

Within a few days of the thirty votes (out of 191 parcels) *yes* on raising the dues from $75 to $125, the board of directors filed another lawsuit against two more parcel owners for covenant violations that were also county law violations. It was disgusting and revolting that thirty present parcel votes could speak as a majority for 199 parcel votes! No ballots were mailed out.

Chapter 22

Fervent Prayer Dispels Anxious Care

We took off, again, for Colorado on July 3. I had forgotten to take my progest cream that I used to keep the estrogen more balanced in my body. Normally, I would start it on the seventh day after my menstrual period, and I would stop it on the first day of the menstrual flow. Since we were going to be gone for eleven days on this trip, I decided to skip the progest cream for an entire cycle. The tumors settled down to their flat stage for ten days before rising again.

Our eleven days in Colorado proved fruitful. Even though it took six days before we got our building permit, we kept busy helping our neighbors finish up their newly constructed house. They were so gracious in allowing us to feel useful while waiting on the paperwork (permits) to start on our own little place in the mountains.

We helped stain the outside of their chalet-style cabin, filled in their well ditch, helped sand and paint the inside of the cabin, and Jerry helped put up the pine-look paneling in their cathedral ceiling. We enjoyed gorgeous weather and wonderful fellowship and laughter.

Another neighbor to us was one who was being sued by the abod. He seemed very nice, but had a very negative attitude. If I had been in his shoes, I would not have been nice in any way. He was being sued by the abod, battling his ex-wife in court, trying to help his daughter combat her cancer, fighting for a decent education for his three boys still at home, and trying to make ends meet on disability and child support. Even though his personal appearance was shabby, his attitude was negative, and it seemed that he was looking for trouble, Jerry and

I were not blind to the man's intelligence in legal proceedings. We felt that the abod was making a very serious mistake taking on this man in court. We also felt that this man would have given the shirt off his back if someone would have asked him for it. It left a sour feeling in our stomachs to know that some of the money that we had paid in road dues was being used against a neighbor.

The Lord used this July trip to help get me unwound from the happenings back home. When we got back from our June trip, our eldest daughter announced that she and her fiancé had moved their wedding date from May 1997 to August 1996! I was upset because Jerry and I had committed ourselves to a contractor in Colorado to start on the basement and shell once the permits were obtained. There were no monies for a wedding in 1996, but our lovely daughter told us that was paying for the wedding herself—she just wanted our love, blessing, and moral support. Since we liked her fiancé and the positive influence that he had on some positive changes in her lifestyle, giving our blessing was easy. It just rankled me that she was footing the entire bill and that she was only eighteen years old. We were thankful that he was twenty-two and a fine, decent, caring young man. We tried to talk them into keeping with the original date, but they wanted to be with each other day and night—not be "live-ins." They felt that they were ready for permanent commitment. We could not refuse them our love or moral support any more than our folks could refuse Jerry and I when we wanted to get married in 1967. Since all concerned were of legal age, there would have been no stopping of either marriage on legal grounds.

We were thankful that our older two kids brought fine mates into our family as our children-in-law. We may not have agreed with their timing or circumstances for marriage, but we liked their selection. We also got fine in-laws who treated our kids great.

Along with the scheduled August wedding, we had signed a sale contract on our house. We had the possession date set for the end of August to cover the wedding and the trips to Colorado to oversee our building project. We needed to start sorting all the material goods for garage sales, storage, and moving.

We had prayed that the Lord would work out all the details, as our move looked like it would be to the upstairs apartment in Jerry's folks' house. They were talking about selling their house, but Dad had not been able to do any maintenance for the past few years. Their house needed work done on it to get the price that they wanted for it. Mom was in need of help in caring for Dad, as he became more difficult to deal with. He had his days and nights mixed up, so she was nearing exhaustion.

We still believed that constant laxatives over many years had contributed to his mental deterioration and that the various long-term drugs prescribed over the years had brought on Parkinson's disease. Even the alternative clinic ignored his laxative dependency (since we had managed to finally get him off the antidepressants).

Mom already had a good renter, so she could not bring herself to say anything to him about moving. We were willing to move into the small apartment if we were wanted and needed, but we were not about to fight for the responsibility and cramped quarters. So we just left it the details for the Lord to work out while we were in Colorado.

Out of three eight-foot holes dug for a septic tank and perk test, two proved unsuitable for the septic system as they filled with water. By quickly leveling the bottom of the third hole and quickly setting a tank in it, we were then able to go on with filling the perk hole back in. We left the other hole as we wanted to see if there would be any water in it by our August trip. If the Lord wanted us to have a shallow well for clean-up purposes, who were we to argue with Him? We roped and ragged the hole to try to prevent any cattle, horses, people, etc., from falling into it.

Our thirteen-year-old, Jeremiah, was given the opportunity to learn to operate a backhoe—for an hour or better—in digging out the footing and foundation area of our soon-to-be-built cabin by our neighbor, friend, and abod member. It was just as thrilling to watch our son moving the dirt with the backhoe as it had been for us to spend the Fourth of July in Estes Park, with more neighbor friends watching the exciting fireworks over Lake Estes.

When we left Colorado for home, our contractor said that he should have the shell up by the time we got back in August. We left Colorado with great anticipation and joy in our hearts that things were finally moving forward.

Chapter 23

No Trial is without God's Blessing

How disappointed we were when we learned from our Emporia realtor that the bank loan was not approved for the couple who contracted to buy our house. We had set our minds to a move, plus we now needed the money to finish the mountain cabin without getting ourselves deep into debt. We felt that more than ever, Mom needed help in managing Dad. We thought that the sale of our house would free us up to help Mom if we were not so busy maintaining our own place.

I ranted and raved to Jerry and the Lord about the house not selling. Jerry was dealing with his own feelings of frustration, so harsh words and lack of tact was the result between us. The Lord's reaction was to prick my ungrateful heart with His word—just as He cared for the birds and flowers of the field, He care for all His children—He wanted nothing but the best for His children, and when He asked for His perfect will in our lives, we could rest assured that nothing was going to come our way that was not the best for us.

The trials were necessary for our growth in Him. With my and Jerry's quick flare-ups, we might have been no use in the situation with Mom and Dad. We might have been easy pickings for being taken advantage of once we had some spare monies from the sale of the house. We could always see places to spend money on our kids in our desire to see that they did not have to struggle too hard in life to make ends meet (sometimes that very struggle is necessary for maturity and growth). And finally, we might have ignored all of our responsibilities in Emporia to head permanently to Colorado.

I became peacefully reconciled to the fact that my Lord was saying, "No, not now." He was in control, and I needed to rest in Him. The mountain cabin and property were His just as everything else that we had in this life. Our desire to use the cabin for a retreat for others (if we could not live there) to draw closer to Him was in His power to see it done.

Since our Emporia home was His also, it was His business to see it sold or not. Our prayers were to be in His perfect will—not His permissive will—as we did not want our self-will to get us into trouble.

God's perfect will stopped us from getting deep into debt from buying a campground in Colorado, Illinois, and Kansas. He had allowed us to manage the campground west of Emporia for a full year (1990-1991). While others have managed to run a campground and raise children successfully, Jerry and I had found it hard to divide our time properly. He still worked his full-time job at the mill, and I still homeschooled our four kids. Even though we loved the campground work and experience, our kids lacked the right kind of attention and interaction for family time and relaxing activities. God's permissive will would have been similar to the weary parent who finally surrenders to the begging child and says, "Okay, have your own way and just suffer the consequences."

The Lord also stopped us from buying a half a dozen houses that would have buried us in drudgery and debt.

Our daughter's wedding arrangements were lovely. She not only took care of everything possible for her own wedding and reception, she also made all the arrangements for the twenty-fifth wedding anniversary reception for her future mother- and father-in-law. The silver celebration took place at the same time and in the same location as the wedding reception. Michelle had made these arrangements so that folks coming from a long distance away could celebrate both important events with the least amount of inconvenience (and it was a surprise silver anniversary reception for the in-laws). The only thing she had forgotten was to appoint someone for kitchen duty, but having been blessed abundantly with fantastic aunts and uncles, they saw the situation and immediately pitched in. Everything turned out beautifully. It thrilled us to know that our daughter was able to think of others and to show that thoughtfulness and unselfishness in sharing the limelight of her wedding day. Her upbringing of being surrounded with unselfish and thoughtful grandparents, aunts, uncles, cousins, and friends had rubbed off on her. We were *very* proud of her.

Our church family reached out to her mate and welcomed him openly and lovingly, just as they did our son's mate. Michelle and Troy attended church regularly, and he seemed to enjoy growing in the Lord's word preached from the pulpit. I looked forward to the day when Ryan and Lisa attended church more regularly for their spiritual growth.

With Michelle handling all the wedding arrangements so smoothly, there was very little stress on my part other than feeling guilty that she was financially footing the entire bill. I should have been praising and thanking the Lord that she had earned and saved the money to be so financially independent.

I would like to say that I handled my stress level well when it came to having the basement and cabin built, but I did not. The contractor had warned us that we would feel like we were being nickel-and-dimed to death, and how right that proved to be! I dreaded his calling because it meant more money for more material that had been forgotten. I ranted and raved, again, to Jerry and the Lord, about a $5,000 Sutherland house kit costing $25,000 just for the lockable, weatherproof shell over a basement! When the contractor ordered $800 worth of unneeded lumber, I flipped. When he put the roof sheeting on and discovered no roofing felt ordered, I flipped. I became a stressful mess, and any delays, such as concrete trucks not arriving until four days after they were scheduled, excavators being a day late, the contractor cutting his hand so badly that it required fourteen stitches, the backfilling of dirt being delayed to the contractor not getting enough gravel for the French drainage system, the trusses and wood laying out in the rain once they arrived just added fuel to my stress level.

I would actually find myself pacing back and forth. I could not concentrate or think about anything but the cabin. I would tell the Lord, "It's your ministry cabin, you take care of the details." Then, five minutes later (or less), I would take it back from Him and try to take care of it myself. "Why aren't you supervising this project better, Lord?" I would ask. Even Jerry tried to be patient with me for a change. It was stressful for him on two counts. (1) He knew the money was running out, and the payment plan on our home equity loan was going to be mighty hard to stick to. (2) He did not like to think what my stress level was doing to my cancer tumors, because he loved me terribly—even when I was flaky from my own senseless worrying.

Another thing that was bothering us was an oversized freckle located on my right shoulder (under the right bra strap when I bothered wearing one). During the summer of 1995, the kids and I had gone to a neighboring town to go swimming. We spent a very hot day swimming in a huge pool with cool, refreshing water and a wonderful waterslide. We had put on sunscreen, but too late or not enough. We all came back with blistered sunburns. After the peeling was over, I noticed several large freckles that I had not had before. In August 1996, the freckle started rising, but there was no hardness under it, as those on my chest. One evening, my shoulder itched, and I just naturally scratched it. I suddenly felt pain, looked at it and discovered it was bleeding. I had a moment of panic, when I remembered Laurie's large tumor on her collar bone area—her tumor and a lot of muscle tissue were surgically removed, adding to her tremendous pain in her last three months of life. But my panic subsided as I ran to the Lord for strength to face another obstacle. I put progest cream on it for three days before I had to stop due to starting my menstrual flow, again. I had used the progest cream on the mole, and I did not know if the cream helped or the Lord just took it away. I do know that without the Lord's blessings on the vitamins, minerals, herbs, and dietary changes, I would not have enjoyed the outstanding health, vigor, and vitality that I was physically thriving on.

I prayed for the Lord's guidance on what to put on the freckle—if anything. While I was praying, olive oil came instantly into my mind, as the healing ointment of the Bible. I was afraid that I might unconsciously scratch the itchy freckle and cause more irritation to it, so the olive oil was to keep the itching minimized. I used the oil every time the freckle itched. It was painful as I gently rubbed the olive oil into the freckle. A crust formed on the freckle and then fell off on August 30, 1996. The result was a smaller, flat freckle until it eventually disappeared like the mole had done.

In the meantime, my chest tumors were really up in arms. Several were sharp and painful to the touch. I knew my stress level was high over the cost of the twenty-four-by-thirty-eightfoot house kit. Common sense should have told me that the cost would be much higher than the kit price, because of putting it on a basement and adding several upgrades to meet county codes such as egress windows. We chose a metal roof, instead of roof shingles, as the strong winds liked to peel shingles off houses. We replaced the hardboard siding with rough cedar, and there were extra costs for stairwell steps, garage door, septic tank, excavation, backfill, etc.

We were nearly broke as to money available to us on our home equity loan. The tumors were the largest they had ever been since the removal of the original three and one-half inch tumor, so I did two things.

First, I gave the cabin to the Lord totally. If He chose it to be for an investment to sell for profit, so be it. If He chose for it to be a glorified tent for the next several years of visiting Colorado, so be it. If He chose for it to get finished and become a ministry cabin for His honor and glory, so be it. It was His to do with as He saw fit.

Second, I started liberally rubbing olive all over my left chest wall. I worked it into each sharp lump, including those around my armpit. By the time September 5, 1996, rolled around, my tumors had calmed down considerably. I had continued remaining on the biological immunotherapy program while doing the olive oil treatment, and the Lord continued blessing the physical well-being of my body.

Chapter 24

Our God is Bigger than Any Problem

Our third week's vacation in Colorado during the summer of 1996 proved to be very hard, but satisfying, work. The contractor was about a month longer getting the shell up than he had anticipated. Some of the delays were not his fault, but some were. We had been delayed ourselves in that Jerry's employers had extended the annual plant shutdown for a couple more weeks. It was not a good thing because the contractor could not have handled our breathing down his neck, since he was not on schedule either.

The cabin shell was completed, weather tight, and lockable. I got the job of putting wood preservative on the rough cedar siding. Eleven-year-old Deb gathered all kinds of rocks for a three-foot landscaping border around three sides of the cabin. Thirteen-year-old Jeremiah shoveled many yards of dirt into the basement area since it was full of holes, and I was afraid that someone might trip in one and break a leg. I also thought it would be better to have a level dirt floor for the concrete poured that we hoped to put in some day.

Jerry had to put the garage door together so it was usable as the contractor seemed to have a problem getting it put together correctly. Jerry ended up putting up the south guttering and all downspouts, but we were glad that the contractor did get the very tall north guttering on. Jerry then completed connecting the plumbing from the septic vault to the basement, where he was able to make a workable toilet system for our use. We had the eight-foot water hole, from which to bail water. We would strain the water, treat it with chlorine bleach in our ten-gallon tank, and use it for bathing purposes. We used the water straight from the hold for flushing purposes. We got our drinking and cooking from our lovely neighbor friends. We did our cooking in the tent camper, which we had set up in the basement. Our modern lighting system was tea candles and Coleman lanterns. It was glorified tent camping at its best, and we loved it!

We did lose some sleep on a couple of nights, however, as a neighbor's dog had, apparently, adopted our basement as a storm refuge. Since the garage door now shut him out, he woke us up trying to dig under the door. It took a great deal of persistence to convince the dog that the basement was now off-limits as a dog house!

On another night, we were awakened by a horrible racket sounding in the rafters. It turned out to be an owl, trying to get a hold on the metal roof and screeching at the same time; it was scratching the metal. What a racket! The owl finally settled for perching on the metal roof of our van. The full moon night just added to the eerie excitement.

The free-ranging horses did not come near the cabin but did graze our property several times, which we thoroughly enjoyed. They were so beautiful, but absolute nuisances to property. They liked to stable around buildings and houses, which meant manure piles, flies, and cribbing (eating the wood siding). They also liked to test the strength of decks and porches with their weight! We knew that we would eventually have to fence the cabin area, since we would not be there most of the year to protect the cabin from the horses.

The hard work helped my stress level to stay under control, and the tumors remained calm for that week. By September 12, they were o the rise again, so I figured I was probably nearing another menstrual period since my hormones seemed to play a part in their rising and falling. The removal of my ovaries was still not under consideration, because of hormone replacement therapies following afterward. The negative of an oophorectomy far outweighed the positive in my understanding, plus I was greedy in not being willing to jeopardize the great physical health and vitality that I had been experiencing for the past two and one-half years (even if I did wear menstrual pads more often than not).

On the home front in the meantime, Mom had finally managed to get Jerry's dad on a good schedule, and he was sleeping all night. The Lord had arranged for our daughter and her husband to rent Mom and Dad's upstairs apartment. Dad seemed to be more coherent and interested in life, and then Dad had to have emergency hernia surgery—his third one caused by being constipated and straining despite long-term laxatives.

With the surgery on September 18, 1996, all the headway with Dad over the past fifteen months since his last surgery, he went down the drug route again. The painkiller, Demerol, had him sleeping constantly for five days. We insisted that the doctors give him a weaker pain pill. He was switched to Darvocet, but (according to the book, *Worst Pills/Best Pills II*, by Dr. Sidney M. Wolfe and the Health Research Group) Darvocet was no more effective than aspirin or codeine, yet like Demerol, it was addictive. When the hospital staff moved Dad from the main unit to the skilled nursing unit, we discovered that the doctor had put him on another addictive drug, Vicodin. Poor Dad! He did not know what end was where! Again, he became mean, rude, and violent with all the drugs going in and out of his system. Mom wore herself to a frazzle, practically living at the hospital with Dad. Several of us took turns relieving her, but Dad would get violent when she was out of sight. When Mom's health broke down for a few days, Dad was nearly unmanageable—hitting and beating on anything or anyone—and raised a royal uproar all night. The staff had no choice but to confine Dad in a geriatric chair near the nurses' station. We requested all medication be stopped except for Tylenol at night. The doctor conceded with Tylenol and Ambien to put him to sleep at night. The doctor claimed it was a nice little pill with no side effects. During the day, Dad still slept a lot and was usually incoherent until the evening hours when he would start to make sense—right before time to start the drug cycle all over again.

On September 30, 1996, Mom was informed that she could take Dad home, even though Dad had not been taken off the catheter or been detoxed off all the drugs. We argued with the doctor that Dad needed detox at the hospital—not at home with his seventy-five-year-old wife! Mom's vigil at Dad's side was taking a toll on her health too. Our kind and well-meaning doctor felt that Dad's mental condition was going to get worse with time. We could not argue the point, but we knew the drugs hastened his mind's deterioration.

Even though the nurses and aides were all very nice, it was hard to get things done the way the family thought best because the doctors were hard to get in contact with at the hospital. We believed that emergency care overall in the United States was good, but the long-term care was sadly lacking in common sense.

I was beginning to realize that I wanted very little to do with most hospitals and the medical community as a whole. It seemed to me that medicine had become so drug oriented that most health problems got hidden under drug side effects.

I had found myself trying to control the situation at the hospital, which was totally out of my hands, so I ran to the Lord again and again.

During all this time with Dad and the hospital drug routine, my right breast nipple had activity going on. It had been crusty for many years, but now the crusty area was slowly turning blackish. It became very itchy, so I put olive oil on it for two to three weeks before the crust disappeared. The crust had come off in the past, too, but as a wart-appearing lump. This time, it just slowly dissolved.

The Lord enabled me to let go and let Him handle Dad, drugs, and doctors. All the Lord seemed to want me to do was bring the situation to the medical staff's attention and to help Mom physically care for Dad.

Chapter 25

When You Turn Your Care into Prayer, God Turns Midnight into Music

We spent the first week of October 1996, at the Lord's cabin in Colorado. The eight-foot-square hole with a depth of nine feet had four feet of water in it. Even though we had the hole staked, roped, and flagged, we were concerned about the danger of someone or something falling into it. After all, horses roamed freely all over the subdivision, and the cattle from Sylvan Dale Ranch got out of their pasture on a regular basis. We hired our abod neighbor friend, again, to scoop all the water out. When he watched the water start filling in the hole again, he suggested we do a simple two-foot pipe in the center and fill the hole with gravel. If, in the future, the spring dried up, we could then have the gravel pulled out for our driveway and dirt filled back into the hole. It made sense to us, as we had no intention of drinking or cooking with any of the water. Of course, we could continue using it for bathing and flushing purposes.

We also decided to put up a fairly tight barbed wire fence around the cabin. Our front porch stoop was already bowed from the weight of a cow or horse standing on it. With horse prints and cow pies all around the south and west sides of the cabin, it was an easy guess as to what happened to the porch stoop. When our friendly contractor saw us putting up the barbed wire, he said, "People around here usually use friendly wire."

After he made the comment a second time, I answered, "I thought we were being friendly by not using a gun and shooting at them like some others have done."

Supposedly, conflicts in the area between men and free-ranging horses had already resulted in shooting horses when one parcel owner was not able to discourage the horses from eating his newly planted sod yard. Another conflict resulted when a rider of a mare in estrus was charged by a free-ranging stallion. Supposedly, these conflicts escalated into gang fistfights and juvenile graffiti by adult men.

It was hard for me to understand getting any animal that was not affordable to feed, maintain, or control. I have had a love for animals since childhood, but because I did love them, I believed it to be my total responsibility for their welfare, if they belonged to me. I have always enjoyed the animals that the Lord created for our enjoyment and dominion over. I believe that the Lord not only wants, but also expects us to be responsible for all that He gives us—not just the animals. It is sometimes hard to put some human beings ahead of devoted pets, but God's word is quite clear that man was to have dominion over the animals—not the animals over man!

We took advantage of one of the beautiful days to hike in the Rocky Mountain National Park. Jeremiah chose the alluvial fan to Lawn Lake trail. We, unwisely, did bother checking out the trail mileage or rating. That was our first mistake. We had already done all the easy trails and half of the moderate trails. For some strange reason (or lack of reason), we thought the alluvial fan was a moderate trail of a couple of miles. Not being in the brightest condition that day, it did not occur to us as we scrambled up over the huge boulders and the steep sides of the cliff running along Roaring River that we were taking on more than we bargained for.

I was huffing and puffing and beginning to doubt my hiking ability about two miles or so up the vague trail we were supposedly following. After much questioning of their so-called trail, we finally came to a log bridge, crossed over the river, and actually found ourselves on a lovely trail of long switchbacks up to Lawn Lake.

I was starting to really enjoy the true trail (not Jerry and Jeremiah's idea of a trail), when my not-so-thoughtful husband decided to forge on ahead of us slowpokes—without telling us of his plans. Jeremiah kept up with him for a while, but then lost track of where his dad got off the trail in trying to shortcut the switchbacks (second mistake). Jeremiah decided to wait for us and when asked if his dad went on ahead, he did not know. The high altitude must have affected his mind, because he thought his dad had gone down along the river to take more pictures. So we called and called and called. I decided that we would go on up the trail and probably find him waiting on us to catch up with him. We went for several miles, calling out many times, but nothing. I was beginning to lose the joy of the trail as I started thinking of the dangers off the trail, such as stepping on a loose rock and tumbling unconscious over the edge; stepping or jumping on a slippery rock near the river and falling into the rapidly flowing water over rocks; falling out of sight unconscious; finding a bear or a bear finding him and running until he was thoroughly lost and exhausted. Of course, I should have remembered that Jerry did not believe in running from animals anymore. He and I had gone hiking in the Wichita Mountains of Oklahoma (we were engaged at the time). We had followed a small buffalo herd for an hour or two when a buffalo cow decided we were too close to her calf. She charged at us, and I ran one way, while Jerry headed into another direction. Suddenly, I heard him screaming! I turned around in horror, expecting to see him being gored and stomped by the buffalo. Instead, he was jumping up and down, waving his arms up and down and screaming at the top of his lungs at her! She turned aside and ran back to the herd. When I ran to Jerry, he gasped, "My shoes wouldn't grip the ground . . . she was gaining on me . . . so trying to scare her was my only option."

Needless to say, the more active my imagination, the less enjoyable the hike. And my imagination was going wild! What if we never found him? How would I explain to Mom the disappearance of her son on a hiking trail?

Jerry set a time limit of 2:00 p.m. for us to turn back down the trail. We had started on the hike at 10:30 a.m., and it was now 2:17 p.m., and we still had not found Jerry or Lawn Lake. He had said that we needed to be sure that we had plenty of daylight to get back to the van parked at the trailhead. We did come across an arrow drawn in the dirt, pointing toward the Lawn Lake marker instead of the Black Canyon trail, but we could not be sure who had drawn it or when. We started calling out again, but no one responded. I learned later that we were only five to ten minutes away from the actual Lawn Lake dam—our former goal. I decided that Jerry would stick pretty close to his time schedule (if he were able), and that we had better not go any further. That was our third mistake.

On the way back down the trail, we met three single hikers at different times. We asked if they had seen anyone fitting Jerry's description of wearing a red plaid shirt around his waist and a red hat (fourth mistake). Until coming across us on the trail, they had seen no one else. As we talked to each hiker, we told them that if they should meet Jerry, tell him we headed back to the van.

We hiked back to the spot where Jeremiah had last seen him and started climbing up and down, along the riverbank, looking for him. We called, searched, hiked, and climbed, over and over, again and again. I was fretting, fuming, and making myself sick with worry. I was made clear through that he did not stay with us on the hike. After all, he was the first one to chasten or rebuke the kids if they got too far ahead or behind us in hiking other places. But I told Deb and Jeremiah that we would probably find him waiting in the van for us. Jeremiah said, "I hope so, because he locked the van up and has the only keys. Our water bottles are now empty, and the water jugs are locked in the van also." That was mistake number five—not carrying any more than I just had to. Each of us had carried our own lunches and water bottles. Jeremiah's had broken his water bottle on the trail, so we all shared our water. I carried my wallet in a belt purse around my waist, but had left my keys locked in the van.

I worried about how to get to a ranger station for help in finding Jerry. I totally forgot that we were in the park during elk-bugling season, where hundreds of elk watchers abounded along the roadsides. Deb took a look at my face and said, "Boy, I'll bet your tumors are really going to get wild, now!"

I foolishly worried about how I was going to get a job that would pay enough to provide a living for the three of us. Who was going to hire a person with cancer, regardless of how healthy and robust they seemed to be?

Again, it took my thick skull awhile to realize that all the stewing, ranting, raving, complaining and worrying were a waste of time and energy, when all I had to do was talk to the Lord. Jerry belonged to Him, just as much as the kids and I did. No matter what happened, all of our lives were in his control—not mine. Just as I was gaining some semblance of peace, Deb shouted, "There's Daddy! There's Daddy!"

Sure enough, there was Jerry (wearing a blue hat) coming down through the forest, grinning broadly. Something snapped in me. On one side of my brain, I was praising God that Jerry was safe. On the other side of my brain, I wanted to throttle him, to smash him, to downright murder him on the immediate spot where he stood smiling! I do not remember how I greeted Jerry, or if I even did, but I do remember Deb saying, "It's a good thing we have a long way back to the van so Mom can cool off."

Jerry's return comment was, "Are you kidding? Just look at how hard she's stomping down that trail!"

We got back to the van at 5:00 p.m. and found hundreds of vehicles parked along the roadsides as drivers and passengers observed the elk herds. We had heard the bulls bugling while we were still a good distance up the trail. I was embarrassed at how foolish I was in not using my head in a logical, common-sense way. I was also angry at myself for not going to the Lord the very first thing and saving myself needless anxiety. I was no longer furiously mad at Jerry, but I was still hurt. As long as no one mentioned Lawn Lake, I was fine, but I would be instantly hurt, again, as soon as the hike was brought up.

Jerry had told us that he had sat at Lawn Lake for thirty minutes, waiting on us, before a hiker that we had met on the trail said, "You're supposed to be wearing a red hat. Your family said to tell you that they headed back down the trail."

Other than being very stiff and sore the next day, we all got over the 12.4 mile hike just fine physically. It took longer for me to get over it mentally, but once I enrolled Jerry in an accidental death and dismemberment insurance policy, I felt much better. Jerry just grinned at me when I told him, "You are now free to hike where and when you please."

Jerry had taken pictures of the broken Lawn Lake dam, so the kids and I did get to see what we missed. However, I made up my mind that one day that I would do the hike again, totally on the correct trail. There is something about hiking in canyons and in the mountains that gives me a feeling of adventure, excitement, and freedom.

Chapter 26

When We Put Our Cares in God's Hands, He Puts His Peace in Our Hearts

By October 18, 1996, Dad was back home, being cared for by Mom and his sister. He was doing a good job of wearing them out at night. Home Health would come to check his vitals and give him a bath, and a therapist worked an hour or so with him each week. Each physical therapy session was $111; each skilled nurse visit was $111 and each aide visit was $91—and people wonder why government health programs are not the answer to the high cost of medical treatments!

My tumors were holding their own ground. I seemed to be at a standstill. It was possible that the second pending sale of our house was a subconscious part of my not being able to make headway on the lumps. We were going to need a three-bedroom house to rent once our house sold. An elderly neighbor had a house that he needed help in fixing up so he could sell it. The rent would be cheap in return for the labor in helping him repair it, so we entered into an agreement with him upon the sale of our house.

Our realtor failed to mention to us that the approved loan of the buyers was a state-subsidized affair for first-time home buyers, which meant time-consuming red tape. We should have known better as anything with bureaucratic fingers involved is bound to get messed up. Again, we just did not put on our thinking caps.

I seemed to be guilty of not thinking through my therapy program also. It was possible that I neutralized the effect of the three months of shark cartilage by taking cayenne capsules at the same time. The shark cartilage was to slow down the blood supply to the tumors, since tumors need blood for nutrients and oxygen and to get rid of toxic wastes. Capillary-grown supply is good for normal development of cells and healing processes, but cancer's abnormal cell division and sprawling capillaries undermine health. My goal was to cut off the tumor's blood supply, thereby cutting off their growth. However, I had been on cayenne of capsaicin capsules to improve the entire circulatory system. Cayenne feeds the cell structure of arteries, veins, and capillaries so they will regain elasticity. According to Ralph Moss's book, *Cancer Therapy: The Independent Consumer's Guide to Non-Toxic Treatment and Prevention*, cayenne is a great herb that stops bleeding on contact. But it was possible since cayenne encourages blood supply, that it was defeating the shark cartilage to cut off the blood supply to the tumors.

I had also tried DHEA earlier in my therapy program. It too may have offset my goal, because DHEA is supposed to encourage more youthful aspects of our organs. It very well could have encouraged more production of estrogen instead of less that I needed since breast cancer feeds on estrogen.

Something I learned personally and read of similar happenings to others' tumors is that the tumors seem to enter a crisis stage (get bigger suddenly) right before they drop again. It is possible that I switched tactics too soon, as patience is not one of my strong points. My immunotherapy program was just like life—for every action, there is an equal and opposite reaction. Of course, I already stated that I personally believe that for every action I take, there will be ten reactions that I did not plan on. Therefore, I am a very poor scientific experiment, as I am inconsistent about the time the second or third reaction hits me. Not being a scientific person, I have as much belief in the placebo (faith) effect of healing the body, as well as faith that heals the soul. I am convinced that many wonderful healthy results occur when a spirit of gratefulness exists, when laughter abounds, when love supports, when prayers go upward, when we have trust in our medical consultants and their treatments and most of all, when we trust that the Lord God only wants what is best for His children. The placebo effect is a large part of everyday life for all of us. If we did not believe that we would arrive at our destination safely, we would not leave our houses. If we did not believe that a doctor could help us, we would save our hard-earned dollars and do our own guesswork. If we did not believe that we would receive financial benefits for our labor, we would not be an employee. Belief (placebo) is a vital part of everyday life and should not be treated as insignificant or unscientific. It seems to be okay with the AMA, the ACS, and the NCI for cancer patients to believe in the traditional treatments, but certainly not for cancer patients to believe in alternative treatments, because the livelihood of the cancer industry would be affected.

A dear elderly lady in our church was diagnosed and treated traditionally for breast cancer in 1988. She was in her eighties when more cancer was found. She was not in pain and she got around pretty well, although her eyes had been bothered by cataracts for several years. She had been on Tamoxifen for eight years, and cataracts are one of the side effects. This lady had total trust and confidence in her doctors even when they suggested she go through radiation treatments at her advanced years! I tried to convince her that radiation was rough on much younger people than she was, and that I was afraid that her quality of life would suffer. However, this dear soul had absolute belief that no doctor would ever recommend anything to her that was not in her best interest. I made noises about the big money involved, but she was notable to comprehend that any doctor would put money ahead of any patient's health. Even when she experienced nausea, dizziness, and extreme fatigue, she believed the radiation would help her because the doctors told her that these side effects worked on killing cancer cells. I did not have the guts to tell her that I thought that the medical establishment was just continuing to make a killing off her Medicare-Medicaid insurance before she died of a complication from the treatment. One of the doctors did tell her that the radiation would probably just slow down the cancer before it came back again but said that she would just come back to see them again! She really had no clue as to what was going to happen to her body in following "proven," traditional treatments. However, this dear lady had a placebo (belief) that the medical profession had all the answers. If it were not for the placebo (belief) effect, millions of cancer patients would not have gone through the horrors of traditional treatments.

No all placebos are right or good, but if the placebo is founded and grounded upon God and His word, then regardless of the consequences in this life, the peace obtained is beyond human understanding.

My energy renewal within two weeks of taking three to five grams of vitamin C and 50,000 IU of beta carotene, however, was not placebo. In the beginning of my cancer treatment journey, I just knew they would not hurt me and might be able to get me through the recommended radiation treatments for six to eight weeks. It was just common sense (not that I claim a great quantity of that precious commodity) that if cancer was in my body because my immune system was down, why not help to build the immune system up? It was not the strategy of the AMA, ACS, or the NCI to build up the immune system but to bombard it with toxic chemicals and burning, in the hope that more cancer cells would be killed than good cells.

The only thing that seemed to take my energy level down fast was looking after young children. I felt my energy level to be equal to anyone's in physical labor, but after a few hours or looking after small children, I was physically and mentally drained. Jerry claimed that it was because I could not relax because I expected kids to get hurt and therefore could not relax around them if I was in charge of them. Accidents and kids go together.

Accidents that occurred around my own family are always in my mind, such as when several of us running round a wagon when my brother tripped over the tongue and broke his arm; several of us running through the cow pasture, when I got the inside of my thigh cut open by the barbed wire; when the kids were climbing in a tire then rolling it down a hill while throwing rocks at it, and my brother got a concussion from being hit with one of the rocks; when my cousin broke his leg while bicycling down a steep hill and lost control of the bike; when we kids were throwing stones up into a cherry tree to knock the cherries off the branches, and one of the stones cut my eyebrow open; and many other accidents when the cousins and siblings got together.

My own four children did not make me any less fearful of children being an accident looking for a place to happen. I was the one at home when Michelle broke her collarbone while playing on a child's swing set. I was the one at home when Ryan punched a hole in his head with a well driller release handle. I was the one at home when Jeremiah slipped on the concrete steps and split his chin open to the bone. At least Ryan was at home with me when Deb tripped over Jeremiah's foot and fell into a wooden shed door, slicing her arm wide open like a wedge-sliced tomato. And, Jerry's Dad did accompany me to the doctor's office when Jeremiah split his chin wide open, again, in a bike accident. It seemed to me that Jerry was a little naïve about kids and accidents, but that might have been because he had more than enough broken bones of his own and looked at accidents as facts of life.

Chapter 27

God Speaks through His Word—
Take Time to Listen

On October 18, 1996, I experienced a very great itching and tightness across my mastectomy scar, where the original tumors were first noticed. The tumors were raised, red, and crusty. Even though I had experienced something similar ten months earlier, I refused to panic this time, as I had done before. Whereas I had changed tactics by quitting the progest cream and green tea and some of my supplement quantities, this time, I decided to keep on doing exactly what I was already doing:

1. Massage olive oil over the left chest wall and armpit daily.
2. Massage progest cream on inner thighs or over the ovaries once daily, one-quarter teaspoon until the arrival of menses, then the rest from the cream for a minimum of seven days.
3. Continuation of the vitamins, minerals, and herbs as follows:

   - Four multiples, without iron and occasionally one with iron.
   - Twenty-four, 1,000 mg tablets of vitamin C (antioxidant required for tissue growth and repair—produces anti-stress hormones and aids in interferon production)
   - Three calcium-magnesium tablets of 500 mg to 250 mg each (important in the maintenance of regular heartbeat and the transmission of nerve impulses)

- Two potassium tabs of 99 mg each (important for a healthy nervous system and a regular heart rhythm, works with sodium to control the body's water balance)
- One chromium picolinate of 200 mcg (maintains stable blood sugar levels through proper insulin utilization—vital in the synthesis of cholesterol, fats, and protein
- One vitamin E, 400 IU, mixed tocopherols (improves circulation, repairs tissue and is useful in treating fibrocystic breasts and premenstrual syndrome)
- Two beta carotene of 25,000 IU each (enhances immunity and protects against pollution and cancer formation)
- Three CoQ 10 of 30 mg each—when affordable—improves cellular oxygenation
- One sod-3 of 2,000 McCord Friderich Units (known as superoxide dismutase—destroys free radicals)
- One B-12, sublingual, 1,000 mg tablet (prevents anemia)
- Two kelp tabs of 225 mcg of iodine (for mineral balance)
- Two Bromelain tabs of 500 mg, 600 GDU each (aids digestion)
- Nine shark cartilage capsules of 740 mg each (enhance blood vessel development in the good tissue, while the bad tissue does not get its blood supply)
- Two red clover capsules of 430 mg each (blood purifier)
- Two garlic tablets of 500 mg each, with lecithin of 500 mg each (garlic is a natural antibiotic and detoxifies the body. Lecithin is needed by every living cell in the body because without it, the cell membranes would harden)
- Two Echinacea of 400 mg each (two weeks on, two weeks off, good for the immune system)
- Three milk thistles tabs—also known as silymarin—of 100 mg's each (some of the most potent liver protecting substances known)
- Three dandelion tablets of 520 mg each (works synergistically with milk thistle in protecting the liver)
- Four alfalfa tabs of 500 mg each (detoxifies the body— especially the liver)
- One chlorella tab at 1,000 mg (the chlorophyll in chlorella cleanses the bloodstream)
- Two acidophilus daily (aids digestion)

- Two zinc tablets of 25 mg each (acts as a spark plug to activate the enzymes that digest cancer cells)
- One selenium tablet of 200 mcg (vitamin E's synergistic partner)
- Water—one-half gallon minimum daily (the human body is approximately 70 percent liquid, so good water is necessary for all the body's function)

My diet remained the same, even with the tremendous itching going on. I ate whole-grain pancakes, breads, cereal and pastas. I ate brown rice, potatoes, tuna, salmon, and a variety of beans. Meat had been cut back to a third, or less, of what we used to consume, due to the growth hormones and antibiotics fed to most livestock and poultry in the meat industry. Growth hormones could have spurred estrogen production, which would have fed the breast cancer. The antibiotics could make the body immune to antibiotics necessary to fight an illness. I wonder if all the antibiotics in milk could be why children seems to be developing immunity to antibiotics besides from the overprescribing of antibiotics by doctors? Since dairy products could be products of hormone-treated cattle, and eggs products of hormone-fed poultry, these items were restricted also in our home—not forbidden—just limited. I treated myself to rich foods at family and church gatherings, but otherwise, simple desserts served our family well. I tried to keep a wholesome diet as daily fare, but still had to rely on the Lord's protection from any chemicals and preservatives on our fresh fruits and vegetables. The cost of organically grown fruits and vegetables was very high.

We did not drink distilled water but boiled our tap water and set it aside to cool down to room temperature. Jerry and I drank green tea a couple of times a day. I wanted to replace it as my main drink, but was hesitant to do so when it had caffeine in it. Green tea was made from the unfermented leaves of the tea plant. Medical researchers had discovered a number of health benefits of green tea, because it contains epigallo catechin gallate (EGCG), which lowers cholesterol and improves lipid metabolism. It also has significant anticancer and antibacterial effects. Green tea is the most helpful of the caffeinated beverages, according to Andrew Weil's book, *Spontaneous Healing*. Green tea has been shown to inhibit tumor promotion in the skin and gastrointestinal tract in mice, so I had no qualms about making it a part of my daily diet. I first started drinking it in October 1995, then had the big tumor uprising by December, panicked, and temporarily stopped drinking it. Another reason for drinking the green tea was because it had chlorophyll in it, as well as the EGCG. Chlorophyll also has anticancer effects, according to Ralph W. Moss's, *Cancer Therapy: The Independent Consumer's Guide to Non-Toxic Treatment and Prevention.*

I had to keep in mind, with the latest uprising of the tumors, to not change what I had been regularly doing. It seemed that my body had benefited whenever there was an uprising and I had allowed it to run its course, so in the October 1996 uprising, I decided to ride it out as long as I could stand the itching.

On October 29, 1996, I saw Dr. Joe, as I just wanted him to document the activity that he saw, so that in the event my tumors disappeared, he would have a medical record of the proceedings. He did not know what to say or to recommend, as there was no visible seepage, but definite crusty redness. We were still learning together about God's fearfully and wonderfully made body. Even though his medical training was traditional, he was a positive-thinking medical man and an encourager. His patients were human beings who needed care, concern, and comfort—not just medical talk. He did not hesitate to show his compassion for his patients. He radiated the desire to help his patients—not play at being a coldhearted medical god.

Let me clarify that I was not a brave person. I simply believed that the Lord was in charge of my life and that He would show me daily what I needed as I sought His guidance with prayer. I might live the rest of my life with cancer—be that one day or many years. If that life was without harsh pain and able to be enjoyed (mentally and physically), it was worth my wanting to stick around. It had been shown to me by watching others, that staying involved in life, having interests and hobbies, and visiting with others was a necessity in good mental and physical health. I had already seen too many loved ones leave life mentally by way of medically prescribed drugs and I wanted no part of the drug scene—legal or otherwise. If I left my world mentally, there was no reason for me to remain on earth. Did I believe in euthanasia? *No!* Did I believe in death with dignity? Absolutely! I wanted no part of resuscitation as long as I had cancer, or if the resuscitation resulted in my being put off life-support equipment for an indefinite time period. I wanted no part of long-term life support equipment for me or anyone as it only benefited the medical community, while draining the mental and financial resources of loved ones.

For me, most pain medication would likely go into mental dementia as it commonly does in thousands of the elderly whose metabolism has slowed down (according to Dr. Sidney Wolfe's, *Worst Pills/Best Pills*).

By November 4, 1996, my tumors were covered with a fine, itchy, red rash. It was similar to a severe case of poison ivy or hives over the entire left chest area—up to the tumors in my armpit, over to the right breast, down to the drainage tube tumor, and back to the left side of my rib cage.

I would place a hot cloth over the area for several minutes (as hot as my hands could stand to handle it). The head was uncomfortable, but the relief it produced for a while was worth it. After allowing the area to dry for fifteen to thirty minutes, I would then massage the entire area with olive oil. It too was uncomfortable, but the relief was worth it. There were a few days when I thought the skin would burst from the swelling of the tumors. Jerry took pictures of the area for our records and to send to Dr. Joe for his records.

Slowly, the tumors started shrinking as the itching became intense. I constantly sought the Lord's help in keeping me from digging into the area with my fingernails. "I can do all things through Christ, which strengthens me." (Philippians 4:13)

"God is my refuge and strength, a very present help in trouble." (Psalm 46:1)

I did not know how anyone could face cancer and its deadly track record in the billion-dollar cancer industry, without the Lord's presence guiding and directing.

By November 9, 1996, the olive oil was discontinued. My chest felt like it was on fire, but not in pain so much as in warmth. The desire to scratch the itching was so strong that I could wrap my arms around myself as tight as possible and just hold myself. I tried A & D Ointment, which helped relieve the itch until time to peel the sticking clothes off. Then, I thought I would lose my skin when I tried to get it to part company with the clothing material. By this time, the rashy chest was not only swollen, but also hot to the touch. I was not sick, feverish, or in much pain, but definitely uncomfortable. I wore loose sweats with my hands under the top to keep the material from touching my skin. But most importantly, I kept busy and talked to the Lord continually, knowing He was in full control.

Chapter 28

The Heavier the Load, the Better the Traction

I kept busy with homeschooling Deb and Jeremiah, and with cleaning up our neighbor's rental house. He had agreed to rent the house to us cheaply, in return for our labor in cleaning and repairing the house and lot upon which the house was located. The original closing date of November 7 was extended to November 30, with possession of December 30, 1996. We wanted plenty of time to shovel and haul over one and one-quarter tons of trash from the rental house and garage. Our neighbor also wanted new roofing put on the back porch, kitchen, and dining-school room.

I scrubbed the food art off the cabinets and walls in the kitchen, scraped and sanitized the bathroom, and helped Jerry shampoo and sanitize the carpet. I was concerned about all the filth and cleaning chemicals coming in contact with my skin, but I tried to keep in mind that I had broken out with the rash before ever messing with the rental house. I did use plastic gloves, because the grease, mice droppings, brown recluse spiders, and human and animal waste were almost more than I could stomach.

It was beyond my understanding how anyone could live in such filth. I am not spic-and-span clean myself, so I know what normal dirt is all about. Most of the filthy homes that I have helped clean up came from overabundance and kids left to their own devices. We are a society that overindulges ourselves in material goods. The sad part to our overindulgence is that we do not even care enough about the material goods to put them away properly or to make our kids pick their overabundance. We compound the desire for material goods by charging the on credit cards that we cannot pay off at the end of the month. We do not appreciate all our abundance, yet we crave more, because we know that something is lacking in our lives and we think that material goods will fill the void. It is selfishness on our part, because we find it easier to buy some new gadget for ourselves or for our children, instead of giving of ourselves and our time to family and worthy causes. We lack order and responsibility in our own lives, so it is hard for us to teach order and responsibility to our children.

The only time I was ever "Mrs. Clean," was when Jerry was serving our country in another planned no-win war in Vietnam. The house and my job kept me occupied so that I would not become depressed by feeling sorry for myself because I missed Jerry so much. Once Jerry was back home, Mrs. Clean left as she no longer had the time, or the inclination, to fill a physical void in her life.

On November 13, 1996, I was forced by the itching to switch tactics, again. I got out the body lotion, which provided relief and since it was non-oily, it did not make my clothes stick to my skin. The tumors had shrunk to being level with the mastectomy scar, but they were still visible in their slight roundness. My menses for November was on schedule but was a heavy flow for nine days.

Since the rash stayed over the left chest wall and ribs, that knocked out the idea of an allergic reaction to food or drink. It could have been possible that the rash was irritated more by the rubbing of olive oil onto the already disturbed area, but only the Great Physician will ever be able to tell me the cause of the rash. As long as the medical profession does not have the freedom to deviate (with patient permission, of course) from standard protocol, cancer cures—using nontraditional therapies—will remain "spontaneous remissions" in the medical field.

I understand that there are a few insurance companies that do encourage and pay for alternative treatments, because they find them less expensive and just as efficient—if not better—than traditional treatments. It would seem that other insurance companies should follow that example, because it should help insurance premiums to go down (or at least remain the same). Many cancer patients want to try new therapies, but cannot afford out-of-pocket expenses, so they compromise their bodies to "approved," expensive, traditional mutilation, burning, and poisoning therapies. My vitamins, minerals, and herbs were approximately $200 a month. The nuclear medicine for the liver test had cost $1,188 for about three hours of my time (counting waiting around for my turn with the technicians).

I feel that there are many things available to help fight cancer and other diseases. Sometimes the Lord shows one person one way and another person a different way. A strong will to live is a big positive force, and we need to guard that will to live from the nasty side effects caused from the drug-pushing medical establishment.

Chapter 29

Keep Focused on God and You'll See Clearly What He Wants You to Do

As I was having twenty-three people to our house for Thanksgiving dinner on November 28, 1996, I was very thankful that most of the rash and itching was over. Most of the ten tumors were in a flattened mode. Three of them still had a sharp, pointed state, but I continued feeling physically fit and was too busy to fret over them. I knew that I was doing what the Lord would have me to do, and the final outcome was in His capable hands.

The Lord said, "Occupy, until I return." I applied this to my breast cancer and lived well each day that I looked to Him for my strength, comfort and guidance.

I would have been quite satisfied to quit the biological immunotherapy program and the more natural diet and just put my health totally in the Lord's hands for healing, but He did not give me that freedom. His still-small voice would counsel me to keep on following the path of biological immunotherapy, to keep on reading of natural healings and to keep in mind that His Word said in Genesis 1:29, " . . . Behold, I have given you every herb bearing seed, which is upon the face of all the earth, and every tree, in which is the fruit of a tree yielding seed; to you it shall be for food."

Thanksgiving food, fun, and fellowship were a good time by all. Even though we were getting closer to the government statistics on poverty level, we realized that much of poverty comes from our attitudes more than our finances. We had each other and everything we needed.

By the first half of December 1996, my tumors were in their flattest mode. When I ran my hands across them, I could barely feel them, but their outline was still noticeable in a mirror. The Lord was blessing the immune-building program, and He was also helping me to deal more successfully with stress. In the past three years, the Lord took me through the following stressful situations:

1. Mammograms, biopsies, cancer diagnosis, mastectomy, invasive tests, three different oncologists, design of a biological immunotherapy program and digestion of conventional versus unconventional treatments.
2. The off and on engagement and then marriage of our oldest son.
3. The purchase of land in Colorado (after an eight-year search and after the cancer diagnosis).
4. The birth of our first grandchild.
5. The surgeries and consequential dementia of my beloved father-in-law.
6. The building of a vacation ministry cabin long distance and very short of funds.
7. The quick engagement and marriage of our eldest daughter.
8. The selling of our home of nineteen and a half years.
9. The clean up and rental of a temporary home for our family for an undetermined length of time.

There was no way that I could figure (short of physical death) how to avoid stress. My only choice in life was to make the best of it with the Lord's leading.

We had another closing date extension for December 18, 1996, which meant we had until January 18, 1997, to get moved into our neighbor's rental house. The continual changing of the closing date and the lack of push on our realtor's part was beginning to turn into bitterness on my part. The Lord had to continually remind me that righteous wrath was okay, but not bitter anger. No matter how much I refused to pray for patience, the Lord was even more determined that I would learn it—not hate it.

I continued scrubbing and painting the rental house, while Jerry worked on shampooing extremely filthy carpets and redoing the roof.

Even if the sale did not go through, we had told our neighbor that we would have then rental in good enough condition to sell—as that was his plan once we were through renting it from him.

On December 14, 1996, we were blessed to have a family gathering of thirty relatives to celebrate the visit of Jerry's sister and her husband. Since they lived in Ohio, we did not get to see them very often. It was also Jerry's Uncle Relden's seventy-third birthday, so a great time was had by all. Jerry's uncle was recovering from arm bone cancer surgery and after many months of therapy, he was doing great and looking great. Little did we realize that he would not see his seventy-fourth birthday, here on earth, as traditional cancer treatments would take his pain-wracked life eight months later. But at this family gathering, he was totally upbeat and looking forward to many more good years with his earthly family. He truly was a joy to be around and a wonderful blessing to all who knew him.

Chapter 30

Smooth Seas Don't Make Skillful Sailors

Our house sale closed on December 19, 1996, and we were moved into the rental house by January 10, 1997. We had until the nineteenth, but I felt that buyers needed to be able to move as soon as possible, as they were expecting their fourth child. They had hoped to be moved in before the baby came, but none of us expected the sale to take four months for closing and possession—the penalty for getting involved in government programs and all the resultant red tape.

The weather held nicely for Jeremiah, Deb, and I to get most of the belongings moved. Jerry and a couple of friends helped move the heavier items. We only had one bitter, cold-blowing, snowy day with which to contend. I was thankful to the Lord for His grace to us in giving us such overall mild weather. After all, we were moving in the wintertime in Kansas—the weather *could* have been a nightmare!

Moving from our three-bedroom home of twenty years with a full basement, two-car garage, a shop, and a large yard shed to a three-bedroom home with no basement, a single-car garage, and a utility porch was an adjustment for us all. Jerry and I were at peace about the move, but it took the kids about two weeks to accept their new environment, as well as the house. Homes should be a secure place for living, but not our security for life. But the kids were just like us—they did not always seek the Lord's leading or appreciate the circumstances He placed them in when they knew He knew best.

By the time we had gotten settled in—about three weeks unpacking and organizing—the kids had our house full of neighborhood kids.

The reduction of space, which then involved the reduction of material goods, seem not to bother them, but I was a little bothered to say good-bye to several boxes of books and some bookcases. Although I had been planning on reducing our personal library of nearly four thousand books to half, whether or not we sold our house, it was hard to decide which books stayed and which went. Deb and Jeremiah were not the readers that our older two were, as we had a TV set by the time the two younger ones came along.

My December period just barely required more than a panty liner, but by the last week of January 1997, my tumors were up in arms, again, in my underarm and around the scars. The tumors located on the mastectomy scar remained in a flattened mode. I had looked forward to the end of my menstrual cycles, but now I wondered how that would affect the tumors. After all, the tumors were notorious for going down considerably after each menses.

As I mentally wrestled about the changes in a human's life over which one has no control, the Lord comforted me with His Word, "What? Know ye not that your body is the temple of the Holy Ghost in you, which ye have of God, and ye are not your own?" (1 Cor. 6:19)

Our dear, elderly friend (see chapter 26) was in severe pain and unable to walk safely by January 1997, after undergoing radiation treatments in the fall of 1996. She was put on pain medication that worked at the same time that her mind was scrambled, and she was put in a nursing home. After the radiation treatment, the bone scan showed cancer throughout her body. Before the radiation treatments, the bone scan had shown some cancer in her underarm lymph nodes.

We, who loved this formerly active and independent lady, were comforted knowing that she belonged to the Lord. She had asked Him to save her many years before and would be going home to Jesus quickly.

On January 30, 1997, my menses started heavily after a fifty-three-day cycle. I came down with a mild cold of a sore throat and stuffy nose. I was a little put out that my body dared to get a cold once or twice a year, when I consumed all those vitamins, minerals and herbs, daily! I guess it was the Lord's way of keeping me humble and keeping me from feeling physically invincible.

Even though the red rash on my chest was over with, I started treating a sore spot on my upper chest with olive oil. It had appeared after the rash episode was gone, and I thought that it was just a sore pimple trying to head out. However, the sore remained painful and itchy until the olive oil treatment.

It was a great day (even with the mild head cold) on February 5, 1997, when I celebrated my fiftieth birthday! Jerry put the announcement on the radio, "Donna is fifty today and going strong." It was such a wonderful blessing from the Lord to have active cancer for over three years and to feel outstanding in physical health. Even though I had asked the Lord daily for healing from the cancer if it was according to His perfect will, He allowed the cancer to remain. I was strong in His strength and blessings, and I had so much for which to be thankful. How great is my God, and how marvelous are His works!

Jerry and Michelle had arranged a surprise birthday party for my fiftieth, and it was certainly a surprise. They had planned on my being in church services while the guests came to the house. Instead, Deb and I had stayed at home with our mild head colds just to keep spreading colds to others. When the doorbell rang, I was quite surprised and pleased to see a dear friend who I do not get to see very often. We had just started visiting when the doorbell rang again. It was Nancy—from my cancer support group—and Michelle. Clueless me! I still did not get the connection of a birthday party. When the doorbell rang for the third time, I was flabbergasted that friends were dropping by on prayer meeting night and all picked the same night to come visit! Just call me extremely dense! When the pastor and his wife showed up, I finally get it all figured out as to what was going on—finally got it through my thick skull. The small rental house held twenty-one people even though it was a bit crowded and a mess of overflowing books, unhinged closet doors, and scattered bathroom fixtures. A good time was had despite unfinished projects and lack of organization due to Deb and I throwing a wrench into Jerry and Michelle's surprise party for me.

After five days of the olive oil treatment, the area around the itchy, pimple-like spot broke out in several itchy lumps. When the itch began to become a nuisance, I stopped the olive oil and put progest cream on it instead. The itch settled promptly. By February 21, 1997, the sore spot was nearly invisible, and the tumors were back to a low mode again. I would go back and forth on drinking green tea, as I could not decide if the caffeine in it had anything to do with the rising and falling of the tumors. I had grown rather fond of green tea on a daily basis, so I decided to use it as a treat, rather than a regular beverage just to see if there was any effect on the tumors. It was hard to give up the hot green tea several times a day, as the rental house was cold, except for the sunny dining/school room. Even with the thermostat set at sixty-three degrees, the bills were outrageous. The house had been built when utilities were cheap and the construction was such that our neighbors' wood smoke came right into our house if the wind was right. I was thankful that the winter of 1997 proved to have a lot of sunny days as the sun streamed into the dining/school room. The heat spread into the kitchen and the utility porch, where we spent most of our daytime hours.

We had no idea of a timeframe for living in the rental house, but we somehow knew it would not be that long. It was just an unsettled feeling—one of marking time while waiting on the Lord to show us where and when. We had a lot of personal preferences, but our prayers were to be where the Lord wanted us for His purposes. He knew the beginning and the end and all the in between.

For a person who absolutely hates patience, I was content to wait on the Lord for a change.

Chapter 31

We Conquer by Continuing

When the weather started warming up in February, I couldn't wait to start doing yard work—raking, hoeing, and shoveling sidewalks that had been buried under sod and gravel over many neglectful years. Of course, I incorporated Jeremiah's strong muscles to help me haul tree limbs and tree trunks to a central area for future burning. He also helped carry five-gallon buckets of soil to the bare front yard, so that I could scatter grass seed on it. Over the years, I did a lot of physical work with the four kids that the Lord blessed us with, but the working with them definitely had its drawbacks. They let it be known in all kinds of ways that they would rather be elsewhere. It never did get them out of the work, but the continual griping did put a damper on my enjoyment of the various work projects. I just had to accept the fact that my griping as a kid with my parents was being repaid twice as much! I warned the kids that their kids would also repay them with triple griping! Of course, my and Jerry's father would never have tolerated chronic griping, as the rod of correction would have been applied to the "seat" of the problem. It certainly never caused us to hate our parents, but reinforced our respect for their authority as our parents. We applied the rod only when absolutely necessary and when talking did not work first.

Our weather bounced back and forth from sixty- to seventy-degree days to twenty- to thirty-degree days. Our outside yard work was as spastic as the weather, but it felt so good to get out of the house. If it hadn't been for the well-lighted dining/school room producing so much heat and light in the main areas in which we lived and worked,

I might have been overcome with depression. I must have been around eleven years old when my family lived in a house that was sandwiched between two other houses no farther apart than a few feet. I didn't mind it then, because it was what my family was used to at the time. Now, the closeness of one neighbor approximately five to six feet away and the other neighbor fifteen to twenty feet away made the rental house seem hemmed in—almost claustrophobic from the front end of the house, so we had the tendency to congregate at the back of the house that had lots of windows to the east and south, and a view that looked out upon our backyard, a neighbor's backyard and the wide-open spaces of the National Guard Armory. My only experience of apartment living was living in a barracks that allowed good views from the windows, not the sidewall of the neighboring building a few feet away. The Lord was gracious in giving us lots of light in our main living areas.

On February 27, I started another menses. Since I had a heavy flow in January, I told Jerry that this one wouldn't amount to much. One day I will learn not to make statements like that as I gushed through two sets of pj's, sheets, and blankets during the night hours. I thought to myself, *If I don't even know my body and the way it works, how in the world can I expect Jerry to know where I am coming from.*

At times like this, I could understand some women feeling as if they got the short end of the stick in creation. With having to put up with monthly menstrual cycles (pads, cramps, and PMS), child bearing (important, but certainly not a fun time), and then menopause to top it all (irregular menses, spastic hot flashes, vaginal dryness), it was fairly easy to get negative about being a female. The Lord would remind me in His still-small voice that he had made women stronger individuals *because* of these trials. He also gave me a greater appreciation of my husband for his toleration (more often than not) of the mood swings. God blessed me with a husband who was willing to be the sole financial supporter of the family so that I (his helpmeet) could be a teacher of good things, a keeper at home, helping to train up the children in the way they should go. A lot of men and women are perfectly content with others raising and training their children (and in my greed for material goods, I would have gone the same route, however, my husband proved to be stronger on following the Lord's guidelines on raising a family than on following the trail of more and more material goods). Some families truly do need the mother working outside the home to make ends meet. Each family has to decide if it is out of necessity or material greed. I certainly am not against women being in the workforce, as long as the family ahs priority over the job. A woman can work an outside job all the rest of her life, but she has only a few short years with her children. I fully intended to work outside the home when all my children graduated, but the job that I would get would have to have similar hours to my husband's and vacation time that agree with his. He—not the job—must be my priority. Even though we had only one middle-class (on the lower end of the scale) income, the Lord saw to it that we lacked nothing necessary in the material world. In fact, He blessed us with many extras.

One of those extras was the property in Colorado. Another extra was the half-acre lot adjoining the house and lot that we did sell. And, on March 15, 1997, Jerry and I bought five lots at an auction in a neighboring town. We have always believed that land is a wonderful investment over the long haul, and there was always the idea that we might build a home of our own around the Emporia area as prices for ready-built houses just continued to escalate. Emporia was rather restrictive in prefab homes to just two local builders, so price ranges were also rather restrictive. Double-wide mobile homes were allowed in mobile home parks only within the city limits, so buying the five lots gave us future options in the neighboring town, which was not as restrictive in the house market as Emporia. Whether the loss of freedom of choice was called the cost of progress and growth, or called protectionism, depending on whether one was on the receiving end of the pocketbook or the spending end.

Shortly after we bought the five lots, we received a call from a rental manager whom we had contacted in the summer of 1996 about the sale of a 920-square-foot house that was being rented at the time, but had been offered to the occupying tenants to buy. The tenants decided to renew their rental agreement for a few more months, as they wanted to look for a bigger house in an affordable price. Six months later, the owners offered it to us.

We really had not been thinking of buying a fix and repair home yet, but we really liked the setting of this little house. With the one-hundred-by-three-hundred-foot lot, expanding it would be easy, if necessary, but the time we were ready to move into it. We knew the little house had problems with a wet basement and most of the renters had been chain-smokers and all had indoor pets.

We told the owner we wanted to inspect the house before making a decision, even though his price was quite reasonable. Unfortunately, the tenant was not in a cooperative mood and installed deadbolts on the doors to keep out the owner. The tenant had lost his family due to his booze mistress making his life one big mess. We had to make it clear to the owner that the tenant was his problem—not ours. We had no desire to be landlords. We knew many fine landlords and tenants, but the few bad one of both categories made us want to avoid both positions, if possible, in the long run. Even though we were presently renting, we still had the memory of the mess we had just cleaned up a few months ago. Our landlord had another house dumped on him in even worse shape, and he was trying to find someone to clean it up for him so he could sell it and be rid of one more burden weighing heavily on his already poor health. He felt that most of his renters were good people, and he took pride in the fact that many of his tenants had been with him for many years.

My own parents had been renters most of their lives. Dad had raised us "to leave a place in better shape than you found it." Poor does not mean trashy or filthy. We moved a lot when I was growing up, so we were not collectors. A four-by-six-foot or four-by-eight U-Haul trailer usually moved all the belongings of our family of seven! We were not heavily burdened with material goods.

Too many material goods is really destructive. We have to spend too much of our short time here on earth trying to protect it from others or hoarding it until maybe we can find a use for it. We have spent many hours at the auctions watching years of collections being sold to the highest bidder so that the proceeds could go to family members who had no attachments to the various collections. One of our neighbors kept his collections in a huge metal building filled to the brim with junk that he might need someday (if he could just remember where he put it). Another neighbor organized his junk in neat rows. A third neighbor had a junkyard completely surrounding his house. The city finally had to get tough with him when the neighbors started complaining—their long suffering had suffered too long! Even Jerry and I had a junk pile on the south edge of our property for many years before we wised up to the useless material goods weighing us down with "someday projects."

After getting rid of a lot our own junk, we noticed that Jerry did not heave near as many headaches because he did not have all the junk around, reminding him of what he was not getting done. The junk pile had been a constant nag, weighing him down mentally and physically.

We have seen marriages destroyed as the material clutter strangled the family so that they brought a bigger house with a bigger mortgage and more room to continue adding more material goods. Instead of recognizing their problem of material strangulation, they added to it financial strangulation. Since the problem continued unrecognized, the bigger house soon overflowed again with material clutter, creating overburdened and overcrowded feelings. Foreclosure and bankruptcy were added to the collecting problem. Divorce was soon erroneously seen as the solution!

The right amount of material goods gives a feeling of security and a sense of belonging. Too little gives insecurity, while too much overwhelms. We need the Lord's wisdom to guide us materially, as well as spiritually.

The Lord helped us to get rid of most of the collecting habit, but we still fought it on the little everyday things, like, bread ties, rubber bands, plastic bags, etc. We stopped going to most garage sales and auctions, unless we were after a specific item that we felt we needed. It was too easy to find treasures, bargains, and more clutter that we could not find a proper place to keep.

Collecting could become as addictive and destructive as any other bad habit that is allowed to become a way of life.

Chapter 32

Death is the Last Chapter of Time and the First Chapter of Eternity

Our eighty-four-year-old friend who had undergone radiation treatments in August and September 1996 for her recurrent breast cancer died in March 1997. She was on morphine that did not always manage to keep her from screaming in pain and agony. From what I understood in talking to her family, her arm joint dropped out of the socket and broke in several places. The family attributed it to the cancer, but I wondered how much bone destruction was done by the radiation. Her death was due to pneumonia, which seems to be a common side effect of traditional cancer treatments.

At her funeral, the first pastor that Jerry and I served under preached her service. In the kitchen, I was helping to get things ready for the funeral dinner when the pastor and I started visiting about each other's children. He and his lovely wife were the proud grandparents of a robust three-week-old grandson, and of course, we both had to pull out the latest photographs of our children and their families.

The pastor made the statement that even though our children were brought up in practicing Christian homes and had to abide by our rules, there comes a time when they must choose for themselves whom they will serve. They have to decide if they will make our God their own personal Lord—not just their Savior. Like Ruth did with Naomi (book of Ruth in the Bible), "Your God will be my God and your people will be my people."

God gives children parents (authority) for an umbrella of protection until they are able to become responsible, independent, self-reliant, and able to choose freely whom they will serve. That is the Lord's perfect plan, but we humans do not always choose to follow His perfect guidelines in His Word, the Bible. We choose to go against Him, then get furious at the consequences of our choices and blame Him for the messes we make.

On March 18, 1997, Jerry and I celebrated our thirtieth anniversary by going out to eat with our children, our son-in-law, and Jerry's folks. Then, the very next day, sixteen of us gathered at Jerry's folks' to celebrate their fifty-fifth wedding anniversary. We did not live in fear—because we all knew that our final home would be in Heaven with our Savior (John 3:16). However, we did want to make sure that we were leaving good memories for those left behind until a later time.

Dad's mental condition was rapidly deteriorating and Mom's health was beginning to fail because of the stress.

On March 24, 1997, our son and his wife celebrated her twenty-third birthday by buying a lovely older home at a fantastically reasonable price in a nice, older neighborhood. We were so happy and excited for them.

Three days later, our eighteen-month-old granddaughter laid her hand on an electric burner grid that had just been turned off. An emergency room visit was necessary. Ashley received excellent care and was also given a stuffed toy to take home with her. Her mother was so thankful that the accident happened while they were visiting her parents. She did not think that she could have coped by herself, but Lisa is a good mother. I knew she would have come through just fine, even if she had to do it alone.

When we saw Ashley two days later, she was her usual bouncing, bubbly self, with a big bandage on her right hand. Being a typically happy child, she automatically started using her left hand to replace her use of the right hand. Children adapt so quickly and find other ways to enjoy life, even under the most painful conditions. There is so much we adults could learn from children about adaptability and forgiveness.

In April 1997, three more of our friends were diagnosed with cancer—one with serious skin cancer, another (Norma) with uterine cancer, and the third (Harold) with a sarcoma lump on his arm.

Another friend, Charlie, had been treated for a slow-growing cancer, after a long series of chemo. He had been pronounced in remission, but the treatments had taken a lot out of him. He was not able to bounce back from the deadly drugs for nearly a year or more. His recent tests now showed the cancer was back, but he decided to wait a few months before undergoing any further treatments. He was finally feeling more like his old self and was not sure that he would go the same route that he had chosen before. However, he did. Not just once more, but twice, and then he died.

I felt as if I were a very poor testimony of the Lord's biological immunotherapy program. These friends knew that I was in outstanding health, with plenty of vim, vigor, and vitality; but they could not get past my active cancer. They believed that I was going to die at any moment, regardless of how good I felt. Of course, that could be true for me or anyone, since only the Lord knows our appointed time. Many friends and family members believed that I was playing with a deadly disease and just being obstinate. Jerry and I had a reputation for standing against the crowd when we felt the crowd to be in error. We had committed our lives to our God, and even though we had to desire whatsoever to be "oddballs," fanatics, or troublemakers, unfortunately, we were labeled such by many who loved us, as well as those who did not.

Jerry's aunt and uncle (who were some of our most dearly loved relatives) had undergone the traditional cancer treatments. She had cancer in her ear, so after surgery, she was radiated from the neck up to the ear and around. For over a year or more, she had no energy or any appetite. Some foods are still tasteless to her eleven years later, as the radiation had destroyed some of her taste buds.

Jerry's uncle had broken his arm shutting a gate. It was discovered that cancer was the culprit, so doctors removed and replaced a portion of his arm bone and put in a new joint. After successfully going through intensive physical therapy, he was doing well. When it came time for his routine checkup, doctors found spots on his lungs. Even though he was feeling good again, he was persuaded to begin the nightmare of invasive tests, surgeries, and aggressive chemo and radiation.

Both had unbelievable faith and trust in the doctors. They took the knocks of life with the attitude that there were others much worse off than they were. Thankfulness radiated from them most of the time, but naturally, there was some depression from the treatment assaults, as well as the idea of leaving loved ones behind.

As I thought of what lay ahead of these loved friends and family, my heart ached for them. The traditional treatments that they were choosing guaranteed them pain, depression, nausea, mutilation, and maybe extended life in quantity, but would the *quality* exist? I did not think so, but I hoped so.

Again, I was so grateful to my Lord for showing me a better way. From all indications of the lumps on my left chest at the mastectomy site, I still had breast cancer. The rising and falling of the tumors indicated activity, even after fifteen years from diagnosis and mastectomy. Yet I had enjoyed nothing but the finest level of energy, vitality, and stamina, once I took myself off the Tamoxifen recommended by the experts and began the natural biological immunotherapy program that the Lord led me to do (I did not count the yearly cold that the Lord used to remind me that I was not indestructible). The Lord blessed the vitamins, minerals, herbs, and dietary changes.

Even though it had been a very stressful fifteen years, with children going astray, children getting married, a grandchild arriving, building projects, moving challenges, failing health of parents, etc., it had also been a very blessed fifteen years. From all indications, it would continue being a stressful, busy life.

We closed on the little 880-square-foot house in our old neighborhood on April 21, 1997, and I started another period (fifty-four days from the last gusher). This one flowed strongly for twenty-four days before even slowing down and then stopped two days later. Even with a heavy flow and being in the middle of remodeling the little house and the rental house—redecorating, patching and repairing, mowing four different places, etc., it was great to continue feeling energetic and vibrant while facing the daily challenges of life on planet earth.

In the meantime, Jerry's uncle was now undergoing surgery and chemo for large tumors under his arm that had been operated on in 1996 for bone cancer. He now had cancer throughout his body, and the doctors felt that they needed to do surgery on the fast-growing lump to try to slow down the cancer. They sued the very aggressive chemo in the hopes that it would kill more cancer cells than good cells. The doctors bound him tightly around his body to help keep the swelling and pain under better control. He was still trying to maintain a good attitude, but it was a struggle. His concern was not about himself, as he knew he would be with Jesus and out of pain.

His concern was for his wife of fifty years, who had battled the ear cancer, prior to his bone cancer. Naturally, he wanted to see his fine grandsons grow up to be as fine as his two sons were. Having been a hardworking farmer his entire life, he still wanted to work the soil that he dearly loved. I had a hard time thinking of this outdoor man having cancer and wondered if the use of insecticides, herbicides, and chemical fertilizers caused it.

Chapter 33

You'll Never Get a Busy Signal
on the Prayer Line to Heaven

About mid-May, I started getting stressed out again (this time over the little 880-square-foot house). It boiled down to the same old rule that I really did not want to claim—that for every action we did to fix up the house, there were ten reactions; maybe a few less). The wiring was poorly done with wires strung everywhere. Termite damage was found in many places under the carpet and linoleum. Thankfully, none of the damage seemed structural. We discovered that the house was build in 1930, so some of the materials used in the construction were just pieced together. We knew that we would have to replace most, if not all, of the doors and windows for security, as well as for the weather. We discovered hardwood floors throughout, but they had paint, water stains, and termite damage. However, we wanted to try and salvage them, if possible, as we desired to stay clear of carpet dust. Carpet was a great noise absorber and a nice foot warmer on winter days, but it also absorbed dirt and dust that was difficult to remove with ordinary vacuuming.

Water was still coming into the small basement, but Jerry helped the air circulation by removing a non-supporting wood wall that had blocked the only workable window in the basement. The small basement would be ideal for nonrusting storables and a storm shelter, if we could get the water seepage under control.

We were madly rushing to get cabinets, countertops, cupboards, closets, ceiling fans, etc., put in by June 15. We were hopefully going to be moving from our neighbor's rental into the little house located in our old neighborhood. The pressures of the following were weighing heavily on me:

1. A self-imposed moving date;
2. The desire to help our married son with their repairs and redecorating challenges of their newly purchased home;
3. The need to help Jerry's folks with badly needed house repairs and maintenance;
4. The need to pass an inspection or two on the Lord's ministry cabin in Colorado;
5. The extra-long flowing period, with irritating pads and marital inconvenience.

The pileup of stressful concerns came to a head after two humid days of temperatures in the nineties. Our married daughter asked her Dad for a loan to enable them to buy a house. Even though she was permanently employed, her husband was not, as he had been laid off. They had not been able to save any money due to owning three vehicles and maxed-out credit cards. I had expected Jerry to reason with them and turn them down, as his Dad had done for us many years ago when we were trying to buy a camper van that Dad felt was not worth the money (the van proved Dad correct). However, Jerry agreed to help them!

God's word says, "Let not the sun go down on your wrath," but I went to bed *furious*! I woke up in the same way. When Jerry greeted me warmly in the morning, I snapped at him like a rabid animal would do. Finally, I burst into tears and the stress seemed to flow away with the tears. I knew in my heart that the Lord would not put on us any more than we could bear. I needed to live one day at a time, trusting the Lord to guide me through each day's trials. I had been back to borrowing trouble and trying to do things under my own weak power. I had prayed for His perfect will in getting the little house—not His permissive will. I needed to realize that the little house was His perfect will for us to buy it, but perfect will did not mean there would be no trials or difficulties! Our daughter and her hubby belonged to the Lord too, and were also praying for His perfect will while they tried various doors.

Their loan fell through, so they decided to move out of Jerry's folks' upstairs apartment and move in with her husband's parents, who had a large house. They wanted to save up money for a down payment on a house of their own.

Jerry's mom then asked us if we would consider taking the upstairs apartment, plus a bedroom downstairs so she could have more help. Deb and Jeremiah would each have their own bedrooms upstairs, as usual, and our family would have our own little kitchen, dining-living and full bath.

We could not consider anything else but helping the ones who had helped us over the years, so naturally, we said we would take the apartment. The pressure of having the little house ready to move into was no longer a problem, since we figured we would be able to work on it at our leisure. Our son and his family were able to get their house in decent order without any help from us, as her parents were able to dig right in. Together, they did a beautiful job.

Our friends in Colorado were awaiting our next trip, so that they could help us get things ready for the rough-in plumbing inspection. The long-flowing period finally ended with no ill effects. The marital inconvenience did not end in infidelity or loss of physical or emotional love for each other.

Since the folks' apartment was fully furnished, we decided to store our furniture in the bedrooms of the little house, as we wanted to finish the living room and kitchen before other rooms were worked on. We were just taking our clothes, cooking and eating utensils, bedding, one bookcase of books, entertainment center and all its electrical components, video cabinets and a baker's rack for the extra storage needed in the little kitchen.

Basically, life proceeded as usual—normally abnormal!

Chapter 34

Compassion is Love in Action

We had just finished helping our son and his family to get moved into their newly redecorated house. We had finished moving Michelle and Troy out of the upstairs apartment and into his parents' home. We finished all of our obligations to our landlord. We moved most of our household furnishings to the little house and the necessities to the folks' apartment so we could assist Mom in the care of Dad, and I started another overflowing period on June 12, 1997! Praise the Lord—it lasted only five days and was over before we left for Colorado again!

Jerry had borrowed a trailer from a friend so that we might move some things out to the cabin basement in Colorado. However, he finally decided that we were not going to move any more things anywhere for a while. We decided to just take our 1986 Aerostar, packed with our clothes, some food and cooking pots, and toiletries. Jerry and I were looking forward to a little less stress and more of a vacation from June 20, 1997 through July 6, 1997.

The kids and I mowed our various properties before leaving for Colorado. We helped Mom get her spare bedroom organized so that Jerry's sister from Ohio would have a place to sleep, as she was coming back to Kansas to help out while we were gone. The folks had celebrated fifty-five years of marriage in March, and I do not think that they had parted with much of the material goods accumulated during that time (including a lot of their four children's junk and clothes).

It is too bad that we Christians (specifically) need so much security of material goods when the Lord has promised to care for our every need. I am not writing about being wasteful or discarding everything not in use to the dumpster. Our move showed me that we were just as insecure as the rest of the family collectors (nineteen coats for two people, clothes closets packed to the brim with more outfits than we would ever wear, two sets of pots, pans and dishes, not counting the boxed china, 550 video tapes, 1,500-plus books still from the original four thousand a year ago, music records and tapes that we rarely listened to and old beta tapes and beta machines.

We decided that every time we bought or were given a new article of clothing, we had to pick out a similar article to give away to someone else or to an organization that helped the needy. That, at least, kept the closets and drawers from overflowing, yet still bountiful and useful.

Our vacation trip in June to Colorado was anything but a vacation! From our arrival time until two days before our departure, we met one obstacle after another. However, every obstacle had a blessing right alongside it.

We drove onto our property and found the driveway and the dirt basement flooded. Neither was usable. Our camper was parked in six to eight inches of water and another six to eight inches of mud. We had stored our bedding mats, sleeping bags, camping cookware, flatware, dishes, cups, candles, and lanterns in the camper. But within a very short time of our arrival, a couple who lived about one-quarter or one-half mile from us dropped by to meet and visit. When they saw our water problem, they immediately started pitching in to help us. They got water hoses to start siphoning the water out of the basement and over the hill. He went to get a water pump from a neighbor of his and a generator from another neighbor of ours. Our good friends in the chalet-style cabin loaned us waders or rubber boots so we could get items out of the camper that we needed.

The neighbor who loaned us his generator for pumping out the unwelcomed water wanted us to keep it for any electrical use that we might have. Once we got all the water pumped out, that same neighbor loaned us his lawn mower and weed eater, because the very wet spring had also brought forth an abundance of tall grasses, flowers, and weeds clear up to the front door. Next, he brought us a camp shower to heat our water in. We would then take the three-hour, sunshine-heated water and pour into our ten-gallon insulated container so that all four of us would each be able to take warm sponge baths each evening after the day's hard labor was done. By the way, this particular neighbor was the very same person who was sued by the abod, who labeled him as a "lazy, welfare recipient who didn't care about anything but himself."

Some of the neighbors who loaned us items and helped bail water had never met us before. Each and every one became special to us (just a couple of the abod members were special to us, even if we did not see eye to eye on the interpretation of the covenants and the spending of road dues). These people acted upon a need—not for any monetary gain or future business prospect. They went out of their way to visit and to meet needs. We hoped that we would not have to go against any of these neighbors or offend them in the stand that we felt the Lord would have us to take in dealing with the abod management of the association. But we had picked this particular week to be here for the annual summer picnic and business meeting so that we could express our displeasure of their wrongful expenditures of road maintenance fees.

Deb and Jeremiah's playmates of last year had moved away. Even though they missed Josh and Jenny, it didn't take long to find other great kids to play with. Even though Jerry and I did not have a lot of spare time for visiting, we did it as often as we could. Our wonderful neighbors who had taken us under their wing last summer (he took us rock rappelling), brought us homemade chocolate chip cookies and a gallon of pink lemonade! She said we needed a break from all of our hard labor of ditch digging and mud mucking. It did not take much persuasion on her part to convince us to relax and visit awhile with her. They are country folk clear through and so absolutely easy to visit with.

Deb and Jeremiah made new friend with the three fine sons of the "generator neighbor." In fact, our two kids practically lived at their A-frame home when we did not have them shoveling mud and hauling dirt. We had met our generator neighbor last year and liked him, even though we thought he seemed a bit radical in his opinion of the abod and their rule on the mountain.

Unfortunately, we too noticed some big problems as the year had passed (see chapter 21). We were still irritated at the lawsuits (using road dues) and the refusal of the abod to accept our proxy letter and *no* votes on raising road dues. So Jerry and I had worked up an eleven-point, three-page letter to read aloud at the annual summer picnic meeting, which was our first reason for the June trip. The second reason was to get the framing and rough-in plumbing inspected.

Neither job proved to be easy, but the Lord provided the strength, support, and endurance to do both. The meeting proved to be a name calling, cursing, shouting match after we verbally presented our three pages of concerns. Some may have cursed Jerry and me, but most of the cursing was to or from board members. The lawsuits that the abod had done were arbitrary, selective, and personal vendettas by a majority of the five directors and a few other parcel owners who believed they had the right to collect road maintenance dues to spend in any way they chose under the guise of enforcing the covenants. Some board members did not agree with the lawsuits, but were voted down, and some were replaced by a vote of the other board members. We could not find any indications that ballots were ever sent out to parcel owners of record for voting on board of directors or raising of dues. Only lot owners present at the annual summer meeting (and in "good standing") could vote.

We had arrived at the meeting before noon, but were not able to get back to the cabin until 6:30 p.m., because various individuals tried to explain to us what was what. Some of the individuals had nicknames such as Tattoo, Volcano, and Rambo, because of their physical or character traits.

Jerry and I were put on the "delinquent dues list," even though we had owned the two lots less than two years and had already paid $400 in dues. The realtor had told us that dues were $75 yearly, per lot, for road upkeep. We reminded him of his statements at least three times the day of the meeting. Our eleven-point letter did offend the abod, and we did not like hurting two of the directors that had been a tremendous help to us our fist summer. We still liked them very much and hoped that one day, they would like us again.

We had tried to make it clear that we were not accusing anyone directly of misappropriation of funds, but of a general lack of financial and legal wisdom, as well as selective prosecution.

One couple had wanted to voice their concerns also, but since they were not living year round in their lovely little cabin, they feared retaliation if they made waves. We explained that our cabin belonged to the Lord. If *He* chose to let fire or vandalism destroy it, it was entirely in *His* capable hands. After all, *He* bought us! "What? Know ye not that your body is the temple of the Holy Ghost, which is in you, which ye have of God, and ye are not your own? For ye are bought with a price: therefore, glorify God in your body, and in your spirit, which are God's" (1 Corinthians 6:19-20).

It hurt us to have some of our neighbors go by a few days after the meeting and not give us their former, friendly waves of greeting, but we knew our stand was the right stand, whether in the minority or not. A lot of the parcel owners did not like what was going on, but they felt it was important not to rock the boat for fear of not being able to go up and down the roads safely. They failed to realize that those thousands of misspent dollars cost them even more in lost revenues from the court decree that filings 1 and 2 were not legally bound to the covenants. Their fear of hazardous roads was coming true from allowing the abod to do wrong.

I could not help but think of the saying, "All that's necessary for evil to triumph is for good people to do nothing." And, that mountain community was filled with many good people who had reached the frustration point, but did not know how to go about correcting errors that had just kept multiplying.

However, even with the association problems, the Lord continued showing us loving, caring neighbors. A lovely family fixed suppers for us. Another invited us to celebrate the Fourth of July with their family. Deb and Jeremiah's three friends pitched in and helped dig and haul dirt. Another new neighbor brought up his tractor and dug a drainage ditch along our driveway. The parcel owner directly south of our lot (he had not yet started to build on his parcel), helped Jerry line out the rough-in plumbing for inspection. Even the county inspector was gracious in stopped by a few days before the scheduled inspection, to see if they were doing it correctly. Jerry had asked the inspector to drop by before they glued the plumbing. There were a couple of big errors, so correcting the mistakes was much simpler since the plumbing had not been glued.

Deb and I enjoyed a day in Estes Park at the Arabian Horse Show that was held each year at the fairgrounds. Jerry and Jeremiah went to the miniature golf course and the go-cart track. Then, we all met in the evening at our friend's camper to enjoy the Estes Park fireworks display over Estes Lake.

Our hearts were uplifted from the show of love and neighborliness radiating from many of the folks on the mountain. It made going back to Emporia a lot easier just knowing the Lord's cabin was under the watchful eye of good neighbors.

Our neighbor who was being sued by the abod was good enough to show us how to look up public records at the courthouse. We did not know what the Lord had in store for us, but we knew we needed to be prepared for a possible court battle, as the abod insisted that we owed $100 in road dues or they would turn our names over to a collection agency. As it was, one abod member told Jerry that he was not a member in good standing, so he would not be able to vote. When Jerry challenged him on that stand, the director told him that Jerry's opinion did not count. The director did not get to eat his lunch until Jerry firmly made him understand that Jerry's opinion *did* count—whether right or wrong—his opinion counted!

Chapter 35

No Force is Greater than the Power of God's Love

Jerry's folks had a huge garage building on their double-lot property. The garage could have easily held several compact vehicles, but due to years of material accumulations, it was only able to house one vehicle. So, when we got back from our June trip to Colorado, I made their garage a priority. Jerry's dad had been an outstanding carpenter for over twenty years and had owned apartment buildings also. Therefore, no scraps of lumber, electrical parts, plumbing supplies, roofing material, carpeting, etc., were ever disposed of; this, not to mention the fact that he was also a mechanic and collected all kinds of vehicle parts. Being a general handyman meant that he kept everything. If he had been an organizer, it would have been a thrifty thing to do, but that was not the case. His garage reminded me of when we used to have a big, twenty-three-cubic-foot chest freezer. I very rarely ever got to the bottom to get frozen food out of it. I just kept buying more good buys and putting the specials on top or in the middle of the food already stored in the freezer. Since emptying the freezer to defrost it was such a nightmare, foods got frost tasting because I did not defrost it. We finally wised up and sold the big freezer and bought a much smaller one. Organization and rotation of the frozen foods proved to be an easy task, as very little food was wasted from old age or frost buildup.

The cleaning out of the garage went slow, but I would put out Sale signs and place items on the lawn by the garage. Mom and Dad lived on a very busy street corner, so they made nearly $120 in two afternoons of my cleaning off a twelve- to fifteen-foot section of shelves.

It seemed to work out well with us living in the same house with Jerry's folks. Dad was not happy that he could not send us to our own home when we would have to exercise tough love on him. For the past couple of years or more, Dad had been used to abusing Mom verbally and threatening her physically. It was a hard thing to keep in mind that even though Dad looked and sounded like the "old Dad," his gentleness, wit, wisdom, and tolerance were generally gone. The shell remaining had a bitter, paranoid, stubborn, cantankerous, demented person I left behind most of the time. It was never easy to tell if Dad knew what he was doing or what he was saying.

On July 1, 1997, our son and his wife celebrated two years of marriage (by God's grace). We could not help but wonder how much longer it would last if they did not put Christ first in their lives. We loved them so much, but we knew the Lord loved them even more. Because of the good qualities that both possessed, we knew that they could have a little piece of heaven in their marriage if they would allow their Savior to direct them. They had such good points to build on, but usually, they only showed each other the bad points. They both loved their little girl, and we sometimes thought our granddaughter was the only "glue" holding them together.

The Lord reminded me that Jerry and I had been in their shoes after eight years of marriage. We had no room for the God of heaven—only room for the god of materialism and self-centeredness. But God's timing for us was perfect. About the time Jerry asked me for a divorce, we had a small baby boy (Ryan), who was about six weeks old. A lot of our messed-up friends came from split homes, and we suddenly realized that we did not want that lifestyle for our helpless, innocent baby. We had told our son that he had saved our marriage because we had to think about what was best for *him*, instead of our selfish selves. In reality, God used an innocent, helpless baby to save our marriage. It took more than two years for us to realize that we're sinners and needed to be forgiven by a Holy God. It took more than two years for us to accept the fact that God the Father sent God the Son (Jesus Christ) to die on the cruel cross for our sins. It took more than two years for us to swallow our vanity, pride, and selfishness to ask Jesus Christ to forgive us and save us from our sins that we might be with *Him* when *He* calls us to our eternal heavenly home from this temporary, earthly home.

Our prayers were that our son and daughter-in-law would surrender to the Lord's leadership a lot sooner than we had done. It would save them a lot of heartache and heartbreak. Even though they both accepted Jesus as their Savior, they were not letting Him be the Lord of their lives.

My menstrual cycles seemed to be doing fine, even though irregular. I spotted off and on between a thirty-two-day cycle and a twenty-one-day cycle then hit a full-flowing period that was finished by August 9, 1997, when we left for Colorado again.

Our daughter and son-in-law had just celebrated their first year of marriage. Their year had been rough financially, and there had been a lot of physical illness between the two of them. Troy was temporarily laid off and then in the hospital twice for different medical problems. Both Troy and Michelle maintained good attitudes toward each other and made the Lord a priority in their lives.

We loved all of our children very much and when they hurt, we hurt also. We would like to have shielded them from all pain and obstacles, but the Lord did not allow us to interfere. Obstacles and trials strengthened them and made the good times even sweeter and more precious.

We knew we could not bail them out of too many problems, because they would not rely on the Lord then. The Lord met every need the kids had and then some.

Jerry's family was always there for us, but they were not able to hold our marriage together. We wanted to always be fore for our kids and their families, but we knew that we could not build strong marriages for them. Only the Lord had the power to lead, to direct, to build and to strengthen their marriages. We tried to help out when possible, without interfering.

Our two younger kids would have loved a lot less interference in their lives socially, and would have loved to get money from us at every opportunity, but we had the philosophy that honestly earned monies built strong character, as well as greater appreciation.

Chapter 36

God's Strength is Best Seen in Our Weakness

Our August 1997 trip to Colorado was enjoyable again, even though it involved a lot more hard work. We waterproofed the house siding for the second year in a row. We also spread ten yards of three-quarter rock in the basement. The sad part of the entire week was when I lost my wedding ring somewhere in the ten yards of gravel distribution. Our neighbor (the one being sued by the abod for back dues and junk vehicles in sight) spent hours with his metal detector looking for it, but to no avail.

I tried not to let it ruin my time in Colorado at the cabin, but I did get grumpy and grouchy when I would think about the ring that I had worn for nearly thirty-one years! It was sentimental materialism mostly, but also symbolic of enduring some hard trials over the years, as well as enjoying many blessings together. The Lord helped me see that the ring was not my marriage. My marriage would go on even without the little white gold band. I prayed that the Lord would help us find it in the driveway, ditches or basement, but He did not see fit to answer my prayers with the finding of my ring, at this time.

It took a few days to experience a peace with the lost ring that I was also experiencing with my cancer. The Lord knows all things, and as a former pastor once told our congregation, "God has a beautiful quilt pattern of our life that we will see the topside of one day, but for now, all we see are the knots and tangles of a fuzzy picture from the bottom side of the quilt."

On August 23, 1997, I started another period that lasted twenty-five days, with lots of overflows. I had no back pains, no headaches, no stomach cramps, no cold, no loss of energy—just lots of inconvenience!

I was now starting into my seventeenth year of homeschooling. Deb was an eighth grader, and Jeremiah was a freshman in high school. I had five more years left to supervise the academic education of our two youngest offspring before both graduated.

I was looking forward to every day the Lord gave me and all the new experiences that He had in store for our family. I also looked forward to starting another new career in life on this earth, if the Lord tarried in calling me home. Jerry was looking forward to a new career too. Even though neither of us knew what tomorrow would bring, we still needed to make flexible plans and goals.

A friend (Harold), who was only sixty-two years old, died suddenly of a heart attack. He had been under a lot of medications for asthma and high blood pressure and had felt poorly for a long time. I remembered reading about a Dr. F. Batmanghelidj who had presented at the Third Interscience World Conference on Inflammation, Antiheumatics and Analgesics in 1989 (*Amazing Medicines The Drug Companies Don't Want You To Discover*, pp. 358-361).

Dr. Batmanghelidj showed that if a person drank eight to ten glasses of water a day, asthma would disappear and not return as long as the person maintained the water regimen. He also maintained that high blood pressure was caused by dehydration. Yet the medical establishment prescribed diuretics to alleviate high blood pressure. Diuretics accelerate the movement of water out of the body, according to many of my older friends who have high blood pressure and have been told by traditional doctors that these diuretics are necessary to lower their blood pressure. According to *Worst Pills/Best Pills II*, a diuretic (water pill) is a drug that increases the amount of urine produced by helping the kidneys get rid of water and salt. Potassium may be lost also, so doctors should monitor their patients who are placed on diuretics. I know of several people who have blacked out from potassium deficiency (they did not have flu symptoms), but they did have blood pressure problems.

It does not cost anything to try the water treatment. It may mean a few more trips to the toilet, but exercise is also good for everyone. I, generally, try to drink a minimum of sixty-four ounces of water daily, counting the use of one green tea bag in two cups of tea daily. When I failed to drink at least that amount daily, I would be reminded rather quickly with bladder infection symptoms. I had the tendency to get so busy on a project that I would forget to drink enough water. In my zeal to organize and clean the folks' garage, I did not take the time to drink as much water. In just a few days, I felt very uncomfortable, sharp-pulling when I urinated. As soon as I got it through my thick head that what was going on, I started drinking out of a sixty-four-ounce plastic squeeze bottle (filled with dechlorinated water) for the next three to four days. The problem cleared up. I boiled my tap water, then drank it hot or at room temperature, depending on the temperature of the day. I also had a filtered pitcher that I used to help provide better water than straight from the tap with all the added chemicals used in most municipal water systems.

Hebrews 9:27 reads: "And as it is appointed unto men once to die, but after this the judgment."

Job 14:5 reads: "Seeing his days are determined, the number of his months are with thee, thou has appointed his bounds that he cannot pass."

God alone knows how many days He has given us on this planet earth. Therefore, I did not believe that anyone could lengthen their days on earth by changing diets, taking supplements, drinking bottled water or exercising so minutes per day. However, I did feel that the "quality" of those days could certainly be better with the addition of some of these changes to our lifestyles. I definitely wanted quality over quantity of my days on earth.

I had so much for which to be thankful and would get so angry with myself for wanting things like less humidity, Indian summer year round so work projects could be enjoyed, Dad's mind to be restored or for the Lord to take him home to heaven, my cancer to be gone from my body as well from the bodies of friends and family, the abod in Colorado to be disbanded so neighbors could be free of the threat of lawsuits and liens, and for everyone to like us!

I was content with where the Lord had me at this time of my life, but that contentment was more of an acceptance of the trials. It did not mean that I had no wants or desires. It just meant adaptability on a temporary basis in my mind.

The irregular and sometimes very lengthy menstrual periods certainly had an impact on my physical love life with Jerry, but so had the mastectomy. We adapted and learned how to fulfill and satisfy each other's physical and emotional needs. Because we cared enough for each other to adapt to these inconveniences, our love life was better than ever—absolutely wonderful. The Lord's determination to teach us adaptability made us better lovers to each other. However, I still looked forward to the ending of my menstrual cycles naturally (not by way of hysterectomy or oophorectomy), even though I knew it would mean adapting to other changes that would then occur in my body when that time came.

I was glad that I did know the future for my family or myself on this earth, yet I was delighted that I did know where their and my eternal futures would be. Life on earth would continue having obstacles (with the blessing right alongside). Just as I wanted only the best for my children, my Heavenly Father wanted only the best for His children. However, unlike myself, who did not always know what was truly best for my children, the Lord always knows what is best for His children.

Chapter 37

God's Warnings Are to Protect Us, Not to Punish Us

It was amazing how therapeutic talking to others with cancer was—even when they, more often than not, disagreed with my cancer therapy program. By the time they finished telling me about their treatments and the side effects they endured, I was more than excited about the Lord's program for me. It could have been possible that the Lord, knowing what a weak person I am, chose this treatment for me, because I would not have "endured." Just as I claimed that the Lord did not allow me to go through morning sickness as being the weakling that I am, the Lord knew that I would do some selfish thing to avoid any more pregnancies if I had to endure continue vomiting and nausea. My Lord knows all my weaknesses!

Another therapeutic measure that I found to be beneficial was reading of other people's cancer battles—those who won as well as those who lost.

A third therapeutic help was writing down the thoughts and happenings from diagnosis, doctors, treatments and daily life. This particular therapy let me know how much I relied on the Lord to keep me straight and balanced (there are some who would argue the balanced part).

Our fourth and final trip to Colorado in 1997, was past mid-September. We arrived in clouds and mist on a Saturday. We did not see sunshine until Wednesday morning. With no heat in the cabin, we were too chilled to work on the electrical wiring. With a rainy mist, it was too wet to work on the terraced slopes that was our planed outdoor project. But the Lord blessed us by giving us the time to visit our wonderful neighbors for awhile each day or evening.

Our camper remained dry in a dry basement (even after nineteen inches of rain since July!). The cook stove kept us warm, while we played our various family board games. Once we snuggled under all the quillows (a quilt that had a pocket sewn on it that allowed the quilt to be folded in a specific way and tucked into the pocket—making a neat pillow!) and sleeping bags, we were toasty warm throughout the cold nights.

The news in our mountain community was that our sued neighbor managed to get ballots to the parcel owners asking if they wanted to keep the covenants or not. Since the covenants gave each parcel owner the right to vote to change the covenants in part or in whole, a majority of filings 3 and 4 voted to get rid of the covenants.

It made for a happy, but temporary, celebration, as the association then became a volunteer organization only. No one could be forced to belong just because they owned a parcel in the subdivision. We knew there would be parcel owners who would not pay a dime for road maintenance, regardless of how often they used the roads. There would be others, like us, who would pay for the internal roads of the subdivision, but not for the public access road to the subdivision. We believed strongly that the public access road needed to be maintained by the county and federal governments, since they claimed it. We paid taxes at the same rate as the other Larimer County residents were also forced to pay. The third group did not want to pay for the public access road, because they (1) did not have the belief or patience to petition the government to take on the responsibility of the public road; (2) feared poorly maintained roads for emergencies or getting to their jobs safely; and (3) feared that financial institutions would recall their loans if there was no association with legal force behind mandatory road fees.

We knew that there would definitely be pangs of change, yet strong doses of pain had already been felt with neighbors being forced to fork over monies to sue other neighbors. There did not seem to be any painless solution, and we knew it certainly would take a lot of effort to get the government to be responsible for its own road for at least two reasons.

The first reason was called *The Code of the West*, a book in which a government employee decided that if people chose to live in a rural or remote areas, they did not need to expect to the government to provide services like police, fire, utilities, or maintained roads. The code might have been considered sensible if the taxes took into account the lack of services provided, but common sense is not compatible with the term "government." The book reads like, "You're on your own if you move into the boondocks." But we must not think for a moment that the code means we can build or live as we please—no way. Just because the county isn't interested in providing services for taxes received does not mean that county rules, regulations, and codes set up or the more populated and serviced areas does not apply to the boondocks resident, because the government really does not mean that we are really on our own.

I know of no more prejudiced organization than big government. Since most citizens in our country look upon government as "Big Brother" looking out for their best interests, they really do not understand that the government is looking out after its own interests—not those of the ordinary citizen. If I, as an ordinary citizen, am murdered on my nonfederal job, the killer may get the death penalty. If a federal employee is murdered on the job, the killer automatically gets the death penalty. The message seems to say that federal employees have more value than nonfederal employees.

When minority groups demand that their unhealthy lifestyles be forced on the majority and the government is the biggest pusher of acceptance of the unhealthy lifestyle, whose best interest is taken into consideration?

Who supports and subsidizes the tobacco industry at the same time that it pushes keeping the addictive and health-threatening products away from vulnerable youth and captive audiences?

What organization continually interferes with parental rights under the guise of protecting innocent children—while it legalizes every day torture and murder of helpless babies?

What institution claims we have the right to choose our own religious convictions, yet when the citizens of a community overwhelmingly want Christianity shining forth openly in their community, will stop such activity under the guise of "separation of church and state? The constitution forbade the government from making any law respecting an establishment of religion or *prohibiting* the *free exercise* thereof. Our local, state, and federal governments ignore the prohibiting the free exercise thereof as they throw God out of the public educational system, Christmas programs, and judicial courts, as often as possible.

Even our local government gets caught up in being "politically correct," regardless of common sense. When a group of minority persons (not necessarily citizens of the United States) were raising fighting cocks that were not only illegal to fight in the state, but also a nuisance to their neighbors because of the noise and the fighting, common sense should have dictated that local authority put a stop to it, with citations and/or removal of the nuisance. But no, our city officials did not want to chance being considered racial or prejudiced against a minority group, so they made a law banning all livestock from the city limits, unless strict guidelines were met. So the law-abiding citizens who were raising hens for eggs and meat and those raising rabbits for their family table no longer had that freedom—all because of a few violators who were of a minority race.

Governments punish the majority constantly, because of the minority offenders, but only when government has something to gain, such as more control over the ordinary citizen. Gun control is an example of a few deaths by crazed individuals (counting on not being accountable for insane or juvenile actions) being responsible for legislative bills to rid law-abiding citizens of their right to keep and bear arms. If the government was really concerned about the senseless killings with the use of firearms, there would be mandatory hard time served in jail and prisons, regardless of the mental condition or the age of the offender (proven guilty of premeditated murder, beyond a shadow of a doubt by a jury of twelve peers). If our government was truly concerned about senseless deaths, then why isn't there legislation to ban automobiles from the highways where greater numbers of people are killed, mangled, and mutilated? Such blatant control over our freedom of mobility would cause an instant revolution.

Our government is made of people, just like us, with sin natures. God is no respecter of persons and neither should our governing officials be. Governments will do right only when the citizens *make* them do right—either through the voting process or through grassroots movements.

The Lord said, "Occupy, until I return." I take that to mean being prepared to stand and be counted for right—regardless of what effort it might cost.

The second reason that the county and state governments might fight over the maintenance of the access road, was due to the fact that the association had maintained it for nearly thirty years—even while forking over tax dollars! And as already stated, governments are not willing to take on any responsibilities that do not benefit the government more than the average citizen. However, more homes with a bigger tax base might be in our favor.

Chapter 38

Duty Can Be a Delight,
if Seen as a Divine Opportunity

My menstrual cycle and tumor activity continued being spastic. Eleven days after my twenty-five overflow days, I started heavy spotting again, for only for six days. I just continued with the progest cream until my twenty-one days were completed. My vim, vigor, and vitality remained good.

On October 2, 1997, Jerry's uncle went home to be with the Lord. After approximately eighteen months of surgeries, chemo, and radiation (up until the day he died), his quality of physical life was horrible for the last several months. He sang "In the Garden," with family members right before they were to wheel him to his final radiation treatment. He did not make it out of the room before the Lord called him home. We were so thankful that he did not have to spend any time in a nursing home—wasting away with mental delirium and agonizing pain. This beloved man was going to sorely missed by friends, family, and neighbors. His good works were known far and wide, as well as his hard work and generosity.

I found myself asking, what happened to common sense in the way of practicing medicine? Is it true that our medical colleges are heavily supported by pharmaceutical companies and that doctors are no longer capable of treating patients without deadly drugs of some kind or another? I looked into the *Journal of American Medical Association* (JAMA) and found page after page of drug ads and decided that there was a great deal of truth in the book, *Amazing Medicines the Drug Companies Don't Want You to Discover*, by University Medical

Research Publishers. They claim that pharmaceuticals control American medicine!

Our daughter and son-in-law decided to move into the little house that we had bought in April 1997. Since moving into the folks' upstairs apartment, Jerry and I had not been able to get back to the remodeling of the little house, so we had just used it to store most of our belongings. Michelle and Troy said they would work with us in getting it livable, if they could move into it afterward.

Jerry and I cleared and cleaned more of the folks' garage to store whatever furniture of ours the kids could not or would not use.

It was slower going than we thought it would be just putting down decent flooring, as we had to scrape up the old linoleum, put down underlayment, and then glue down the new vinyl flooring on the kitchen floor. That took an entire weekend for ninety square feet of space! The kitchen cabinets took ten days to put on the walls, since we had a difficult time finding studs to nail into. It meant leaving Mom to care for Dad alone, except for Jeremiah's helping her to lift and move him to the pot. We were trying to get the kids into the little house by the November 1.

On October 17, 1997, we were upstairs in our apartment working on our academic lessons, when we heard a crash and Dad screaming, "My back, my back!" We rushed down the stairs to find Dad on the floor and Mom trying to get him up. He had just blacked out, and his dead weight had hit solidly on the floor. For the next day or two, he complained about being stiff and sore, and he would not move much. Getting him to move in a certain position or place was even more difficult than usual, and getting him to the bathroom was nearly impossible.

A friend loaned us a wheelchair after Dad fell a second time within forty-eight hours. Dad quit using his right side in any controlled manner, but his speech was very clear as he yelled and cursed us for the pain he felt when we had to move him. His unsteady gait was possibly the cause of the falls, but he could have been deficient in certain nutrients also. His laxative dependency made him a prime candidate for loss of vital nutrients to his body.

With a great deal of physical maneuvering, three of us could usually get him in and out of bed, in and out of the recliner chair, and up and down on the bedside toilet (when he told us that he needed it). We had to clean up his messes, endure his screams and cries, diaper him, feed him, and try to keep a sense of humor through it all. One moment he was sweet, gentle, and thoughtful of others. The next moment, he would curse, physically fight us, and call us all manner of names. We fought to remember the former man whom we loved.

We had to exercise tough love in encouraging him to help himself and us in any way that he could so we could avoid sending him to a nursing home, if possible. Mom and three of the four offspring had checked out a few of the nursing homes already at the doctor's advice, as well as Home Health's advice, as they could see that Mom's health was starting to fail. We kept Dad informed in the hope that it would help motivate him to try to work with us, to keep exercising his body by moving about. Each day seemed as if he tried less and less.

There were days when I thought that Mom would not be able to handle one more day. She had been struggling with an arm and shoulder pain and numbness for several months. The Home Health nurse had been trying to get Mom to see a cardiologist for nearly a year, but Mom attributed (as we did too) the pain to pulling, pushing, and lifting solid Dad so much. Since I had also put my back and shoulders out a couple of times in lifting Dad, I thought she was right on target. However, her numbness bothered us, so when we had to take Dad to the family doctor, we brought the numbness to the doctor's attention. He set up an appointment for her to see a visiting cardiologist two weeks later, so Mom would not have to go out of town for an evaluation or consultation. We all left the doctor's office feeling easier of mind and somewhat relieved that she was also going to get a thorough examination.

Chapter 39

For a Healthy Heart, Give Your Faith a Workout

On the evening of October 26, 1997, Jerry and I were upstairs, talking before he and the kids headed for evening church services. I was staying home to help Mom move Dad around, should it be necessary. Deb suddenly yelled up the stairs, "Mom! Mom! Come quick!" I rushed down the stairs, thinking that Dad had fallen again. Instead, I found Mom moaning in a chair. In a low voice, filled with pain, she said, "Donna, get me to the hospital quickly, I'm having a heart attack."

I yelled for Jerry and started grabbing coats as we helped her into the van. I was afraid to call for an ambulance for fear it would take too long. I prayed, "Dear God, You promised that You would not put any burden on us that was too great to bear, so give us the strength to handle this. We need Mom so much, but if You want to take her home to be with you now, so be it. I don't know how we will cope without Mom, Lord—especially Dad—but Your perfect will be done."

The doctors pronounced her heart attack as a mild one, and they stabilized her in the ICU wing. Jerry came home about 10:00 p.m. and helped me get Dad ready for bed. By the time we got him cleaned up from having soiled himself, I knew that I was going to be talking with the Lord again, as I could hardly keep from gagging. I hated being so weak stomached (after all, Mom had put up with it for some time), but I knew that I would not be able to handle the stress physically or mentally. I despised my mental weakness.

In the morning, Jerry went on to work as usual as Home Health was sending over a young man to help clean Dad up and get him dressed for the day. Dad was familiar with the young man and liked him for his teasing, fun-loving character. Mom just called him the Bath Boy, and he was always singing his praises as he had worked with them for several months and could usually get Dad to do things that she or we could not get him to do. But the morning after Mom's heart attack, Dad was untouchable. He screamed and cursed at both the bath boy and at me. I ran to the Lord with this prayer:

"Please, Lord, if it's wrong of me to try to place Dad in a rest home until Mom is fully recovered, please slam the door quickly. If it's okay with you, please let Dad understand and be at peace with it. If it's the right thing to do now, please let it go smoothly."

When I called the Home Health office, they had all the papers necessary, the right people to contact and Dad's favorite nurse came to talk to him about the nursing home. She helped him to understand where Mom was and the rest and care that she would need. Dad's sister came over to see if he really understood what was going on. Dad told her very clearly, "I love her, and I will go so she can get better." We were able to get a private room for him and took some home items to decorate his room.

Mom was transported eighty-five miles away to Wesley Medical Center in Wichita for tests and a subsequent angioplasty, after the tests showed a clogged heart artery. With everyone's busy schedules, life did not slow down any, but definitely picked up a faster, more hectic pace. We were no longer able to slip away and help the kids work on the little house that they wanted to get moved into.

It was strange, however, that even though we were like chickens running around with their heads cut off, the Lord gave us peace about most of it. I was fretful and concerned about Jerry coming back late each night from Wichita, because I feared that six hours of sleep nightly might catch up with him while he was traveling 70 mph on the turnpike. However, the Lord always had another sibling with him who did not seem to get as sleepy as he did.

Jerry's younger sister always amazed me at how well she handled stress. She just did not seem to let stress bother her, and she could find her way around any major city, such as Topeka, Kansas City, and Wichita, Kansas; St. Louis, Missouri; Columbus, Ohio; and Pittsburgh,

Pennsylvania. The Lord had blessed her with talent galore, a great big, generous heart, and a sense of direction that wouldn't quit!

Mom was able to come home about a week later. She had several severe bouts with diarrhea (probably from the dye that had been injected into her system or medications that she had been pumped full of). She would get dizzy and very sleepy. Jerry and I questioned why she was put on a beta blocker if the angioplasty was successful. She did not have high blood pressure, chest pains, irregular heart rhythms, or migraine headaches. Mom had been under so much stress for so many years in caring for Dad that we could not be sure if the medications were responsible for her sudden tiredness or if her body was just letting down. She was feeling guilty that Dad was in the nursing home and she was relieved not to have to take care of him for awhile.

Dad seemed to adjust to the nursing home routine just fine while Mom recovered. He did ask friends to take him home sometimes, but we tried to explain to the friends and his siblings that Dad had been asking or yelling at us for nearly a year or so to "take him home"—this would be while he was sitting in his own recliner in a home that he'd lived in for over thirty-four years!

At this time in the nursing home, Dad was not yelling, screaming, or cursing the caregivers, as he had been doing to us. The staff got him up regularly (which we had not been doing, as we savored the peace and quiet for as long as we could get it). He was made to take part in the planned nursing home activities—if not as a participant, as an observer.

It was disgusting how much static Mom took from friends and relatives (of Dad's) to get him back home and under her care. We noticed that none of *these* people offered to help her care for him or to take him into *their* homes until she was fully recovered from her heart attack. It almost seemed as if they thought that her heart attack was a "put on" so that Dad could be put into a nursing home. Jerry and Mom were patient and more understanding about it than I was. In fact, I failed the tests of patience and long suffering, constantly.

Jerry's sister from Ohio was able to be with Mom in the hospital, as well as for a few days after Mom came home. In the thirty-one years that I had known Mom, I never saw her cry when one of her children left her home to return to their own home and responsibilities. The day Sis left for Ohio, Mom clung to her and cried. It really tore us up to see Mom in this state of mind. When Jerry came home for lunch, he found Mom still crying. We had appreciated Sis being able to be here as it not only comforted Mom to have her near, but it also allowed Jerry and I to help Michelle and Troy finish the little house so it was livable for them.

With all that had been going on, I was amazed that I had the first "normal" menstrual cycle for the year. With the cooler weather, I was back to drinking green tea (one teabag daily). My tumors had been up and down daily for nearly a year. They might be raised up by evening and down by morning or vice versa. I was still on the same program of twenty-four grams of vitamin C daily in four divided doses, plus the other vitamins, minerals and herbs previously mentioned (see chapter 27). I had stopped taking the CoQ10, SOD, red clover, and shark cartilage, due to budgetary reasons.

I did not spend a lot of time listening to the daily news, but I admit to a great irritation at how often the news media would bring up vitamins, minerals and herbs needing to be regulated by the noxious FDA. Granted, I had experienced a few mild side effects such as the lower body poison ivy coming out of my system after taking green barley supplements. There was also the great chest rash, but I could only guess at its cause—maybe green tea combined with the olive oil rubbed over the tumors daily. I have since used both again, but not as heavily. There was minor crusting, but no itchy rash.

According to the news media, the FDA and the ACS, the NCI and the AMA, I should be dead by now or at least hospitalized for clinically significant side effects from the large quantities of "unregulated supplements" that I have been taking daily for over fifteen years. Since it is a fact that the supplement market is taking a big chunk out of the profits of some large pharmaceutical companies, could it be that the pharmaceutical companies have bought the FDA, ACS, NCI, or even AMA officials to put the screws to the unregulated supplement market?

Brenda and I went with Mom to her internal medicine specialist for a checkup in a couple of weeks after her angioplasty. We all asked why she was on the beta blocker, and if that could be responsible for the stomach problems that she had been experiencing since coming home from the hospital. His reply was that the recommended daily aspirin was probably the culprit, but he did not want her to go off either medication or even lower the dosage being taken. Instead, he gave her another medication (Prilosec) to add to her system.

We went home and looked up Prilosec in the book *Worst Pills, Best Pills*, by Dr. Sidney Wolfe. We found the medication was recommended for ulcers or Zollinger-Ellison syndrome. She returned the sample to the specialist. Instead of taking her one big dose of aspirin daily, she divided it into two doses. She stuck with the same dosage prescribed for the beta blocker.

When she went to the heart specialist two weeks after seeing the internal medicine specialist, the heart specialist tried to get her on cholesterol medication, even though she did not have high cholesterol. Mom let him know what she thought of drugs being pushed on patients for anything and everything and nothing! She told him of the side effects that several friends had undergone on high cholesterol medications. He admitted to the side effects but thought she ought to take it anyway! When she refused his advice, he said he would write to her primary physician to see if he could persuade her differently. After all, side effects from one medication can be overcome with another medication being prescribed to combat the first medication's side effects. And, if side effects result from the second medication, then a third medication can be prescribed on top of the first two! The vicious circle can keep being added to until someone wises up or the patient is deranged or dead.

Mom had told both doctors about having had gallbladder problems for years. Did either check it out for gallstones or the like? *No!* It seemed as if they were just interested in pushing the pill of the month or some such medication. It sure made me wonder what the drug companies were offering physicians for their incentive program.

Was it any wonder that 37 percent of older adults were using five or more different prescription drugs, according to *Worst Pills, Best Pills* and that older adults made up one-sixth of the population, but used almost 40 percent of the prescription drugs filled (650 million filled a year)?

Chapter 40

No Burden is Too Heavy
for the Everlasting Arms

The holidays were celebrated with mixed feelings. Mom was feeling generally better, so we decided that we would have Thanksgiving dinner as in the past. But with Dad not being present and Jerry's uncle having gone on to be with the Lord, there was a definite sadness and loneliness. We older ones knew though that it was important to keep good traditions going for the next generation and their families. We did have a good time and we began looking forward to another gathering scheduled at Jerry's brother's home.

Since they now lived in the eastern part of Kansas (after living several hours' drive away from most of his family for nearly thirty years), Bill and Irene decided to have a pre-Christmas gathering, as their son and his family were going to fly to Alabama for Christmas with their daughter-in-law's family. We gathered at their lovely new home and had a grand time with nearly thirty friends and family. Irene fixed three varieties of rich, tasty soups and everyone else brought various trimmings. Needless to say, we enjoyed good food, fun games, and fine fellowship.

Mom, however, was being eaten up with guilt that Dad was not home yet, but she still had very few good days herself. When Dad was finally allowed to see Mom—she was brought into his room in a wheelchair—he became very agitated with everyone else. He wanted Mom back at his side, at his beck and call.

The nursing home foolishly let an experienced pregnant aide attend to Dad, by herself, when he was in a highly agitated state of mind. He butted the aide in her stomach, and she had to go home. The administrator's social services director called us to tell us that we might be held responsible! We put the blame squarely back on their shoulders! A few days later, Mom was called to get her approval of a chemical evaluation for Dad in Topeka. We all jumped at the idea that medical science would be able to find a chemical imbalance in Dad that could be corrected once identified. It took three days to get all the paperwork signed and to get Dad delivered to the Stormont Vail psychiatric-geriatric unit, where we understood he would undergo tests for chemical imbalances.

There was an error on Dad's chart from the rest home. It stated that Dad was on Librium for agitation. That was *not* true, because when the nursing home staff had called Mom for verification of her approval, she let them know that Librium was one of the drugs that had messed up Dad's mind in the first place. She flatly refused to approve the drug's use on Dad, again. They sent the drug back to the pharmacy but not clear it from his medical record. The staff in Topeka saw it on his meds record and saw Dad's agitated state upon arrival in Topeka, so they immediately ordered it for him! From past years' experiences, Librium had caused Dad more agitation, so we learned to keep him off of it totally. Imagine our consternation when we discovered, in talking to the Topeka staff, that Dad was back on it and very violent! He became more aggressive, shaky, and demented. What was their solution, even after we told them why we had taken him off the drug? They added Ativan—the same drug family as Librium! Dad went wild! Next, they added Risperdal to take away his aggression (instead of stopping the meds proven to add to his aggravation). As if all those medications were not enough, the neurologist added Requip as the second Parkinson medication for Dad.

In the meantime, we were having a confrontation with the hospital staff, as we were hurt and furious about the deception of getting Dad chemically evaluated (when sedation seemed to the primary goal).

I tried to reason with the psychiatrist (Mom could not understand his foreign accent very well), but he classified *me* as hostile to the medical community! He then threatened Mom with shipping Dad back to Emporia for her to care for (the local rest homes did not seem inclined to want him because of his aggravated agitation). I definitely became hostile, as he let us know that he knew what he was doing, and if we did not trust his judgment, then he was washing his hands of the case. (translated: "If you do not let me keep him sedated, you can have the mess that I have made out of him.")

Poor Mom was about to have another stress heart attack. I felt as if I was about to join her. I was thankful that I was not physically near enough to the man to get my hands on him. I think I could have shaken the medical stuffing out of his educated, but not sensible, head.

Mom was in tears as she told him that she would let his judgment stand and that she wanted Dad to remain in his care. I was frustrated and furious, so I ran to the One who has all the correct answers. The Lord listened and gently reminded me with His Word that He was still in control.

A couple of days later, we received a call from the staff in Topeka that they were finished with Dad. They wanted to know where to send him. I told them that they would just have to keep him until we located a facility for him, since they had not seen fit to give us a timeframe to make prior arrangements.

Mom was totally stressed out and had been since talking to the Topeka psychiatrist. I started calling around as Mom wanted Dad to be in Emporia, close by for easy visiting once her strength returned. After three turndowns because of the psychiatrist's diagnosis that Dad had aggressive dementia, some Parkinson's and some Alzheimer's (we already knew that before he ever went to Topeka, because of other doctors' diagnoses over the years), the smallest and oldest nursing home accepted the care of him.

Dad was brought back to Emporia, and from day one, he seemed to be pretty much at peace just to be back in Emporia. He actually seemed to enjoy the quieter environment. His first nursing home had been lovely but loaded with busy activities and little time to spend in his room. We had thought that was what he needed. Even though Dad was accepted only in the smallest and oldest nursing home, and even though the cost was not as expensive as the first home was, the service was just as adequate to care for his needs.

The staff psychiatrist put Dad on another drug called Aricept, to see if it would help improve his memory. Of course, we had no idea what all the meds were going to cost as reality had not yet set in.

In December 1997, Mom received the Medicare bill for the therapy that Dad had received at the first nursing home. We had, ignorantly, authorized physical therapy to keep his muscles in condition, as he had stopped walking after the two falls at home. It never occurred to us that his continuous pulling and pushing in the recliner chair was all the physical therapy that he needed to tone muscles.

To our dismay, the first thirty days billing was $10,855.68. The second for one-half a month was $5,683.54. The total bill for fifty-one days was $16,539.22. ($324.30 daily average for physical, occupational—Dad was eighty years old—and speech therapies.) We had not gotten any indication of these outrageous charges until Dad was taken to the second nursing home. Medicare paid these outlandish charges, with no questions asked. No wonder social security, Medicare, and Medicaid will not exist for my generation—not as long as big brother government encourages payments to those who take advantage of the infirmed.

We found out from the physical therapy unit at the second care home that they charged $175 an hour. The charge was from zero to sixty minutes. If the therapist showed up at Dad's door and he did not want any physical therapy, the charge was $175! If Dad only lasted five minutes into the therapy session, the charge was $175! It was quite the rip-off scheme to the taxpaying public. When Mom stopped the therapy for Dad, the staff reminded her that it was not costing her, as Medicare paid for it. She reminded them that her baby boomer children might someday like to use the system themselves, since they were forced all their working lives to pay into it also. Even friends and family members reminded her that it was not costing *her*! How blind and ignorant has become John Q. Public!

Bill and Irene opened their doors again and hosted the family Christmas gathering on Christmas Day. They felt that it might be an easier transition for everyone to make, considering the absence of Dad and their uncle. It seemed to make a difference in the new environment of their lovely, very spacious home. Again, their gift of hospitality was greatly appreciated. It let us take a break from the ongoing, everyday troubles that we were all going through.

Mom was billed directly for Dad's medications prescribed by the medical practitioners in Topeka and Emporia. The first eight days billing was $269.49 from December 23 to December 29. I questioned the bill for 124 laxative-stool softeners and eighty-five Requip (Dad was to be taking one laxative daily and three Requip daily). The nursing home management assured Mom and I that it was common practice for the pharmacy to bill ahead as well as sent the next month's meds to the nursing home. It seemed presumptuous to me that any pharmacy would bill ahead, but I did not question it any further.

The January billing took our breath away! It was $439.37. I, again, questioned the bill, mainly pointing out that the 153 Requip when we discovered that Dad was only supposed to be taking *two* daily, instead of the three that we had been originally told he was to get. The nursing home staff told us to bring them the bill, and they would clear up the matter with the pharmacy. We were so trusting and naïve, still, when we called the pharmacy and informed that the nursing home was returning several med packs for credit and that we would pay the bill as soon as they caught up with each other.

When the February bill did not come, we called the nursing home to see if all the meds had been sent back, and we asked for Dad's total med program on paper. We then called the pharmacy and were told that there were some returns, but they had not credited them to Dad's account yet.

Imagine our chagrin when Mom got the March billing of $963.92, including $8.99 finance charge! Another test on long suffering that I failed. I was not nice to deal with, and it was another two weeks getting the nursing home and pharmacy records reconciled. Mom ended up paying for the lost fifty-five tablets of Requip that Dad did not use, according to staff records, nor did they get returned, according to the pharmacy. Regardless of who got the Requip, Mom had to pay for the waste, drug abuse, or erroneous record keeping! However, the bill had been reduced to $580.64, including the finance charge. We paid the bill (minus the finance charge) and explained by letter to the pharmacy how we felt about a company that was so busy that it could not find the time to monitor what was being sent out (the same prescription for the same person for the same week, for the same address for a total of three and one-half times the prescribed amount!).

Needless to say, we changed pharmacies again. The first pharmacy did not give full credit for returned or erroneous meds, and they gave no credit if the meds were under five or six dollars, as they claimed it cost them that much to handle the returns!

We were disgusted with the general outlook that it was acceptable to take advantage of the infirmed—sock it to them! We were also disgusted that the quiet nursing home did not check to see if there was already an open med pack before they opened another. We talked to them about it and were assured it would be brought to the attention of the meds nurse.

Dad was taken off most of the drugs that had been prescribed for him in Topeka, and the staff psychiatrist at the nursing home took Dad off the Aricept also, as he felt that there had been no improvement in Dad's memory.

I was amazed that my tumors did not get any bigger than they did, with all of the turmoil and hassle trying to get Mom's pharmacy bills straightened out. As much as I tried to rely on the Lord, I still found the obstacles a struggle to get over. I just had the peace of mind though that if I fell down, the Lord was there to pick me up.

Chapter 41

It's Always Darkest before the Dawn

On February 18, 1998, I was awakened at 2:00 a.m. by sounds coming from Mom's bedroom. She was having terrible pains across her abdomen. She had me get her a 7UP from the refrigerator, and the pains were a little less by the time we both decided it was safe to go back to bed. She slept for another couple of hours, then Jerry and I were both awakened by her painful moaning. By 6:00 a.m., she and I were at the Emergency Room. Finally, at 3:00 p.m., Jerry's sister and I were told exactly what her problem was. Mom had gallstones. Apparently, one had escaped into her duct work. It then blocked her pancreas as well as her gallbladder, thereby making one a very physically ill Mom. It took nine days to get her pain and the infection under control before the doctor could remove her gallbladder. We brought her back home on February 28.

No one could tell us if the pains that Mom had been complaining about since she went on the beta blocker were due to the gallstones or not (since the doctors did not take any blood tests at those times).

Mom's surgeon made comments about how good Mom's health must be, because she was only on a beta blocker at the age of seventy-six and that people in that age bracket usually had several medications going into their bodies. I will give him credit for not once trying to put another med in her system when she was released to go home.

Mom was very slow in recovering, and she fought with depression again because she thought she ought to feel better sooner than she did. It took nearly six weeks before she was about to get out and about. She tired very quickly, but was having more good days than bad ones.

We started to breathe a little easier, then I got a call from Jerry's boss on March 25, 1998. He said that Jerry was in the hospital with a broken arm. It turned out to the same one he had broken six years ago when we were roller skating. This time, he had missed a step on a ladder that was on a steel platform and about two feet above a concrete floor. I remember saying to the Lord, "I really thought that we had enough going on in our lives already, but I guess You feel that we can handle a little more." I didn't feel angry or bitter, just numb.

At the hospital, Jerry and I laughed and talked to each other as well as the medical staff. He requested the same doctor that had worked on his crunched and broken wrist before. This break was worse in that the radius had two breaks. It took four hours after Jerry's arrival before the bone doctor arrived (due to surgeries). The medical staff had tried to give Jerry pain medication, but he refused it. He would not tell them that he had a far greater fear of needles than he did of pain. When the doctor put the deadener into Jerry's wrist, the doctor was surprised at Jerry's grimace of pain! The nurse then informed the doctor that Jerry had refused any painkillers. All of them felt bad by this time. The doctor said that Jerry was the second man to pass out in a lying down position while being given an injection of deadener. Jerry said that he did not pass out completely, but I sure was glad to see the greenish yellow color turn back to pale white.

The Lord was gracious in letting Jerry have the same doctor as before. This doctor believed in manipulation first then surgery as a last resort. The Lord was also gracious in not allowing too much temptation before us with late spring—warmer weather. We would have then been tempted to draw disability pay and then head to Colorado to the cabin to recuperate—leaving our responsibilities in Emporia to fend for themselves. But by allowing the accident to occur in cooler weather (no heat in the cabin), that temptation was more easily passed.

The Lord also motivated the doctor to give Jerry the work permission slip to return to work the next day when Jerry asked him for it. Jerry was scheduled to work on a job that required the use of one hand only and no ladder climbing, but the final decision (even with the doctor's permission slip in hand) was up to his company's management. One boss did say no, but the boss over that boss was moved to say okay.

It was very tempting for Jerry to just stay home and get some one-handed jobs done while drawing disability, but Jerry did not want to be responsible for lost time incentive rewards being taken from the rest of the maintenance crew with whom he worked. He felt that once the safety award incentives were taken away from the whole crew, it would create an atmosphere of "Who cares? What difference does it make, now, since we have already lost out on the safety rewards?" Jerry did not want to see anyone hurt because of loss of the rewards, due to his accident.

We had made plans shortly after Christmas 1997 to travel to Oklahoma to visit my sister and her husband over the Easter weekend. We all wanted to go, but I admit that it came as quite a shock to hear Jerry tell our brother-in-law that I would have to drive. I started praying to the Lord for the strength and wisdom driving through Oklahoma City. I enjoy driving on the highways, but big cities have always proven to be a nightmare with me—whether or not I drive.

In thirty years of driving, I had only driven in three huge cities, and it took a lot of faith on Jerry's part to trust me because of the following incidents:

In 1969, I was driving through Indianapolis after dark. I suddenly felt my seat being pulled back by my sister, who was traveling with us in our 1968 Mustang. I was just about to ask her what her problem was, when she said to Jerry, "What's she doing?" I quickly glanced over at Jerry and saw alarm written all over his face in the oncoming car lights. Suddenly, he yelled at me, "Are you going around that car or through that car?" I swerved around the car and was surprised to find how close I had been. Later, we learned that I could not judge distances very well at night. It was called "night blindness," with no known treatment at the time. However, the driver's vehicle department required that I wear glasses when driving even though the eye doctors said that glasses did nothing for night blindness.

In 1970, I had to drive to downtown Kansas City to the airport to pick up Jerry. He was coming home from Vietnam. It was daylight, and I took my young sister-in-law with me. Neither one of us caught on to my getting into a construction area where I apparently was not supposed to be. I suddenly saw this man in a bright orange jacket waving frantically at me, then he made a quick dive off the edge of the road. When I glanced back in my rear-view mirror, he was standing up, shaking his fist at me. To this day, I still do not know how I managed to find my way through the maze of traffic and construction coming and going around that crowded, busy airport.

About seven or eight years later, I was driving a full-sized van on I-70 in Columbus, Ohio. I had it on cruise control and had planned on pulling over before the traffic became too congested. Jerry would then take over the driving. However, I found myself with a convoy of school buses on both sides of me, as well as behind me. I panicked, yelled to Jerry to take over, and I left the driver's seat. Jerry grabbed the wheel, as he yelled, "You could have let me get into position first!"

We had both been content for many years to let me read stories aloud to everyone in the vehicle, while Jerry negotiated driving around and through big cities.

The Lord was again so gracious in helping me drive through Oklahoma City. The time of day was perfect for lighter traffic, and I was able to maintain speeds of sixty-five to seventy miles per hour, even though most vehicles were passing me by. I picked the center lane as much as possible, so Jerry and the kids could give me plenty of warning about left or right directional road changes. There was a quick crisis when I suddenly found myself facing a wooden pallet or skid in my lane. I had only enough time to look on each side of me and behind me to know that I was hemmed in tightly. My only option at sixty-five or seventy miles per hour was to attempt to straddle the pallet with our small wheel-based Aerostar. As soon as we got over it, Jerry let out his breath and said, "You did real good, sweetie." I thanked him for the compliment, but I let him know that it wasn't me. The Lord got us over that pallet because the full-sized van behind us just barely had room to straddle it, and I'm still not very good at judging distances, lengths or widths. We felt badly that we could not stop and remove the dangerous obstacle, but we did see the driver of the truck who lost the pallet pulled off to the side of the road. We could only pray that no one would get hurt before the pallet was retrieved.

Our time with my sister, Ginger, and our brother-in-law, Ralph, was wonderful! They gave us a 386 monitor, keyboard, and printer.

Ralph had set it up with Windows and Word processing so that I might be helped in getting this book written and published.

Of course, the first miracle was getting it typed. The second miracle was learning to operate the computer (Ralph made it user friendly as much as possible and gave us *Windows 3.1 for Dummies* 1 and 2 by Andy Rahrbone). The third miracle will be getting this book published. But my God is in the miracle business, and it was my sincere desire that this book would be according to His perfect will. If it could help someone to enjoy every day, cherish every blessing, and recognize trials draw us closer to our Lord (who suffered great pain and humiliation for each and every one of us with our sin-scarred natures), it would be wonderful!

I had not reached my fifth year anniversary of being "cancer free" or "in remission," but I would not have traded my health, my energy, or my well-being to go through the torture offered by the cancer establishment for a small chance that I might live a few more quantify months or years. I was not brave, bold or a glutton for punishment. I was not a macho gal. I was just an average person whom the Lord loved and care for most graciously and with much long suffering.

I looked forward my life on earth for however long the Lord saw fit to keep me functioning here. I also looked forward to the *grand reunion* with family and friends who went on before me to be with the Lord and those who would join me later when the Lord called them home.

It was a comfort to know that Jesus had died for my sins and that my going to heaven had nothing to do with any good works that I might have done. I was going to heaven simply because I believed that Jesus died on the cross for my own sins, because that is exactly what His word tells me. (John 3:16, Acts 16:30,31, Ephesians 2: 4-6, Romans 5:8, Titus 3:5, I Corinthians 1:21)

The Lord is my strength and comfort in time of need.

Chapter 42

This Life is But the Childhood of Our Immortality

Sometime in February 1998, I had been called by a neighbor of Patty's (see chapter 8). About three years after Patty went through the traditional treatments, she had a lump show up in her remaining breast. A biopsy revealed it to be a benign lump, and Patty went on with her very busy, stressful life. Now Patty had a lump on her shoulder, so she went for another biopsy, but this lump proved to be malignant. After the bone scan showed cancer throughout her body, the medical profession said her only hope was a bone marrow transplant.

In March, she was flown to Baltimore, Maryland, to the John Hopkins cancer facility to begin very aggressive chemotherapy. She was blessed with friends and family who looked after her husband who had a major stroke after being on prednisone for nearly two years. Her boss's wife took her to Kansas City International Airport to catch her flight each time she had to go to Baltimore for another round of chemo.

About mid-April, when the friend showed up to take her to the airport, Patty's behavior was abnormal. Patty was a first-class organizer, but now she wasn't even packed or dressed to go! At first her friend had thought that Patty was being silly and teasing, but the friend soon realized that Patty's mind was "glitching" in and out. After calling Patty's oldest married daughter to see what needed to be done, the family and Patty's doctor decided to send her on to John Hopkins for evaluation.

In a matter of a few days, Patty's family was told that they would have to come to Baltimore to get Patty, as she was not able to fly back. John Hopkins claimed that Patty was not totally free of cancer, but now she had Pick's disease (a loss of nerve networks and atrophy in areas involving language, memory storage, and through processing, with speech disturbances common). So much for her quantity of time offered by the cancer experts. Of course, the experts said that the chemo had nothing to do with the Pick's disease, and she was now cancer free!

It was comforting to me to know that Patty knew the Lord personally, and it was tremendous testimony of His love and strength. I wasn't concerned about Patty's life after death, as I knew she would be in heaven with her Lord and Savior. I was concerned about the family coping with another tremendous hurdle, yet I knew that the Lord would provide for their needs. Patty's youngest child was to graduate in May 1998, and she had already purchased the dress for the special occasion.

Even though we had not heard much about Pick's disease, we knew the Lord could heal her if it was according to His purpose. The "if" was not lack of faith on our part, but complete trust in His will for her life. Of course, we prayed for healing of this loved friend, but always with "according to Your will, Lord, not mine." We are limited in what we see, and limited in scope, but the Lord is all knowing.

By May 4, 1998, Patty could only speak in very simple sentences, and she had to have help in everything, including personal hygiene. It seemed as if things were going downhill fast for her. Then, I called over to Patty's to see if I could volunteer to sit with her. I was shocked and delighted to talk to a very normal Patty. She gave all the credit to the loving, caring prayers sent to the Lord on her behalf.

In my readings, it seems that various nerve signal malfunctions can and do occur when our body has a bad reaction to certain drugs. We have believed for years that Jerry's dad and a great-uncle suffered with nervous disorders due to mainstream prescription drugs, and eventually, these disorders became full-blown dementia.

I believe that the chemo drugs definitely affected Patty's nervous system, causing it to malfunction. I believe with all my heart that if she were to undergo any more chemo, her life quality, not quantity, would be shortened. Patty does not feel that way and would possibly go through it again if cancer reared its ugly cells again, but I am positive that her body sent out as loud of a warning as it possibly could.

I am not saying that Patty will die before I do. Only the Great Physician has our appointed time, and until that time comes for me, I deliberately choose to stay clear of man's chemical drug routes. Of course, that does not include the Lord's vitamins, herbs, and minerals, regardless of whether the government tries to call them "unregulated drugs" or not.

Chapter 43

Give Sin an Inch, and It Will Take a Mile

In the continuing saga of the Colorado parcel owners versus the board of directors, we received five pages of changes for the covenants, the by-laws, and the corporation. They lost their court case with our physically disabled neighbor (who had proved their illegitimacy as an association with power to force collection fees). They had ignorantly believed that a physically disabled was somehow *mentally* disabled also. It was hard to believe that anyone in their own right mind could believe such a thing.

Since the abod did not want to give up their desire for power and money, they sent out ballots to the parcel owners to vote *yes* or *no* on legitimizing the abod. In bold print on the articles of amendment to the articles of incorporation, we read, " . . . and to levy and collect assessments as established by the board of directors." They were trying to eliminate the parcel owners having any say over the amount of dues to be paid.

On the amendment of by-laws, we read, " . . . to maintain and operate roads (both interior and access)." The abod still wanted all the parcel owners to pay for a federal and county-claimed public road, nothing to indicate any plan to petition the county to maintain the road under its jurisdiction. The abod was jeopardizing every parcel owner's property, should a lawsuit occur due to an accident on an improperly maintained public access road. The three subdivisions could not reasonably pay enough road fees to meet government road standards.

Jerry and I could not just "roll over" and accept these attempted, dictatorial changes. We not only voted *no* to such despotic desires, we sent our third mailing to all the parcel owners, asking them to also vote *no* and to join with other filings (that had been liberated from the covenants and the abod in a previous ignorant lawsuit, see chapter 21) in signing a petition to the county to take over its own road. We hated being labeled "troublemakers," "chronic complainers," and "the most negative people," by folks that we personally liked as neighbors but not as abod. We hated offending them, but we had to take a stand against the wrong doings.

The abod still maintained that they had all the parcel owners best interests and investments at heart. The abod letter stated that there were no pending lawsuits or any being considered. Unfortunately, we had heard those words before when they used the need to repair the roads to raise the dues from $75 a lot to $125 a lot; and when the small majority of *present at the meeting* voted on a Saturday to increase the dues for two years only, a lawsuit that was served on two more members the following week.

They never saw fit to tell the results of the one lawsuit against the neighbor with a truck camper on his wooded lot. However, they were forced by the court's ruling of their illegitimacy to tell the results of the lawsuit against our disabled neighbor. They also failed to inform the parcel owners of how much money it cost in road funds to pursue the prejudiced lawsuits.

As I talked to the Lord about (1) our offending of people who had helped us, (2) about the time, effort, and money to send out the protest letters to all the parcel owners (a lot of whom could not see any wrongdoing or were afraid to "make waves" for fear of abod retaliation, plus they were concerned about loans being pulled due to no road association and property values dropping). They did not seem to realize that property values would increase more on a county-maintained road, and (3) about wanting to lie at peace with all our neighbors, the Lord's word comforted and strengthened me.

"Therefore to him that knoweth to do good, and doeth it not, to him it is sin." (James 4:17)

"And have no fellowship with the unfruitful works of darkness, but rather reprove them." (Ephesians 5:11)

"When the righteous are in authority, the people rejoice; but when the wicked beareth rule, the people mourn." (Proverbs 29:2)

"Hate the evil (not the evil doer) and love the good, and establish judgment in the gate" (Amos 5:15).

"Righteousness exalteth a nation, but sin is a reproach to any people" (Proverbs 14:34).

These words were for Jerry and me to examine ourselves by also, and to ask the Lord to keep us from unrighteousness ourselves. It would have been very easy to send nasty letters and call names in retaliation to some of the letters and phone calls that we received. But, the Lord also sent letters and calls of encouragement.

We were not going to be able to attend the proposed business meeting at the end of June, but neighbors said they would tape the meeting, if possible.

Chapter 44

God is Big Enough to Care for Our Smallest Need

Before leaving for Colorado for our first trip of the 1998 summer season, I called Patty to check on her progress. She was doing very well in her communication and memory skills, but was still physically unbalanced at times, so doing stairs by herself was a no-no. She was very upbeat. Neither of us knew if she had just been misdiagnosed or if the Lord intervened with another spontaneous remission miracle. Again, Patty gave full credit to the Lord for blessing her with wonderful friends and family who were willing to give of their valuable time and resources to help care for her and her husband.

Since we had decided to take the Aerostar on the first Colorado trip of the season, it meant driving straight through six hundred miles or staying overnight in a motel. With the night temperatures in Kansas being in the forties, yet we opted for a reasonably priced Budget Host in Burlington, Colorado. It was an older motel, but roomy, clean, and decorated nicely in Southwest décor. We had stopped a couple of newer motels first, but the $75 price tag sent us on down the road.

It amazed us every year how much the Loveland/Fort Collins area grew. The Lord's timing emphasis in 1995 on buying the tow lots was now or never as the real estate prices continued to skyrocket. The prices in the Rocky Mountain region were definitely out of our price range now.

The contractor, who had put our basement in and framed the cabin for us, had built a little spec cabin next to our second lot. The young couple who bought it were a delight to our family. We were sad to know that our homeschooling friends in the chalet-style cabin were going to be moving out of state, as they wanted to farm on a bigger scale than mountain conditions would allow. We were going to miss seeing this lovely family of five—soon to be six. Our mountain community was filled with warm, friendly people, and it still disturbed us that there were so many hard feelings regarding the abod management of road funds over the past years. One family, who had protesting the abod for years, had recently had someone shoot into their home! It was possible that a hunter (not in season) or target shooter (not a very good aimer) did the shooting accidentally, but with the hard feelings running amok in the mountain community, it was highly suspicious. Praise God that no one was physically hurt.

We contracted in early March with a licensed Colorado electrician to put in all our electrical wiring. He told us that he should be able to get it done by the end of April. By May, he still did not have it in. We called him to tell him that it had to be in and inspected by the first week of June, as we had to have the insulation done and inspected by the first week of July. When we arrived, the cabin had been wired, but no trench wiring to the utility pole! The electrical inspector had passed the house wiring. Our electrician arrived a couple days after our arrival and dug the trench. He was having a terrible time with the mud and muck clogging the trencher.

Jerry went up and asked him how he was doing. He said, "Terrible! I need some help from God." Jerry told him that were going to eat lunch and asked him if he would care to eat with us. He thanked Jerry, but told him that he skipped noon meals. So Jerry came into our camper in the cabin basement and told me that the trencher was clogging, and the electrician said that he needed help from God. So we bowed our heads and asked God to help him. After lunch, the electrician told Jerry that within a few minutes after Jerry left him fighting the trencher and the mud, he suddenly hit the nicest, driest dirt possible, and the trencher just took off! We told him that we had prayed that God would help him. He said that he had not hesitated to thank God as soon as he hit the nice dirt!

On June 11, 1998, we officially had electricity in our cabin. It was so nice to have a light bulb to shine after dark, without having to put up with the smelly fumes of our lanterns. We did feel a bit bad about the REA men who had to come out to do a simple, quick job of putting the meter on the pole and of hooking the line to the transformer. Unfortunately, when they backed onto our sloping lot, their heavy truck sank into the boggy soil by the pole. They had installed the pole while the ground was frozen, so they had not encountered the soggy soil of springtime. They tried using a road grader to pull them out, but the line just snapped. They had to call for a big tow truck, and it was an hour or two getting to them. The tow truck was not able to hold steady while pulling, so Jerry went after the road grader, again. Several hours later, with the road grader acting as a "dead man" to the tow truck, the tow truck, using four winch lines, managed to pull the REA truck out of the bog. The ERA men had kept their sense of humor. They teased me by saying they hoped I enjoyed our new "swimming pool" and built-in slide! They also said that the REA would come back to fill in the holes at a later date. I hope that I would not have to call the REA on our next visit to keep their word. It is pretty easy to forget small jobs in the midst of very busy schedules. We had already experienced moving a lot of dirt dug up by the various utility companies in Emporia that they just never got back to finishing.

No one from the abod stopped by to talk with us, nor did we stop at any of their homes. We knew they were as busy as we were and feeling foolish about the lawsuit pie in their face (which Jerry and I had spent several hours trying to get them to back off from the lawsuits). We had warned them that they would lose in court because our physically disabled neighbor was quite intelligent about legal matters, and he had thoroughly done his homework on the abod.

Jerry had to make three trips down the mountain to get all the insulation that we needed. All four of us managed to get most of the insulation up, even though we ran out of staples and decided to finish up on our next trip before the inspection. I used the time (while Jerry and one of the kids went down the mountain) to go through abod records and court transcripts to prepare for a possible lawsuit involving us. Our best defense was being prepared with the facts from the abod's own records. On this first trip, I had spent a few hours in our gravel driveway pulling up weeds and wild flowers. I admit to searching very carefully the gravel, dirt, and roots for my lost wedding ring, but to no avail. I wondered who would find my ring one day in the future. I wondered if it would be in my lifetime or not and if the cabin would even belong to our family anymore. Even though I was again disappointed to not find my ring, I did not let that ruin my time in God's beautiful Rocky Mountain region. I was looking forward to the cabin being used year round, as a retreat to draw closer to the Lord, to be encouraged and uplifted by those in need of different scenery and a quit haven of rest.

Of course, my menstrual cycle hit me that week, and I had one big overflow night. Otherwise, the period seemed quite normal. The weather was very cold at night, and we had lots of clouds with just enough sunshine to warm the cabin during the day hours. As we progressed on putting up the insulation, the cabin became much warmer, so nighttime sleeping was more comfortable. We found that two covers were sufficient, instead of the five or six that we used before installing the insulation.

On our way back to Emporia, we stopped at Colby, Kansas, for the night. The town was filled to the brim with hundreds (maybe thousands) of classic hot rods cruising all about town and filling all the motel, restaurant, and service station lots. I had never seen that many beautiful older cars at one time in my life. It was wonderful, but there was a sad note too because many of the owners of those gorgeous vehicles were loud, crude, and drunk, not just naturally high spirited. Instead of being able to concentrate on the make, model, and year of the fantastic vehicles, a sour memory emerged of pie-eyed, vulgar individuals ruining an event that could have been a cherished memory. Of course, not all of the classic car owners fell into the disreputable category, but unfortunately, our motel was full of the bottle spirits kind.

My chest tumors were still doing their daily rising and falling. Sometime in May, a lump rose on my left upper temple. I pointed it out to Jerry, and he suggested that I see the doctor about it as it appeared ugly and angry looking. However, I knew with my active cancer that a doctor would insist on removal or biopsy of it or both. I asked the Lord to show me what to do about it, if anything. By the next day after discovery, I stared rubbing virgin, naturally-pressed olive oil onto it and praying for the Lord's anointing of the oil for the removal of the disturbing lump. It took nearly six weeks before the lump was entirely gone. It had shrunk a little bit every day. Then, in mid-June, another larger lump appeared lower on my left temple, and I automatically started using olive oil again, as I asked the Lord to anoint my rubbing of the oil into the lump. I had no headaches, and my poor memory did not deteriorate or improve for that matter.

When we arrived home, I made painting a priority in our upstairs apartment. It had been years since the stairway walls had been painted with a flat, off-white paint. My goal was to get the stairway and the living room ceiling done before our next Colorado trip in July.

Chapter 45

Asking God for Miracles is No Substitute for Using God-Given Means

I achieved my goal of texturing and painting the ceiling and walls of the apartment stairwell as well as the living room ceiling and walls. I even had time to tear out an old closet before it was time for our next excursion to the Colorado cabin.

We were able to leave before 7:00 a.m. on July 3, and we drove straight through, except for the normal pit stops of exercise, relief, food, and gas. We arrived at the cabin at 7:00 p.m., still feeling energetic. We unloaded the van, plugged in the electric lights, and headed for our friends in the chalet and A-frame cabins to make arrangements for celebrating the Fourth of July with them in Estes Park. This was our third year of celebrating the Fourth together, and even though they were soon going to be moving out of state, we all made plans to meet in Estes again for the 1999 celebration, Lord willing. The weather was truly superb, and a good time was had by all as we played some miniature golf and did some shopping before the fireworks began over Lake Estes.

We passed the insulation inspection and made a final decision on how we were going to finish the ceilings. We chose tongue and groove, beetle-kill, pine boards for the vaulted ceiling, but the wood would not be available to us until our August trip. We still were able to keep busy by mowing and weed-shipping the tall grasses around the cabin. We did not like the idea of yard maintenance, as we wanted a more natural environment about the cabin, but we discovered that mowing was a safety net for the cabin, should a forest fire ever break out.

I decided that it was a good time to put more plastic around the south and west sides of the cabin and to put our rock collection (for the third time) against the outside basement walls for decoration and splatter protection of the wood siding. It appeared that the dirt was finally settled, and we could pull out the tall weeds and plants for our final grading and sloping of the hand back-filled area. Since the wild flowers and weeds were just as determined to stay as we were that they go, I had to use a potato fork to encourage some of the bigger plants to give up their claim in my future rock garden. Jeremiah was using a cement hoe to get the proper grade and smoothness that would be needed under the plastic. We were on our second day of the landscaping when we came across a really tenacious plant. It was very well rooted, so Jeremiah was bent over guiding me to where the tines needed to be to discourage the plant's stronghold, when he suddenly yelled, "Wait a minute, wait a minute!" Since we were always studying interesting bugs, rocks, and animals, I prepared myself to look upon one of the lord's strange creations.

Imagine my utter shock and delight, when he pulled my wedding ring off the plant roots that had grown through and around it! What a happy moment! I grabbed Jeremiah and my ring, shouting and dancing, hugging and kissing him, and praising the Lord over and over! Jeremiah was happy that he was able to be the Lord's instrument in making me happy, but he was having a difficult time extricating himself from my tight hug! He finally managed to struggle loose, so I ran into the cabin to show Jerry. He was as happy as I was, he told me that he had been making plans to have his matching wide wedding band cut in half and sized to fit me. Even though I had made the statement several times over the past year that I did not want any other ring (because I had not given up on the idea that it might be found someday), I thought his idea was a beautiful thought, and I would have gladly accept half of his band.

Jeremiah was the hero of the day, but it did not get him out a couple days more work. With his strong muscles pushing the wheelbarrow and shoveling dirt, we completed the terraced steps on the northwest corner of the cabin. The terraced steps on the southeast corner that we had put in last fall were doing fine.

A young couple with five little children walked about a quarter of a mile or so up the road just to make our acquaintance. Their oldest was eight years old, and their youngest member was thirteen months. They were very active Christians and homeschoolers. They invited us to a cookout at their home the next evening. We knew everyone at the gathering, and we all had a great time.

Our generous neighbor that had put in our driveway drainage ditch, put in a new drive off the main road for us. The road grader has pushed a lot of the road base over onto our property, thereby making an embankment that we could not drive over. Then, this same neighbor welded our lawnmower deck that had split by the wheel. He even painted the weld a bright red to match the color of our lawnmower! He has never allowed us to pay him for any of the work that he has done for us.

We spent our last evening on the mountain with the newlyweds, who were our closest neighbors. We all viewed the video tape that had been recorded of the summer meeting. The video showed some positive steps in wanting to get all the subdivisions and filings together on petitioning the county to maintain its claimed road, and it was a calm, peaceful meeting. The negative part to the meeting was that the abod was supposedly legal now, as they claimed that they received enough votes to legalize the association (no proof of such was offered). The man heading the meeting announced a couple of times that there were not enough people from filings 3 and 4 to make a quorum, so a business meeting could not take place. Then, they discussed what the dues should be. Even though it was suggested that several choices be given to all of the parcel owners (dollar amount and how the money was to be spent), it ended up with the $125 per lot yearly dues. Since many of the people in attendance were not required to pay dues because they had been freed from the covenants under a previous prejudiced lawsuit, it flabbergasted us that some of these people voted for us to pay $125! Another idiosyncrasy was the ex-abod was still arguing to spend monies for the continued maintenance of the county-forest service road.

It was with a great deal of pride that we watched our disabled neighbor very calmly and quietly explain the legal ramifications of jeopardizing all of our properties in the event of a lawsuit, due to an accident on the road from wrongful maintenance. The county was immune from the loss of property, but we parcel owners (as members of the road association) were not.

The meeting ended with the plan of sending out ballots for people to vote for association board of directors whose names would appear on a prepared list. We would also be able to vote on the $125 fee, either yes or no, with nothing in between.

Jerry and I figured that we would have to write another open letter to all the parcel owners. We felt that we needed to be on the offensive, this time, instead of the defensive, after they sent out their letters. So we wrote up another letter, but the Lord did not give us peace about the matter. We wrote up another, but again, no peace, so we decided that the timing or wording was not right. The Lord would show us which in His time frame. It was important that we not jump ahead of the Lord.

Chapter 46

A Merry Heart is Good Medicine with No Bad Side Effects

By our August 1998 Colorado trip, the second lump on my left temple was just a flat, remaining blemish. My menstrual cycle had been forty-two days from the June 1, so I did not have to contend with that inconvenience on this trip.

We left Emporia at noon. After making six different stops for gas, food, and restroom breaks, we arrived at the cabin at 10:15 p.m.

My chest lumps still remained in the flattened mode that they had been in for nearly two weeks. My energy level remained great. I found myself fretting over the Kansas governor's race and had to remind myself that the Lord only expected us to do our best in getting information of the candidates to friends, neighbors, and family. We had been very busy putting up yard signs and handing out information sheets for the Kansas primary election before we left for this Colorado trip. It was usually a difficult thing for me to do, as I would get so angry at the apathy over candidates. I would get downright furious at friends and family who thought higher of party politics and finances than they did of God's Biblical standards! I knew that we would all stand before the Lord one day and have to answer for our votes—either for His principles or against His principles. Therefore, I had to rest the matter in His capable hands. Our job was to be watchmen and to warn of accountability of our votes for moral politicians or immoral politicians, nothing more.

Having electricity in the cabin helped to speed along the unpacking and setting up of beds, as well as getting water ready for bathing and flushing. We had to get our bodies in gear early in the morning, so that we had plenty of time to get our beetle-killed pine boards from the small lumber company located at the bottom of the switchbacks. It took us two trips up the switchbacks to get the 152 boards to the cabin.

We had a quick visit with our wonderful friends who lived in the chalet cabin. We were blessed to help them finish. They were delighted that the cabin had just sold. She was due to deliver their fourth child any day. They returned our spare cabin keys to us and introduced to us the young couple who had just purchased their chalet. Our friends had gotten too deeply into debt, thereby forcing him to hold down two jobs to make ends meet. Therefore, he saw very little of his growing family and had very little time to enjoy their mountain paradise. After much prayer, they decided to sell out and move to a different area with more reasonable housing and greater opportunities for raising livestock and farming. Their goal was to become debt free—a very worthwhile goal for us all. I believe that it also pleases the Lord as His word tells us that when we owe money, we are actually in bondage to the money lender. It takes sacrifice and self-control to be debt free, which explains why today's society is in financial bondage. Society lacks the two necessary ingredients: sacrifice and self-control. Jerry and I have been both routes. We admit that it has been harder to live on one less salary, but the blessings have been much greater.

Besides putting up the ceiling boards in the open living-dining-kitchen area, Jerry, Jeremiah, and a good friend from Emporia were able to also do the stairwell and hall ceilings. Deb and I finished placing rocks around the west side of the cabin and on the terraced steps. Jeremiah and I were also able to put in steel posts to mark the boundaries that the surveyors had found, staked and pinned. We did not get the posts as deep as they should have been, because we only had a thirty-two-ounce ball-peen hammer to pound the posts into the soil. I would stand on the v-crossbar of the steel post, while Jeremiah hammered. Our method may have been unconventional, but it accomplished our goal. Of course, the first free-ranging cow or horse that rubbed up against any of the posts would find scratching the itch short lived.

We decided to go to church in Estes Park as the Lord had been convicting us. The lumber mill operator (from whom we bought our beetle-killed pine boards) did a fine job of adding to the Lord's convicting us to seek a Bible-preaching church in the area. We usually had our own miniservice, under Jerry's leadership. We thoroughly enjoyed his short lessons and singing hymns and praises to the Lord.

We enjoyed the church service so much that we decided to stay in Estes for the day, because the church was having an evening meeting to discuss Y2K (year 2000) problems that might arise. There was no sense of panic but a sense of preparedness. Because all branches of governments, utility companies, financial institutions, and a majority of businesses are computer controlled, people need to be aware of Y2K happenings.

We were asked questions, such as (1) If your electricity is off for a week or more, do you have any back-up system for lighting, cooking or heating? (2) Is your water system dependent on electricity or computers? (3) If your grocery stores are closed down for a week or more, do you have enough food on hand to get you by for a while? (4) What if your bank closes its doors for a couple of weeks or more, what are your options?

We were told to think of basic needs—food, shelter, water, and waste disposal. Sensible preparedness might include a water storage tank, candles, lanterns, canned goods, barter goods, etc. Not everyone would view a need in the same way, which is why the bartering system could be back in our society. Those folks with septic tanks, leach fields, and lagoons would not need to consider a portable toilet or outhouse facility. Those of us in the cities might find those items to be a necessity.

There were some at the meeting who believed that the Y2K was nothing more than a scam to get people to buy new computers. Another felt that the government and industry would have all the Y2K problems solved—what faith he had in our government looking out for us! One man felt that he Y2K scenario was similar to the bomb shelter scare of the fifties and sixties—a waste of time and money in building them. After the meeting, I did feel inclined to inform him that some of those bomb shelters proved to be excellent storm shelters. Preparedness is never a waste of time when done in a sensible manner.

Jerry and I determined that we would rather be on the giving end of necessities than the not so comfortable receiving end. We did not plan on blowing the budget or going into debt to prepare ahead, but buying an extra package of toilet paper or a couple of cans of vegetables instead on one or an extra package of batteries every week or two was not hard on the budget. Should Y2K not be solved in 1999, then we will be in a little better position to help ourselves and others. Should the Y2K problems not come about, praise the Lord. We should not have to buy non-perishables for a few months. Should the Y2K scenario come to pass, praise for Lord for directing us to heed the warning of His Y2K watchmen.

The pastor did stress listening to the Spirit of God through His word. Our dependency is upon the Lord and the pastor shared many comforting and strengthening verses like these: Isaiah 41:10, Isaiah 42:24, 1 Peter 5:8, Hebrews 4:16, Psalms 99, 37:5, and 55:22, Proverbs 16:3, and 1 Timothy 6:15. Since God is the Blessed Controller of all things, we are not to get anxious or stressed over Y2K. We must be concerned about the future, plan for the future, but not anxious about the future. The Lord told Noah to prepare for the flood many years before it took place. He told Joseph to prepare for the seven-year famine that was coming after the seven years of plenty.

The pastor even suggested that we study Mary and Martha closer, that we might be a combination of both—wanting to be with Jesus spiritually (Mary) and wanting to prepare food for the physical well-being (Martha).

Just as I cannot let Y2K be a single focus in my life, I also cannot let cancer be a single focus in my life. Both need wise preparation and faith in God's direction and leadership.

We were grateful to the Lord for convicting us to attend a Bible-preaching, Bible-teaching church in Estes like we do in Emporia. Even though it was a much larger church than ours, we found friendly folks in the Sunday school class that we also attended. We felt that we could recommend this church to our friends on the mountain, as well as to any folks staying at the Lord's ministry cabin.

My health was great, except for a bad headache due to a lack of sleep from visits with friends and neighbors until the wee hours of the mornings. Since I knew the cause of the headache, I just took one willow bark and one feverfew capsule before going to bed earlier than I had been. Again, I realized that just as proper rest, nutrition, and exercise is necessary for the physical well-being of the body, our spiritual bodies need the same ingredients—rest in the Lord, exercise in prayer and spiritual food from His word.

As far as the abod saga went, several committee people from all of the filings were distributing, mailing, and gathering signed petition cards to deliver to the county—requesting them to take over the maintenance of their claimed road. The former abods made it clear that they did not think much of the petitions. However, it did appear that positive steps were being taken to develop good community spirit in working together for a common cause (a willingness to forgive).

Chapter 47

Gratitude is Always the Right Attitude

I was reading an article taken from the April 14, 1998, issue of the *Journal of American Medical Association* (JAMA). It was about adverse drug reactions (ADRs) in U.S. hospitals. ADRs are defined as any noxious, unintended and undesired effect of a drug occurring at doses used in humans for prevention, diagnosis or therapy. A serious ADR was one requiring hospitalization, prolonged hospitalization, permanent disability, or death. The authors estimated over two million hospital patients experienced a serious ADR (I could not help but remember my reaction to the drug given to me to combat the hives reaction that I had to another drug—see chapter 3). The authors also estimated 106,000 deaths were caused by ADRs in the United States in 1994. While the length of hospital stays were decreasing (due to increased costs and insurance companies refusal to pay), the amount of drugs per day were rising to compensate.

I was thankful that the Lord gave me a body system that tolerated very few drugs of any kinds—be they painkillers or relaxants. I had several friends whose lives were emotional and mental basket cases from their dependency on antidepressants, back pain pills, relaxants, diet pills, etc. These items became their gods, as they became totally dependent on these mind-altering drugs. I was thankful that when I had tried prescribed nerve pills (when my marriage to Jerry was on the crumbling rocks instead of the Solid Rock of Jesus), my body declared them totally off-limits. My Lord had made my body super sensitive to drugs and how thankful I learned to be for that. Otherwise, I might have been tempted to go the poisonous route in treating my cancer.

It was true that thousands survived that type of cancer treatment, but thousands also did not. And thousands that do survive have long-term side effect that they have to learn to live with. These include permanent edema, paralysis, other cancers, damaged hearts and lungs, and liver damage. My friend, Patty, who had been sent home with Pick's disease diagnosis after her chemo treatments preparing her for a bone marrow transplant, was seemingly doing fine once her mind came back to her. She gave credit to the Lord and the chemo, but I gave credit *only* to the Lord and His mercy in not keeping her in mental deliriums and deterioration.

Our home pastor had commented several times that good things and bad things happen to Christians and non-Christians alike. Too often, Christians get offended when trials come their way. Jesus also felt hunger, thirst, cold, heat, anger, humiliation, sadness, rejection, extreme physical pain, and loss of loved ones. Saved and unsaved have felt the joy of a birth, the sorrow of a death, the happiness of a loving marriage, the sadness of a divorce, the recovery from a deadly disease, the disability or death from one. How we react to those trials is more important than the trials themselves.

We do need to examine our lifestyles, habits, and thoughts in light of God's word, because some of the bad things that come our way are due to our own choices. If our self-examination shows that we need to change some items in our life, then changes we must make. But we also need to accept what we can do nothing about and leave it in the Lord's hands. That has been a very tough lesson for me, even though I was introduced to the Serenity Prayer many years ago while attending Al-Anon meetings. It goes like this:

> God, grant me the serenity to accept the things I cannot change,
> Courage to change the things I can,
> And wisdom to know the difference.

The Lord insisted that I learn this lesson over and over. I truly had not comprehended just how much of a fretter and worrier I was until after the mastectomy and the appearance of the tumor under my skin. Those chest tumors were a loud visual indicator of stressful fretting and worrying. How thankful I became to the Lord for giving me visual reminders to lean on Him—not myself.

Our daughter and her hubby obtained a loan on a house of their own. Their closing date was in the last week of August 1998. Since Mom's health was much improved and since we had lived in their upstairs apartment over fourteen months, we were looking forward to moving into our own home too. It was not a great deal bigger in floor space, but the taller ceilings and many windows made it appear much spacious and roomy.

Mom had already gotten a couple of appraisals on her house, as she was considering selling it and moving into an apartment complex with which she was familiar. Several of her friends had lived in the high-rise complex over the years. Mom had pretty much given up the idea that Dad would ever be able to come home again. He, both mentally and physically, continued to decline, even with Mom hand-feeding him at the nursing home. He was still over drugged (in my opinion) and would attempt to bite and strike out when agitated. Of course, the nursing home staff and the doctors found him easier to deal with when he was sedated. Mom just did not have the willpower to fight against standard medical procedures. I too backed away, because as a daughter-i-law, I had no authority. I could not fight Mom, Dad, the nursing home staff, the medical community, and well-meaning friends and family who believed totally in traditional treatments for everything. It was another serenity lesson that I had to give to the Lord.

We did not plan to move immediately into the little house once the kids moved into their own home. They had told us that the bathtub had a soft-floor problem, so we decided that it might be better to repair and remodel the entire bathroom before we moved in. We figured it might take us two or three months to get the job done right. We still wanted to get some work done on Mom's house before she put it on the market. We still had another nine-day trip planned for working on the Colorado cabin, and we still had several lots to maintain due to the abundance of moisture that the Lord had sent. It was indeed strange to see green plains in western Kansas and eastern Colorado in the month of August!

I finally learned to ask the Lord to prioritize us.

Chapter 48

Write Your Plans in Pencil, but Give God the Eraser

My supplement program was still being blessed by the Lord. The second lump on my left temple was smaller and pink instead of red. However, since it was still very tender, I decided to continue on with the olive oil. I noticed that my nose seemed to be having a sudden outbreak of little pimples and tiny veins showing forth. It reminded me of rosacea. I decided to put olive oil on it also.

There were a few changes in my supplement program due to prices and availability. I still relied on olive oil for lumps, but I would also substitute tea tree oil, if the olive oil seemed to reach a point of no further improvement. I no longer used the progest cream daily but every other day instead, until the onset of menses. Then, I rested from the cream for seven days before starting back up. I no longer drank a gallon of water daily, but tried to make sure that I drank a minimum of sixty-four ounces of water and green tea throughout the day. I dropped back to one, 25,000 mg capsule of beta-carotene, as my orange palms showed me that I could finally lower the dosage. I was taking two chlorophyll tablets daily, but decided to go back to the alfalfa tablets, as the results seemed the same, and the alfalfa tablets were less expensive. I no longer took SOD-3, COQ10, shark cartilage, red clover, garlic, cayenne pepper, or chlorella. Some had become hard to find, while others did not seem to make any changes in the tumors to warrant their cost. I had added a few other supplements that I had tried at the beginning of my therapy program when Dr. Joe and I actually witnessed the shrinking of the thumbnail-sized tumor down to a pinkie-nail-sized tumor before he surgically removed it in March 1995. These supplements were the following:

DMG—sublingual (pure N, N-Dimethylglycine) 125 mg, twice daily—it is a very powerful antioxidant.

Calcium pangamate (B-15) 150 mg, once daily—it is another antioxidant and liver protector.

Chaparral—500 mg, twice daily—a powerful antitumor activity. However, I was on this for about three weeks when I started having trouble focusing my eyes. Since the chaparral was the latest added supplement, I immediately stopped taking it to see if the eye problem would clear up. Within three days, the eye focused properly, but I also discovered that I had a sinus blockage when I bent over and immediately felt as if my head had been put into a vise. After taking Echinacea, four capsules daily for a couple of days, the sinus passages opened up. Not knowing if the sinus blockage or the chaparral caused the eye problem meant that I would try the chaparral again at a later date.

I stayed with the rest of the supplements listed in chapter 27. Even though there were hectic or forgetful times when I missed one of my four divided doses of vitamins, minerals, and herbs, I thrived anyway. Missing an occasional dose was not a life-or-death situation. Most supplements of vitamins, minerals, and herbs taken orally are slow reacting, not like the chemical drugs that hit the body with a wallop and can have very quick reactions, both good and bad.

We started our school year on August 17, 1998. This was my eighteenth year of homeschooling, and I was excited about their new subjects again this year. Their curriculum publisher seemed to get better and better. Over the years, I had learned to relax about the children's academic progress. I knew that if they could handle ABeka curriculum, they could handle any curriculum in their educational future.

It was always hard to get back into the school routine and lessons after the summer break because it meant that we had to discipline our time from other work and interests to academic studies that sometimes were not as motivating for us. I am not a person with exciting ideas, but I found over the years, that my children learned despite my lack just as other children learn in spite of their teachers' lack.

We generally tried to keep the same schedule as the government and Christian schools in our area. Naturally, we had no reason to schedule "in-service days" or parent-teacher conferences. However, we usually tried to schedule a fall field trip vacation as the weather anywhere in the United States was usually great. Our plans were to go to Rocky Mountain Park again this year. I wanted to take another hike to Gem Lake as this first trip was spoiled by one of my self-pity parties. We also wanted to see the golden aspens and to hear the bugling elk, plus we needed to winterize the cabin and make sure it was tight against weather and varmints.

On August 24, 1998, I sent a letter to Focus On The Family Publishers, asking for their help in getting this book published of my cancer journey (with the prayer, "if the Lord wills it").

On august 25, 1998, I spent four hours talking to two elderly aunts and an uncle of Jerry's. Uncle was eighty-eight years old and had recently been diagnosed with breast cancer. Uncle had lost his mother to cancer, as well as a sister to breast cancer. He was well aware of the horrible pain and suffering that they went through with chemo and radiation treatments. Uncle had already gone through the surgical biopsy on August 3, 1998. Even though the surgeon had gotten all of the small lump, he told Uncle that he had seen a "gelled mass" under the tumor and wanted to go back into the site to remove Uncle's armpit lymph nodes and the gelled mass. The surgeon had also sent Uncle to see Dr. C, who recommended that Uncle start taking Tamoxifen.

When Uncle asked me what I would do in his place, I flat out told him that I would not let anyone touch my lymph nodes ever again, due to the lifelong irritating consequences of their removal. I told Uncle about edema and about the importance of the lymph nodes to the immune system. I told him about my experience with Tamoxifen, and I read the pharmaceutical fact sheet to him. When he asked me what I used to combat the hormones, I told him about the progest cream. Uncle asked me about my therapy program, but he made it clear that he was not going to take that many supplements, as he already took some antioxidants. He was in excellent overall health. His biopsy was nearly healed already, and he wasn't feeling bad at all, when he went in to have the lump checked out. His sisters insisted that he go regardless of how good he felt. He was on supplements in the hope that they would help his memory, as he did have memory problems.

I tried to get the aunts and Uncle to see the need to get all the information they could so that they could make informed decisions, but I probably overwhelmed them. I also assured them that Dr. Tim was a very good and conscientious surgeon who would not push Uncle to do anything that he did not want to do. I had found Dr. Tim to be warm, congenial, and a good listener to his patients, as he had done hernia surgery on Ryan (over three years ago) and gallbladder surgery on Mom (in February 1998). From my understanding, Dr. Tim had also been tutored by Dr. Joe, so he had wise medical mentoring to imitate. Even though Dr. Tim did not believe in vitamins, minerals, and herbal supplements, he still rated high in my opinion. He scheduled Uncle for bone and liver scans on August 31, and for surgery on the remaining mass on September 1, 1998.

On August 28, I had a blood test to check protein levels, liver functions, iron levels, and anything else that showed up in a blood profile test. Then, I would discuss the results with Dr. Joe in September. It had been nearly two years since my last office visit with him.

Uncle's mass was removed with lymph nodes intact. He came through surgery fine, but while visiting him at the hospital, his eighty-four-year-old sister collapsed. Tests revealed a lack of oxygen to the brain from clogged veins or arteries in her neck. She had enjoyed good health for many years (even after the stress of losing a beloved mate to leukemia), until she went to the family doctor for a routine checkup. He declared suddenly that she had osteoporosis (at eighty-two years of age) and proceeded to write out a prescription for the current "drug of the month," which happened to be for osteoporosis! Since four different women I know, personally (ages ranging from sixty-two to eighty-two), went to their family doctor for their yearly checkups. All came home with prescriptions for the same osteoporosis drug. I am making an educated guess that a big pharmaceutical company was running a big incentive special to doctors. Two of the women developed serious eye problems after being on the drug a few months.

There are many fine doctors in our medical community who are deeply for the welfare of their patients, and then there are some to whom medicine is just a lucrative job. Doctors need to ask themselves if they are prescribing a drug for pharmaceutical reward or for the patient's best care. Doctors need to know if the prescribed drug will solve the problem or just cover it up. That, of course, would entail that they have a desk manual, such as *Worst Pills/Best Pills* on their laps, so they can read the possible side effects before prescribing a drug to a patient. Patients too, need to be on the alert for side effects and drug interactions as they might prefer the ailment over the side effects.

Uncle's sister remained in the hospital over a week, but he was released from the hospital in the care of his younger sister (seventy-three years of age). However, on September 6, 1998, that sister was confined to bed, due to temporary paralysis, and my beloved mother-in-law found herself taking care of them both! Uncle pretty much took care of himself, as Mom had her hands full with the bedfast sister, until the sister's daughter was able to come to Emporia to take her mother home to the Kansas City area. Actually, Uncle would have driven himself home from the hospital, but he was under medical restriction for driving until his doctor said different. Uncle was also waiting for his new eye glasses that he had ordered a week or so before his tumor mass removal.

On September 7, Jerry and I were able to start remodeling the back portion of our little house in our beloved old neighborhood. Michelle and Troy were moved into their own home and were busy settling in. Within three weeks of their loan approval, Troy was temporarily laid off his job. They were a little discouraged, yet they were also thankful as the layoff could have happened before the loan approval. Michelle still had her job, and there were a lot of little jobs to do on their home while he waited out the temporary layoff.

On September 15, 1998, I had the pleasure of seeing Dr. Joe for a follow-up exam on my progress with my biological immunotherapy treatment and to discuss the blood profile report. He was very pleased to see smaller tumors than what he had seen two years previously.

Even though I had a slight cold, I was feeling fine. If I had not started my period at the same time that I got the cold, I would not have paid much attention to the cold. However, each time I coughed, I could feel the blood spurt onto the pad, which made me a little fearful of an embarrassing run over.

Regarding the results of the blood profile test, Dr. Joe stated, "Donna, it just doesn't get any better than this." We discussed pap smears, liver scan, and mammograms. I reiterated why I wanted nothing to do with the Pap smear or mammograms. X-rays mutate cells, and I already had enough crazy cells with which to be concerned. Since scraping the cervix usually left me bleeding for three days, I wanted my immune system to concentrate on my cancer—not on an internally inflicted wound. With the blood profile showing that the liver was functioning fine, a liver scan would have been a waste of time and money, and I did not want any nuclear medicines in my body.

Dr. Joe took a couple of picture of my chest as a comparison to the photos of two years before. Even I was impressed! The biological immunotherapy program was not a quick fix, but seemed to be a slow, steady-wins-the-race over cancer therapy. We do not just wake up with cancer over night. It takes years in our compromise immune systems before it is noticeable. Why do we think that we should be able to rid our bodies of it overnight? That type of attitude is one reason that the primitive, barbaric treatments of poisoning and burning are still prevalent today and at an exorbitant cost. One day our society will look back to traditional cancer treatments over the past fifty years and shake its head in utter disbelief that such barbaric practices were routinely accepted. It will look upon today's traditional cancer treatments like it does now on bloodletting leeches and failure to wash the hands between patients—with absolute horror!

In the meantime, more friends, family, and acquaintances will be diagnosed with various cancers and sent to the cancer experts for "expert treatment." Our friend who had been diagnosed with the slow-growing cancer that required mild chemo, was diagnosed with a rapidly growing cancer, requiring aggressive chemo (within a few short months after the doctors pronounced him in remission). He just got out of a two-week stay in the hospital—after several of the aggressive chemo treatments—because his blood count was so low that the only way the doctors could get it back up was with blood transfusions.

Another friend who had major heart problems was recently scheduled to start radiation treatments. All I could think about was my brother's beloved mother-in-law (who had undergone radiation treatments for breast cancer, even though she also had heart problems). She was gone in less than a year.

I have met several people who have survived traditional therapies, but I have known many more who have not. I know only a handful of people who have tried non-traditional cancer therapies, but they are all still alive and in better health than their peers.

Chapter 49

Trusting God can Turn a Trial into a Triumph

On September 21, 1998, I received a very nice letter back from Focus on the Family, regarding the publishing of my book. Even though they turned me down, they were very helpful anyway in sending me information of who else I might contact and how to go about it.

On September 26, 1998, we received more information on the abod saga. "The good ole boys club," as they were called on the mountain, was back in business, as the landowners supposedly voted them back to legal status. Of course, there was no proof offered of signed ballots or how many votes. The letter consisted of a list of candidates for the new board of directors—some of the candidates were from "the good ole boys club." The ballot also included voting on the dues amount. We found it interesting and irritating at the same time. Colorado statues called for thirty days written notice on corporation ballots and votes, from what I could remember reading in my research on corporation legalities. The former abod gave us until October 1 to get the ballots back—less than a week. Also, there was no identification of parcels or parcel owners anywhere on the ballots, making filing of false votes quite easy. For an organization steeped in professional shenanigans, the former abod was appearing to us to try to pull the wool over our eyes still.

We left on October 2, 1998, for our annual fall field trip vacation. We saw gorgeous aspen that looked as if they were on fire beside the evergreens and pines. We encountered light, falling snow in Estes Park, while attending church services on the fourth, but most of our days were with bright sunshine, warm temperatures, and very hard work. We had bought seven hundred square feet of white pine from our friend at the lumber mill. It took us two trips again up and down the switchbacks to haul it to the cabin, but the Lord blessed the 1986 Aerostar's use as a lumber truck.

Since we had put the colorful beetle-killed pine on the ceilings, we decided to put white pine on the outside walls for variety. We did not want to overkill the beautiful beetle-kill pine effect. Our good neighbors over the hill from us had the beetle-kill throughout their smaller cabin, and it was great, but we feared that our larger cabin would be too much for total beetle-kill look.

We stayed warm and cozy in our newly insulated cabin. With the loan of a 1,500 watt electric heater, we were quite comfortable, even when the temperature dropped to twenty-eight degrees one night. Our mountain friends were always looking out for us flatlanders.

We all remained in good health with all the energy we needed to get the tongue and groove wood installed. One morning, I decided to get an early start on setting some nails that I had not gotten set the day before. I sat on a stack of boards, bent forward while holding the nail set in my left hand and the hammer in my right hand. I hit the third nail with the nail set when suddenly I was hit with a sharp pain in my back left side. This automatically wrenched a cry from me. Jerry, Deb, and Jeremiah thought that I had hit my thumb again. My back rib muscle hurt so badly that I could barely breathe, much less move or talk. However, the Lord had blessed Jerry with the ability to pull my back again into proper alignment, so that I was able to function in a few hours. Sudden twists or turns were limited to slow, careful movements to avoid any more sharp pains. Deb took over the job of nail setting—with a willing spirit—while Jeremiah took over the nailing—not so willingly. However, Jeremiah was such a powerful nail pounder that when he missed, he left impressions in the wood. I finally reached the point of not being able to handle any more impressions, so I took the job back.

Our dear disabled neighbor friend laughed at the way I maneuvered my body to keep from turning or twisting my back while nailing the boards into place. He wasn't laughing at me so much as with me since he too had back problems (from an on-the-job injury years before). Most of his sleeping was done in a reclining position in a chair, as lying in a bed seemed more painful.

My back did not go out often anymore, but when it did, it got immediate attention. I might turn to look at something or be painting or maybe lifting, when my back or neck would suddenly be in a painful bind. I was nearly thirty years old the first time that my back went out. I had been playing with our firstborn on the bed in our bedroom, which had a concrete floor. Ryan had jumped toward me when I then realize that he was going to miss me and go over the edge of the bed, onto the concrete floor. I grabbed for his propelling body, but as his solid body weight hit me, I lost my balance and went over the edge of the bed with him on top of me. I landed on the back of my head and neck. It took several days before I could walk, sleep, eat, drink, or talk without feeling any pain. For the next several months and years, my back could be fine one minute and out of order the next. One day, Jerry suggested that I let him pull me over his bent back until my feet were off the floor. I would put my arms up over his shoulder, he would grasp and hold my wrists as he bent forward. As I went over his curved spine, my bodyweight lifted off the floor, causing my back to stretch. It was usually painful, but brief in duration. Sometimes, it took more than one or two body stretches during the day, but it usually put me back together properly.

When Jerry had hurt his back on the job, the Emergency Room doctor had just him home with two high-priced and high-powered pain relievers. Of course, Jerry did not take the drugs. Instead, he borrowed an inverter from a friend. With regular exercise on the inverter and a back brace on the job, Jerry's back was soon back to normal. All the pain relievers would have done was mask the pain to the point that he could have ended up doing permanent injury to his stressed back as the warning pain would no longer have been felt.

High-powered pain relievers can also alter the mind. Over the years, we have seen family, friends, and acquaintances become mentally and physically addicted to pain relievers. By the time they realized their problem of addiction, their lives and families were out of control.

Even with my slower pace of nailing, we managed to get most of the two hundred boards put on the outside walls inside the cabin before we had to go back to Emporia on October 10. We did not accomplish all that we had wanted to get done to the cabin before the summer ended, but we were thrilled at each accomplishment.

We were going to miss seeing our mountain friends, but we were thankful for telephones and postal services to keep us in touch.

We stopped at a preacher friend's home in Salina, Kansas, on our way back to Emporia. He gave us information sheets on another candidate for the Kansas governor's race. The candidate was not of either major party, but that did not make any difference to us. We are not party people. We vote for the candidate who appears to uphold Biblical morality. When enough other people do the same, then Americans will see their country respected again. We were disappointed that our choice in the primary race was now backing the incumbent, simply because he was of the same party. Never mind that our primary choice knew the incumbent was against his and our Biblical beliefs. The party was all that mattered. I was glad that the Lord did not allow our primary candidate to win the party nomination, because his biblical principles took second to party politics in his final stand. Only biblical standards will turn America back on the road to decency and respect, not the democrat or republican parties!

Our preacher friend also gave us more information on Y2K that he was sharing with his small congregation. He felt that as a watchman, he needed to warn of any danger lurking on the horizon to the Lord's flock of sheep. The cost of preparedness was trivial compared to being caught unprepared for hard times when there had been plenty of warnings.

We do not hesitate to plan for the future for education funds, building funds, a new home or vehicle or retirement. Why should we hesitate or delay to plan for the problems that could arise from a big computer malfunction due to a little two-digit error?

Once back in Emporia, we stared in earnest on revamping the back porch area of our little house. The new windows had already been installed, but the caulking job had to be redone by the window contractor. In looking over the redone work, we noticed that one of the new windows was warped. The contractor ordered only the bottom portion, instead of the whole window. Jerry had withheld a third of the contract price, due to the lack of good workmanship and poor communication on the contractor's part. Jerry was determined to encourage the contractor to see the job to a satisfactory finish, even though it made Jerry uncomfortable to have to "ride" anyone about their workmanship. The contract had been signed in May, and the windows were to be installed three to four weeks later. It was July before we had the windows and then it took two more months to get half of the replacement for the warped window unit! As of mid-November, we were still waiting for the window, and the contractor was still waiting for his final payment.

Jerry and I did not like to be a thorn in anyone's side, but it sure seemed to be our destiny for the late 1990s!

Jerry and Jeremiah were able to get the leaky, airy back door and windows replaced with a six-foot patio unit. Deb and I took on the job of picking out and delivering the new paneling for Jeremiah's room, as well as the utility area. There wasn't a straight wall or level floor to work with. Deb and I worked on putting her and Jeremiah's crews-quarter beds together that had been bought for them nearly two years before. The beds had been in storage in Mom's garage for that length of time. Deb and I also put together a corner TV cabinet to replace our larger entertainment center for which we no longer had room. We got so good at putting things together that we purchased a wooden dresser for Deb's room. It gave both of us a wonderful sense of accomplishment in putting together practical, but good-looking furniture pieces. We did not feel helpless or frustrated waiting on a very busy Jerry to do these jobs for us. Twenty years ago, I watched Jerry install cup hooks for my chinaware. This time, I installed them. I took on the job of installing the pad and carpet in our closet and started on the installation of our curtain rods. However, the brick chimney proved to be more than I could tackle—another project for Jerry.

The tumors remained fairly calm during this stressful time. They were not gone, but they were smaller. They were not gone, but they were manageable. I also had a sense of accomplishment with the tumors as the Lord put the care of my body in my puny hands as far as taking His biological immunotherapy supplement program.

With the arrival of daylight savings time, it seemed our days were suddenly much shorter. Of course, I have never cared for the government-mandated daylight savings time. Even as a young school girl, I did not swallow the propaganda that it protected school children. Adjust the school hours by one hour made far more sense. All daylight savings time has ever done for the majority of folks is throw off their bodies internal clocks, causing a sluggish feeling. But, as stated before, government and common sense are oxymorons.

I continued functioning in my normally abnormal way, with plenty of energy and physical stamina. My full-flow menses was thirty-three days from the last cycle, which was fine. Mentally, however, I was tired of all the reactions to every action we took, but I no longer railed at Jerry or the Lord. I tried to find other ways to deal with my frustrations. When the patio door had to be taken out several times for adjustments due to crooked carpentry of past years, I found great pleasure in seeing how many pesky mosquitoes and other insects I could squash. Since they were intent on bugging me, I felt it to be a valid war. I knew I was cheating some poor bird out of dinner, but taking my frustrations and aggravations out on the insect population was a calming experience. I'm sure that Jerry and the Lord appreciated the change!

It was slow work—remodeling and building—with a great sense of satisfaction and accomplishment over each improvement achieved. The Lord's biological immunotherapy program gave me the same sense of accomplishment and satisfaction in rebuilding my body.

Chapter 50

We May Not Know What the Future Holds, but We Can Trust the One Who Holds the Future (five years after and still going strong on alternative therapy)

November 1, 1998, came and went with no moving on our part. Even though I was ready to be back on the quieter eastside of town and in my own house, I was also content to live each day doing what needed to be done and enjoying it. Our homeschooling was moving right along, on schedule. Mom's health was vastly improved from a year ago. Mom was also beginning to accept the fact of our preparing to move out of her home after being with her for seventeen months. It looked like the first of the year would be the time for us to move, so Mom was entering into thoughts of where she wanted to be—whether remain in her own home of thirty-five years or in an apartment complex that she had already turned down in October. If she remained in her big house, she wanted someone else to live in it with her, even if just in the upstairs apartment. Preferably someone she knew so that there would be interaction between them.

The Emporia area received over eleven inches of rain in a ten-day time span, so there were a lot of flooded homes and basements. We were blessed to have properly working sump pumps for our leaky basements. Approximately three inches of water was in part of Mom's huge garage. Only the sweet potatoes got wet, and we had been planning on moving them to the basement on airy pallets, so we just moved them sooner than planned.

The first week of November proved to be very busy, with every evening being taken up with ushers' dinner, missions' conference, and missions' banquet. Therefore, work on our house came to a halt that week. We were only able to work on it in the evenings or on the weekends. Since Jerry needed to use his table saw for cutting most of the boards and paneling, and since his table saw had to be used outside to cut the four by eight-foot sheets of paneling, he needed dry weather in which to work. The week of damp, drizzling weather after the torrential downpours slowed his remodeling projects, considerably.

We managed to get our bedroom closet finished, and Jerry was able to start building a closet for Jeremiah's room. Jerry also discovered that our bathroom plumbing leaked profusely, as no one had ever soldered the joints! We wondered why the basement crawl space remained damp, even after two months of dry weather, so we found the answer.

With all the interruptions in getting our house ready, we were thankful that there was no rush in moving out of Mom's house. Even if we did not enjoy all of the rain, we did enjoy the food, fellowship, and missionaries during the missions' conference. I do confess that we were only interested in seeing and hearing the missionaries talk about their mission fields. We would not have attended the conference just to hear a stateside preacher preach on giving to missions. We needed the motivation produced by the presence of the missionaries themselves as they shared their exciting work, people, cultures, and places of God's creation. The missionaries gave us a personal view and feeling for the mission field. This mission conference was even more special and precious to us, because our former pastor and his family were missionaries to New Zealand and were present at this conference. We enjoyed the slide presentation of the missionaries from Paraguay and Japan, but we were disappointed in not getting to hear more from them as the stateside preacher had been scheduled to do most of the preaching each night. After an evening service ended, we were blessed to have our former pastor and wife over for popcorn and fellowship.

We were saddened to hear of the death of a missionary who had honored us (with his wife and three sons) in sharing our home for a week of missions' conference several years ago. His wife was deaf, and their three sons also had hearing problems. So the family used their affliction to reach other deaf people for the Lord in Zambia, Africa. Our missionary friend had contracted malaria about six months before his death. The various medicines prescribed for him did not seem to help, so they decided to come back to the United States on a medical furlough. He had felt more tired than usual on a Saturday evening and decided to lie down on the sofa for a while. His wife and sons went on to bed, as usual. When she awakened in the morning, she discovered that her husband had gone on to be with the Lord. It was a shock for everyone. Since they had already planned on leaving for the States on November 14, and since her parents had already rented a house for their use while in the United States, she was able to continue on more smoothly.

I found great comfort in hearing how the Lord had the details already set in motion to care for the missionary's family. This is something that I have had to realize many times over the past five years. Even though I did not fear the hereafter for myself, I did fear the present for my family without me. Not because I am indispensible, but because they would need another "chief cook and bottle washer." I feared who they would find to fill that position. The Lord has shown me that they belong to Him, too, and He will take care of them also, as He has taken care of me, so there is no need of my worrying about their care. My job is to take care of the present, with a little future planning—written in pencil, of course, with an eraser at hand.

None of us know what today to tomorrow will bring. It may be sunshine or rain. It may bring happiness or sorrow. Death may be on the horizon with a car wreck, an airplane crash, a flood (Hurricane Mitch took the lives of thousands in November 1998), a heart attack, etc. It seems to me that the very first priority in our life should be preparation for eternity. It should head the list of things to do today if we have not already taken care of our final destination. God's word tells us that there is a Heaven and a hell, and we choose which one for our eternal destination.

When I read John 3:16, "For God so loved the world that He gave His only begotten Son, that whosoever believeth in Him should not perish, but have everlasting life," I knew I wanted that everlasting life with the Son, Jesus—not perishing in everlasting flames of hell. John 3:18 reads, "He that believeth on Him is not condemned; but he that believeth not is condemned already, because he hath not believed in the name of the only begotten Son of God." When I decided there was a real God and that He was perfectly capable of preserving a book about Himself so that I might know Him better, I accepted a new life in Him. I became a new creature in Him—but not a perfect creature, to be sure.

I look forward to heaven, but I will cling to this troublesome earth until the Lord says, "Come home, Donna." I will cling in the most comfortable way that I can, cancer or no cancer. I know there will be more trials in this life, but the blessings will be right alongside the trials.

There will be more fun, food, and fellowship gatherings with family and friends; more building, remodeling, and repairing of dwellings; more hiking of God's beautiful creations of mountains, deserts, forests and plains, graduation, wedding, and birthday celebrations; and hundreds of other blessings.

There will be more challenges to face and overcome with the Lord's help, such as more abod shenanigans, possible Y2K lifestyle interruptions, attempts (through FDA mandates) by the AMA, ACS, NCI, and big pharmaceutical companies to control or curtail the supplement market (as it cuts more and more into their billion-dollar industries), the continued care of Dad as affordable nursing homes close down, my own Mother's seriously deteriorating health and the continual battles incurred while occupying this earth.

Society is beginning to "wake up" to the fact that the majority of mainstream medicine is a "practice." If society was not beginning to medically awaken tot that fact, the supplement market would not be doing as well as it is. It is exciting to see quality natural supplements, right alongside the laboratory chemical copies in grocery stores, discount stores, and drugstores. It is wonderful to see health food stores in most towns and cities now.

I pray that just as Americans are turning to more natural foods, supplements, and medicines, they will turn toward moral, rather than immoral principles. I pray that society will no longer view abortion, homosexuality, adultery, pornography, child rearing, education, health, and welfare as political issues only. I pray that more churches will have pastors, preachers, priests, and laymen speaking out on these important moral issues.

My intention is to continue with my diary of life with cancer for however long I have cancer or however long a life that the Lord gives me. My prayer is that this chronicle of the past five years of living well with active cancer will benefit others who have or will be diagnosed with cancer; that this chronicle will help relieve some of the deadly fear that causes panic decisions, instead of prayerful and researched decisions. I pray that this chronicle will be beneficial to my daughters, my daughter-in-law, my granddaughter, my sisters-in-law, my nieces and grandnieces and friends who have personally seen the Lord's biological immunotherapy program in action at work on me.

Life can be good, even in the midst of deadly disease, if one looks to the Great Physician for strength, comfort, and direction. I am not strong (as anyone reading this chronicle can attest), but God is. I am not wise, but God is. I am not an easy person to love, but God is Love. (I John 4:8)

I do not know what the future holds for me on earth, but I am excited about it because He holds my future. The Lord Jesus will never disappoint me, even though I have and will disappoint Him many times. He will never leave nor forsake me. (Hebrews 13:5)

I am His. I was bought with a price when He gave His only begotten son to die on the cross for my sins and your sins, too. Since Jesus voluntarily gave His all for me, it seems reasonable that I should live for Him to the best of my limited ability.

I believe having the Lord as my Savior is an essential part of my treatment; that taking supplements and eating as healthy as possible is an important part of my therapy and that sharing my cancer walk is helpful to others, as well as myself.

May the Lord Jesus be very real to you as you look to him for direction, strength, and comfort in your total life and health.

Epilogue

Life went on, and the Lord continued working on teaching me patience. The little house in town sold, and we became friends with the couple who bought it. She also was dealing with cancer. She had gone through all the standard treatments and entered in a clinical trial, using interferon. She was usually upbeat and kept busy with church activities, swimming, and good works in the community. She lived abundantly, serving the Lord and loving her family until she grew too weak. Her husband and her family rejoiced that her suffering was over when the Lord finally called her home.

Jerry and I and our youngest two children moved to our true homeschool called Harmony Hill. Our Colorado cabin sold. We were then able to make a nice home and gathering place for our growing and expanding family, friends, and neighbors.

The Lord led us step by step, inch by inch. Nearly seventeen years after my Stage III breast cancer diagnosis, life continues being normally abnormal. Three of our four wonderful children have married and brought three more fine children into our family, and together, they have blessed us with five gorgeous grandchildren!

I still have breast cancer, but the Lord and His biological immunotherapy program (natural supplements) allow me to live a full and rewarding life here on earth until He calls me to my Heavenly home.

My desire is greet all of you in heaven in His time.

I desire a better, that is, a heavenly country.

Therefore, God is not ashamed to be called my God, for He has prepared a place for me. (Hebrews 11:16)

Suggested Reading

American Cancer Society. *Unproven Methods of Cancer Management*, (ACS's blacklist of alternative treatment), 1988

Balch, James F. and Phyllis A. Balch. *Prescription for Nutritional Healing*, 1997, Avery Publishing Group, Garden City Park, NY

The Bible

Bishop, Beata. *My Triumph Over Cancer*, 1985, Keats Publishing, Inc., New Canaan, CT

Cameron, Ewan and Pauling, Linus. *Cancer and Vitamin C*, 1979, Linus Pauling Institute of Science and Medicine, Menlo Park, CA 94025

Day, Lorraine. *Cancer Doesn't Scare Me Anymore*, Rockford Press, P. O. Box 952, Rancho Mirage, CA 92270

Forbes, Alec. "The Famous Bristol Detox Diet for Cancer Patients," 1984, Keats Publishing, Inc., New Canaan, CT

Greenfield, Louise. *Cancer Overcome By Diet: An Alternative to Surgery*, 1987, Author-Publisher, Livonia, MI 48152-2017

Griffin, G. Edward. *World without Cancer*, 1974, American Media, Westlake Village, CA 91359

Lane, William I., and Comac, Linda. *Sharks Don't Get Cancer*, Avery Publishing Group, Inc., Garden City Park, NY

Livingston—Wheeler, Virginia and Addeo, Edmond G. *The Conquest of Cancer: Vaccines and Diet,* 1984, Franklin Watts, NY

Love, Susan M., with Karen Lindsey. *Dr. Susan Love's Breast Book*, 1990, Addison-Wesley Publishing Co., Inc., Reading, MA

McMillen, S. I. *None of These Diseases*, 1963, Fleming H. Revell Co., Old Tappan, NJ 07675

Morris, Nat. *The Cancer Blackout*, 1977, Regent House, Los Angeles, CA

Moss, Ralph W. *Cancer Therapy: The Independent Consumer's Guide to Non-Toxic Treatment and Prevention*, 1992, Equinox Press, 331 W. 57th St., Ste. 268, New York, NY 10019

National Cancer Institute. *The Immune System* (pamphlet)

Quillin, Patrick, with Noreen Quillin. *Beating Cancer with Nutrition*, 1994, The Nutrition Times Press, Inc., Tulsa, OK 74170

Richardson, John A. and Griffin, Patricia. *Laetrile Case Histories: The Richardson Cancer Clinic Experiences,* 1977, American Media, Westlake Village, CA 91359

Stone, Irwin. *The Healing Factor Vitamin C against Disease*, 1972, Grosset and Dunlap, NY

Swope, Mary Ruth, with David A. Darbro. *Green Leaves Of Barley*, 1987, Swope Enterprises, Inc., Phoenix, AZ 85082-2104

University Medical Research Publishers. *Amazing Medicines the Drug Companies Don't Want You To Discover*, 1993, Tempe, AZ 85281

Walters, Richard. *Options: The Alternative Cancer Therapy Book*, 1993, Avery Publishing Group, Garden City Park, NY 11040

Weill, Andrew. *Spontaneous Healing*, 1995, Knopf Publishers, 201 E. 50th St., New York, NY 10022

Wigmore, Ann. *The Wheatgrass Book*, 1985, Avery Publishing Group, Garden City Park, NY

Willner, Robert. *The Cancer Solution*, 1994, Peltec Publishing Co., Inc., Boca Raton, FL 33431

Wolfe, Sidney M. and Hope, Rose-Ellen. *Worst Pills, Best Pills II*, 1993, Public Citizen's Health Research Group, Washington, DC 20036

SECTION III

A DISSERTATION
Submitted in partial fulfillment of the requirements
for the degree of Doctor of Philosophy
Clayton College of Natural Health

by
JOSEPH E. BOSILJEVAC, JR

BIRMINGHAM, ALABAMA
July, 2009

DEDICATION

Thank you, God, for the human machine and for the opportunity to broaden my knowledge to help others.

Contents

Abstract

There is an increasing acceptance and use of CAM, particularly among women with breast cancer. A detailed review of CAM modalities used by the patient in the case presentation fails to reveal a "magic bullet" However, the same can be said for most allopathic treatments. Instead, the information gathered supports a holistic approach. Providing the body with the necessary substrates leads to healing using innate physiological pathways. Biologic plausibility can be seen even if solid scientific evidence is not established at this time, Much of this results from an incomplete knowledge of complex physiological pathway including the hormonal ads. The same criticism used as far as lack of scientific evidence for CAM can also be applied to the current use of Evidence Based Medicine. Many approaches used by the "health care industry" suppress curiosity, observation, and experience, which are considered basic tools used by the clinician-scientist to advance scientific knowledge.

List of Abbreviations

ACTH	Adrenocorticotrophic Hormone
ASCORBATE	Ascorbic Acid (vitamin C)
BMI	Body Mass Index
BRCA	Breast Cancer Gene
CAM	Complementary and Alternative Methods
DFI	Disease-free Interval
DFS	Disease-free Survival
DHEA	Dihydroepiandosterone
DNA	Dioxyribonucleic Acid
EBCTCG	Early Breast Cancer Trialists Collaborative Group
EBM	Evidence-Based Medicine
EGF	Epithelial Growth Factor
ECOG	Eastern Cooperative Oncology Group
ER	Estrogen Receptor
FGF	Fibroblast Growth Factor
G 1/G 2	Phases of mitosis
GF	Growth Factor
GH	Growth Hormone
GI	Gastrointestinal
HEGF	Human Epidermal Growth Factor
HER	Human Epidermal Receptor
HGH	Human Growth Hormone
HIF	Hypoxia Induced Factor
IFN	Interferon
IGF	Insulin-like Growth Factor
IGF-I	Insulin-like Growth Factor I
IGFRP	Insulin-like Growth Factor Receptor Protein
IGFBP	Insulin-like Growth Factor Binding Protein

IP-6	Inositol hexaphosphate
M	Phase of mitosis
MGN III	Modified arabinoxyline from rice bran (Biobran)
mRNA	Messenger Ribonucleic Acid
NK	Natural Killer
NCRP	National Council on Radiation Protection and Measurement
NSABP	National Surgical Adjunctive Breast and Bowel Project
p 53	Human Gene
p 73	Human Gene
PAH	Polyamine Hydrocarbons
PDGF	Platelet Derived Growth Factor
PR	Progesterone Receptor
PUFA	Polyunsaturated Fatty Acid
ROS	Reactive Oxygen Species
SPF	S-phase Fraction
TNF	Tumor Necrosis Factor
TK	Tyrosine Kinase
VEGF	Vascular Endothelial growth Factor
VGF	Vascular Growth Factor

Case Report

D. S. presented at the age of forty-six with a lump in her left breast and was diagnosed with an infiltrating, lobular carcinoma. As her history was reviewed, she noted the following:

"I always felt my left breast was different. The nipple was inverted since adolescence, and I had been treated for fibrocystic condition. After marriage, I started on birth control pills and then noticed before my periods I would have tender lumps under my left axilla. These would become sore and then regress between periods. In general, my medical status was one with lots of reactions to medications. Many times, side effects were worse than the symptoms that were being treated.

"At age twenty-eight I had my first pregnancy. The pain in my left breast would not leave. I was concerned about breast cancer but was told I was too young. At that time, I ate a lot of fat and junk foods. By my third pregnancy, the lumps had disappeared, but then I had begun taking care of my body since I was thirty-five years old (after my second pregnancy).

"During my fourth pregnancy, there was concern about the development of the baby's heart. I felt a lot of stress during that pregnancy and noted that the lumps under my left axilla returned. I also remember that this was a rather difficult labor for me. I came to the hospital dilated to seven centimeters, and a male nurse was assigned to attend my delivery. I did not feel comfortable with him. Another nurse came in and checked me, and the cervix was back to five centimeters dilated. I told her I was not comfortable with the male nurse, so she took over my care, and I soon started making progress with the delivery again. It was almost as if my body said, 'I am *not* having a baby with a male nurse present.' Following this, I delivered quickly."

D. S. was diagnosed as Stage III-B breast cancer following a modified, radical mastectomy. The tumor was estrogen receptor (ER) and progesterone receptor (PR) positive. The mastectomy was accompanied by a right breast biopsy since the histologic diagnosis was lobular carcinoma. Several recommendations were made after the mastectomy.

The first was to have a hysterectomy and bilateral salpingo-oophorectomy. D. S. felt that "if it ain't broke, don't try to fix it," and did not feel that these additional operations were justified.

Radiotherapy was also recommended. From the onset, she had poor rapport with the radiotherapist and felt that she was being treated as a number rather than a person. She prayed to the Lord to show her what she should do. In preparation for the radiotherapy sessions, skin tattooing was performed. After this was completed she rose up and felt very dizzy. Polaroids had been taken of the left chest wall following her mastectomy. When she looked at them hanging on the wall, she said they looked like "slabs of meat" and at that time made up her mind that she would refuse any radiotherapy.

No chemotherapy was offered, but hormonal manipulation was another recommendation. Subsequently, she was started on Tamoxifen and had a lot of side effects. She tried progesterone cream, which seemed to balance some of these effects. However, she discontinued the Tamoxifen and utilized the progesterone cream alone on an intermittent basis depending on her signs and symptoms.

Shortly after the refusal of radiotherapy and her experience with the above, she happened to hear a radio program regarding natural medicine. Her comment was, "Could this be God speaking to me?" She also had been reading a copy of Dr. Susan Love's *Breast Book* as well as multiple natural medicine books (see references used by the patient in her recovery). It had been suggested to take some additional vitamin C and beta-carotene to tolerate the radiotherapy. Despite not proceeding with the radiotherapy treatments, she found that the vitamin C seemed to help with her energy level. She then initiated a regimen that included seven grams a day for the initial seven years after her diagnosis. About one and one-half years following the diagnosis of breast cancer, skin metastases appeared in the chest wall at the mastectomy site (see appendix A, photo 1). She felt she was under a lot of stress in her life at that time.

She went to the Cancer Centers of America and was offered the following recommendations:

1. Buffered (Ester-C) in higher doses that were much more tolerable without GI upset (7 g/day)
2. A short course of intravenous vitamin C up to 100 g/day
3. Increased vitamin B which helped with anxiety and her nerves
4. Nutritional recommendations were made. These included smaller portions of protein of all sorts and hardly *any* red meat. It was also recommended to decrease dairy products (for possible hormone content) and eat lots of fresh fruits and vegetables. She did not necessarily choose organic fruits and vegetables, but washed the ones she bought with soap and water. In addition, she tried to watch the amount of refined sugar in her diet. These changes made her feel much better
5. She also started on a detoxification program. She had read that certain herbs were anti-tumor to slow the growth of cancers. She used milk thistle and dandelion root for liver detoxification. In addition, she took red clover as a blood cleanser (alterative) and felt that this also helped balance her hormones.

Despite these measures, the skin lesions became worse (see appendix A, photo 2) and a biopsy demonstrated metastatic breast cancer with both estrogen receptor (ER) and progesterone receptor (PR) positive, and a 100% diploid DNA pattern. At that point she tried shark cartilage but said the skin lesions became worse as if they developed a *better* blood supply. She initiated DHEA with the same results. She then attempted a poultice as a topical treatment which was recommended by Weir (see references used by patient in her recovery). D. S. found this was difficult to keep in place and remain active. At that point progesterone cream was utilized as well as an increase in red clover and green tea intake. The skin lesions subsequently improved.

Approximately one year later the skin lesions worsened, which she attributed to additional stress in her life when a close friend died. She continued her same regimen and added intravenous hydrogen peroxide treatments. After eight sessions she did not notice any difference. She increased the vitamin C to 100 g a day (intravenous) and with this dosage saw regression of the lesions (see appendix A, photo 3). At the same time, she was also working on her spirituality and the management of stress in her life. She affirmed that she did not want to consider any conventional allopathic treatment.

Very little was heard from D. S. for almost eight years. There was occasional contact for bloodwork and chest x-rays. Basic lab work consistently came back within normal limits. She continues to follow a fairly rigid program that includes daily:

1. Vitamin C, 7 g for seven years (except for the period of a few months when she increased to 100 g daily, which included intravenous infusion) but is currently down to four grams a day for maintenance
2. Vitamin B complex
3. A multivitamin twice a day
4. Calcium 1500 mg-vitamin D 750 mg complex
5. Beta-carotene 50,000 IU
6. Vitamin E, 800 units
7. Bilberry
8. Flax seed
9. Progesterone cream for hot flashes, generally used only one time a week
10. Dandelion root
11. Milk thistle
12. Red clover
13. Acidophilus

In addition, she follows a diet of lots of fresh or frozen fruits and vegetables, soy products, green tea, no red meat or dairy products, and very little refined sugar. She and her husband celebrate once a week with pizza or hamburgers on a "liberation day."

She also relates that she has tried MGN-III with no benefit. About four years ago she was highly stressed when a nephew was killed in an auto accident and noted that the skin metastases grew. She eliminated almost all of the sugar from her diet and started on IP-6. At that point, the tumors shrank. IP-6 is rather expensive, but she has added this to her regimen in the dose of seven capsules a day.

She gave other examples when she felt the nodules were out of control. As part of a jury in a manslaughter case, she could not share the stress she felt during the trial, even with her husband. Her main concern was that she saw a man who may or may not have been guilty, but who could be separated from his daughter. Once the trial was completed, the nodules rapidly regressed with no other change in her regimen. Another example was the death of a close friend, with progression of the skin lesions, followed by regression when the grieving process had been completed.

Using recommendations from Siegel (1986), she has found guidance to help her with a more positive outlook, and did not read newspapers or listen to the radio for that reason. She also believes strongly in her faith in God. She tries to give any worries or stress to God, praying that His will be done. D. S. states, "I have a responsibility to listen to God and follow his instructions." This spirituality is the essence of her primary stress management program.

In summary, when asked "what were the most important aspects as far as her overall program," the following was her response:

1. Ask God, "What am I worrying about?"
2. Watch the junk food.
3. Continue to follow the regimen or program that she has developed over the years.

The final photograph is the most recent, taken sixteen years after the diagnosis of breast cancer (see appendix A, photo 4).

SUBSEQUENT INTERVIEW WITH THE PATIENT:

D. S. confirmed that she is taking 4 g/day of vitamin C, and at that time she was taking 100 g/day included intravenous therapy. Although she used soy, red clover (two capsules a day) and progesterone cream were preferable for hormonal modulation. The progesterone cream is used approximately weekly when she notices hot flashes, but it has been used sparingly the past year. She drinks two cups of green tea daily. The IP-6 costs about $35 for two weeks. Her main protocol consists of stress management through prayer and spirituality, no junk food, and many supplements that are useful for detoxification.

References Used by the Patient in Her Recovery

Dailey, T. J. (1998). *Healing through the power of prayer.* Lincolnwood, Il: Publications International.

Editors of Prevention Magazine Healthbooks. (1997). *Drug-free healing.* Emmaus, Pa: Rodale Press.

Ferguson, E. R. (1990). *New frontiers in medicine. Healing, health, and transformation.* Chicago: Lavonne Press.

Goldberg, B. (1994). *Alternative medicine. The definitive guide.* Payallup, Wa: Future Medicine Publishing.

Griffin, E. G. (1974). *World without cancer. The story of vitamin B-17.* Westlake Village, Ca: American Media.

Griffin, L. (1979). *Please doctor, I'd rather do it myself . . . . With vitamins and minerals.* Salt Lake City, Ut: Hawkes Publishing.

Johnson P. (2987). *Spiritual secrets to physical health.* Waco, Tx: Word Books.

Livingston-Wheeler, V., and Addeo, E. G. (1984). *The conquest of cancer. Vaccines and diet.* New York: Franklin Watts.

Margen, S. (1992). *The wellness encyclopedia of food and nutrition.* New York: Rebus.

Morris, N. (1992). *The cancer blackout.* Los Angeles, Ca: Regent House.

Nichols, P. (1937). *Cancer. Its proper treatment and cure.* Kingsport, Tn: Kingsport Press.

University, Medical Research Publishers. (1993). *Amazing medicines the drug companies don't want you to discover.* Tempe, Az: University Medical Research Publishers.

Weil, A. (2995). *Spontaneous healing.* New York: Alfred A. Knopf.

Werbach, M. (1993). *Healing through nutrition.* New York: Harper Collins.

Willner,R. E. (1994). *The cancer solution.* Boca Raton, Fl: Peltec Publishing Co.

Chapter One

Introduction to the Problem

Statement of the Problem

Breast cancer in women is a prevalent disease in Western cultures. The survival rate for patients with metastatic disease has not significantly increased in the past thirty-five years. Skin metastases (locoregional recurrence) are associated with a very poor prognosis. Complementary and alternative methods (CAM) have increased, particularly in women with breast cancer. This paper will look at CAM use in a woman with locoregional recurrence (skin metastases), evaluate its place in the treatment of breast cancer, and link scientific and theoretical literature to support a possible scientific basis for these methods in the treatment of breast cancer.

Background and History of the Problem

This is not meant to be a comprehensive synopsis on breast cancer, but an overall understanding of the disease, epidemiology, risk factors, and treatment enable insight into relevance of CAM and its place in the prevention and treatment of breast cancer. Although a broad background of information is presented, this will be narrowed down in chapter 4 (Results and Findings), and chapter 5 (Conclusions, Implications, and Recommendations for Further Research) to a detailed discussion of specific areas of CAM used by the patient presented.

Epidemiology

Carcinoma of the breast is a prevalent disease in women in Western society (Brinton, Lacey, and Devesa 2002; Newman and Sabel 2003; Ries et al. 2000). Veronesi, Boyle, Goldhirsch, Orrchia, and Viale (2005) report there were 1,150,000 new cases in 2002, and point out that incidence and mortality rates increased from 1951 to 1990, then decreased in western Europe, North America, and South America. Breast cancer rates are lowest in Japan, China, Africa, and Central America and highest in western Europe and North America (Brinton et al. 2002; Pisani, Park, Bray, and Ferlay 1999). Although the incidence of invasive breast cancer stabilized during the 1990s, ductal carcinoma in situ (DCIS) continued to rise sixfold (Emens and Davidson 2003). In addition, invasive tumors greater than 3 cm in diameter decreased 27% since 1990, but the number of invasive tumors less than 2 cm in diameter doubled in number (Emens and Davidson 2003). This demonstrates a trend for earlier diagnosis from increased screening (Newman and Washington 2003). Five-year survival rates improved from 75% in the mid-1970s to 86% in the early 1990s (Ries et al. 2000). Newman and Washington (2003) state the decrease in mortality is probably due to increasing numbers of women undergoing screening, resulting in treatment of earlier lesions. Disease-free survival (DFS) in Stage I breast cancer has been reported at 82% for ten years and 78% at twenty years (Emens and Davidson 2003). A meta-analysis of randomized trials in early breast cancer conducted by the Early Breast Cancer Trialists Collaborative Group (EBCTCG) shows that adjuvant radiotherapy decreases local recurrence but does not increase overall survival (1995). These statistics are also supported by the American Cancer Society (2002) and Greenlee, Murray, Bolden, and Wingo (2000).

Breast cancer is elusive. Clinicians are well aware that some patients predicted to have recurrence and die do not, while others considered cured die from the disease. Multiple factors are involved in the prognosis, and despite efforts to predict outcome and survival, the aforementioned unpredictability occurs. No one reports complete cure, but terms such as disease-free interval (DFI) and disease-free survival (DFS) are common. There are very few statistics for survival without treatment (Christensen, Anderson, and Storm 2001), which, in general, is considered unethical. Rush (1982) mentions a mean survival from over 1000 untreated cases collected in the literature at 38.7 months. He also states that the aim of therapy is to improve the quality of life and the length of survival, but not as yet to provide cure. Greenberg et al., (1996) point out that there is a small group of patients with metastatic breast cancer who can achieve a durable remission with systemic treatment. However, for most patients with metastatic disease, the treatment goals are palliation of symptoms and prolongation of DFS (Andre et al. 2004; Crown et al. 2002).

The most comprehensive study of breast cancer recurrence rates after initial therapy analyzes the clinical course of 3,585 pre and postmenopausal breast cancer patients enrolled in seven completed Eastern Cooperative Oncology Group (ECOG) studies of adjuvant therapy for primary operable breast cancer (Saphner, Tormey, and Gray, 1996). Most of these patients had positive axillary nodes at the time of diagnosis and 45% developed a recurrence, peaking in the second year after diagnosis. Estrogen receptor (ER) negative tumors recurred more commonly than ER positive tumors during the first five years. Six to twelve years after diagnosis ER positive tumors recurred more commonly than ER negative tumors. Saphner et al. (1996) base this on the fact that most estrogen receptor negative tumors that recurred did so early, and the data further suggests that evaluation for relapse is probably most useful in the first five years, particularly the first two years after diagnosis. However, the risk of recurrence clearly continues up to twenty years after primary treatment (Charefare, Limongelli, and Purshotham 2005; Fisher 1999). In other words, there is no definite time in which a breast cancer survivor can be considered completely cured. Saphner et al. (1996) state that the risk of recurrence clearly continues up to twenty years after primary treatment and further emphasizes that there is no definite time at which a breast cancer survivor can be considered cured.

Environmental factors

Genetics

A familial or genetic predisposition has been recognized, but this actually occurs in only a small proportion of individuals with breast cancer, estimated at 5% (Allain, Gilligan, and Redlich 2002; Coughlin and Piper 1999; Dunning et al. 1999; Narod and Offit 2005; Ziyaie,

Hupp, and Thompson 2000). Genetics do not play a part in the patient presented, but a relationship to DNA mutations and other effects on a cellular basis may be important to support a scientific explanation for some CAM modalities. Separate from familial breast cancer, there are multiple environmental conditions that have been analyzed as predisposing factors for the development of breast cancer (Armstrong 1976; Brinton et al. 2002; Hall 1974; Jackson 2008; Kelsey 1993; Kelsey and Bernstein 1996; Talamini et al. 1997). The following sections present some of the primary ones.

Cancer Risk and Radiation Exposure

A carcinogenic effect of radiotherapy on the lungs of women treated for breast cancer is suggested in population-based and case-controlled studies from cancer registries (Emens and Davidson 2003; Saphner et al. 1996; Veronesi et al. 2005). Other retrospective studies from individual institutions comprising large numbers of breast cancer patients treated with radiotherapy after breast-conservation surgery show conflicting results (Sigdestad, Spratt, and Connor 2002). A relationship between radiotherapy for breast cancer and development of subsequent lung cancer is uncertain, but a higher incidence of primary lung tumors, both ipsilateral and contralateral, is found in the National Surgical Adjuvant Breast and Bowel Project (NSABP B-06 trial) after post-lumpectomy breast irradiation (Deutsch et al. 2003). Vena, Graham, Hellman, Swanson, and Brasure (1991) look at the use of electric blankets and notice a slight increased risk of breast cancer in postmenopausal women.

This leads to reports that evaluate early-age and lifetime radiation exposure as an initiating factor for DNA mutations and development of subsequent carcinoma of the breast (Baral, Larson, and Mattsson 1977; BEIR V Report 1990; Bennett 1999; Boice 1979; Lan 1995; Tokunaga 1987), and includes information regarding routine diagnostic medical imaging where there may be a latency of twenty to thirty years. The amount of radiation exposure to the United States population is reported by the National Council on Radiation Protection and Measurement (NCRP), and the current amounts of radiation received in routine medical imaging is reported as 154 millirad (mrad) for mammograms, 10 mrad for a two-view chest x-ray, and 1000 mrad for a conventional CT (computerized tomographic) scan (NCRP 1987). Mattson (1980) points out an increased incidence of breast cancer that occurs after a latency of sixteen years in patients following radiation therapy for benign disease.

It is also expressed that a combination of exposure to radiation and smoking are additive (Boice 1979; Veronisi et al. 2005). Folic acid ensures that a cofactor is available to facilitate DNA repair (Haas and Levin 2006) emphasizing that antioxidants and a diet that includes sufficient folic acid may lessen DNA damage from exposure to irradiation (Valtuena et al. 2008). Radiation exposure cannot be definitely implicated in the case presented, but the significance of cumulative radiation from routine medical imaging as well as the amount of radiation received in treatment needs to be considered in the response and prognosis of some patients. Some CAM modalities (vitamin C) may ameliorate side effects of radiation treatment (Gerber, Cholz, Reimer, Briese, and Janni 2006).

Alcohol

The literature reports conflicting results on the nature of the relationship between alcohol consumption and the risk of breast cancer (Ferraroni 1998). Multiple studies indicate there is questionable impact from alcohol intake, except as it may affect the immune system, folate levels, or from contaminants in the alcohol. However, these reports all show a dose-response curve with higher alcohol intake associated with a higher incidence of breast cancer (Howe et al. 1990; Katsouyanni et al. 1994; Longnecker et al. 1995). The biologic mechanism is difficult to assess (Tseng 1999). Katsouyanni et al. (1994) suggest a late-stage growth enhancing factor, and shows an increased risk with three or more glasses daily, although a lower dose has confounding effects. Yu and Berkel (1999) propose an interesting mechanism involving IGF (insulin-like growth factor) as far as a role in cancer development and progression. This is supported by Li et al. (1998). Both studies find that moderate alcohol intake increase IGF levels, whereas heavier use decreases the same. Alcohol intake may cause alterations in endogenous estrogen (Zaridze, Lifanova, Maximovitch, Day, and Duffy 1991). A causal relationship between alcohol consumption and breast cancer has not been clearly established, but the effect on hormones and a possible mechanism involving IGF are interesting hypotheses which will be developed.

Obesity, Dietary Fat Intake, and the Risk of Breast Cancer

A study of a relationship between obesity and breast cancer is difficult because an association between dietary fat, total kilocalorie intake, and obesity is complex (Albanes 1987; Freedman et al. 1993). The presumed relationship of breast cancer with a high-fat diet, particularly animal protein, and a body habitus containing increased body fat is that these factors elevate female sex hormone levels, alter insulin resistance, and causes multiple, complex effects on the hormonal axis (Freedman et al. 1993). Promoting lifestyle changes to improve insulin sensitivity may favorably affect the risk of breast cancer (Lajous, Boutron-Ruault, Fabre, Clavel-Chapelon, and Romieu 2008; Li, Hilsenbeck, and Yee 1988; Stoll 1999; Yu and Rohan 2000). Although the literature is controversial, a large case-controlled study demonstrates that subjects in the top quartile of body mass index (BMI) have a 40% higher risk of breast cancer than those in the lower quartile (Trentham-Dietz et al. 1997). Additionally, this has been studied with regards to risk in pre and postmenopausal groups, showing a higher risk relationship in the latter (Huang et al. 1997). Hu (1997) further relates increased BMI and lack of physical activity with a higher breast cancer risk.

Obesity and high-fat intake in women with breast cancer also demonstrate some increase in second primary cancers of the endometrium and ovary, and possibly melanoma, colon, salivary gland, and thyroid (Brinton et al. 2002). A large study by Kelsey and Bernstein (1996) from the Women's Health Initiative assesses the impact of a low-fat diet on the risk of breast cancer. Other case-controlled and prospective studies (American Institute for Cancer Research 1997; Armstrong and Doll 1975; Cho et al. 2003; Hebert and Rosen 1996) fail to find any significant relationship between breast cancer and a diet high in fat. Types of fat are important with a protective effect from monounsaturated fats, such as olive oil, and omega-3 fatty acids (Cade, Thomas, and Vail 1998; Favero, Papinel, and Mantella 1999; Gago-Dominguez, Yuan, Sun, Lee, and Yu 2003; La Vecchia, Favero, and Francheschi 1998). Saturated fatty acids relate to increased risk in three case-controlled studies (Cade et al. 1998; Favero et al. 1999; La Vecchia et al. 1998).

Animal protein, especially red meat, may cause oxidative DNA damage in blood, and the quantity of beef and pork intake in a group of women at high risk for breast cancer is evaluated by Cho et al. (2006) and Djuric et al. (1998). Eunyoung et al. (2006) implicate higher red meat intake as a risk factor for ER positive/PR (progesterone receptor) positive breast cancer among premenopausal women. The risk associated with red meat intake may be decreased when fresh vegetables are eaten on a daily basis (Hirayama 1990). This is also demonstrated by Gandini, Merzenich, Robertson, and Boyle (2000) in a large meta-analysis.

Although some implications are made that high-fat intake during adolescence may increase risk (Armstrong and Doll 1975; Baer et al. 2003; Cho et al. 2003; Linos, Willett, Cho, Colditz, and Frazier 2008), Potischman et al. (1998) find no relationship. In addition, diet or nutritional causes are implicated on a hormonal basis for the disease (American Institute for Cancer Research 1997; Armstrong and Doll 1975; Blot et al. 1993; Boehnke-Michaud, Phillips-Karpenski, Jones, and Espiritu 2007; Cade et al. 1998; Hebert and Rosen 1996; Howe et al. 1990; Yuan, Koh, Sun, Lee, and Yu 2005). This may be an important factor in the case presented.

Fruits and Vegetables

The protective effect of fruits and vegetables is likely related to the protection from cell damage by various antioxidants contained in these food substances (Agudo et al. 2007; Blot et al. 1993; Gaudet et al. 2004; Haas and Levin 2002; Holmberg 1994; Kavanaugh, Trumbo, and Ellwood 2007; La Vecchia, 2002; Valtuena et al. 2008; Watzl 2005). Smith-Warner et al. (2001) report that consumption in adulthood is not significantly associated with decreased breast cancer risk, although amount of intake is not defined. In a prospective study of 285,526 women between the ages of twenty-five and seventy, van Gils et al. (2005) find no relationship between the amount of intake and risk of breast cancer. Freedman et al. (1993) show the benefit of water-insoluble fiber in lowering the risk with a high-fat diet. Large meta-analyses demonstrate a lower risk associated with fresh vegetable intake versus manufactured nutritional and vitamin supplements (Cho et al. 2003; Gandini et al. 2000). Shanon et al. (2005) review botanical groupings of foods with relation to risk of breast cancer. A meta-analysis of case-controlled studies shows a significant protective effect of vitamin A (Zhang et al. 1999). A stronger relationship for carotenoid A from fruits and vegetables versus preformed vitamin A (retinol) from animal sources is presented by Howe et al. (1990). Vitamin E is more difficult to assess as far as the amount in nutritional consumption (Haas and Levin 2006). Selenium is an important component of the antioxidant enzyme glutathione peroxidase that inhibits cell proliferation, although the extent of the relationship of selenium and the risk of breast cancer remains to be defined (Hunter et al. 1990). High glycemic load is presented by Lajous et al. (2008) as a risk factor in the development of breast cancer.

The antioxidants found in fruits and vegetables are vitamins C, D, and E, carotenoids, selenium, folate, lutein, xanthin, and some types of dietary fat. These are all shown to modulate cell proliferation and differentiation (Fairfield and Fletcher 2002; Warner 2006). Antioxidant-rich foods also lower DNA damage (Haas and Levin 2006), measured by monitoring blood levels of five-hydroxy-methyluracil in healthy women (Falk et al. 1999).

Isothiocyanates are compounds that may inhibit carcinogens at multiple cell sites (Auborn et al. 2003; Ambrosone 2004 2006; Brandi et al. 2005; Fowke et al. 2003; Smith-Warner et al. 2001). Examples are the cruciferous vegetables broccoli and cabbage. Broccoli will shift estrogen metabolism to alternative hormones, such as hydroxyestrone, which do not exhibit estrogenic properties in breast tissue (Auborn 2003; Brandi 2005; Fowke, Longcope, and Hebert 2000; Gaudet et al. 2004; Smith-Warner 2001). It may require high levels of broccoli intake to cause this shift. In addition, cruciferous vegetables tend to produce a bitter taste that is worse in patients with cancer which may explain why these foods are sometimes avoided. Folic acid ensures that a cofactor is available to facilitate DNA repair (Haas and Levin 2006; Valtuena et al. 2008), and was discussed in conjunction with radiation therapy. Good nutrition is always a part of health, and significant diet changes appear to play a major role in the recovery of the patient presented.

Vitamin C

Several case-controlled studies find an inverse relationship between the amount of fresh vitamin C intake and the risk of breast cancer (Assouline and Miller 2006; Cho et al. 2003; Loria, Klag, Caulfield, and Whelton 2000; Ronco 1999; Zhang et al. 1999). Vitamin C is a well-known antioxidant which may block the formation of carcinogenic nitrosamines associated with red meat intake (Asplund 2002; Djuric et al. 1998). Paddayatty et al. (2007) demonstrate vitamin C secretion from the adrenal gland in response to ACTH, which is one of the hormones released during stress. Meta-analysis from nine research studies shows that vitamin C intake lowers the risk of breast cancer (Gandini et al. 2000).

Increased mammographic breast density is increasingly used as an indicator of breast cancer risk. Vachon, Kushi, Cerhan, Kuni, and Sellers (2000) find an increase in mammary gland density in premenopausal women who supplemented their diet with vitamin C. Berube, Diorio, and Brisson (2008) further show that regular use of multivitamin/multimineral supplements may be associated with an increased mean breast density among premenopausal women. The significance of this as a possible risk factor not completely defined (Ingehom, Pederson, and Holek 1999).

Ever since Cameron and Pauling (1976; 1978) reported the use of supplemental ascorbic acid (vitamin C) in prolonging survival in terminal human cancer there has been extensive study of vitamin C with controversial results. There are reports showing the beneficial effect of vitamin C in cancer patients (Arrigoni and de Tullio 2002; Cameron 1991; Chen et al. 2005; Padayatty and Levine 2000; Padayatty et al. 2003 2004 2006 2007; Yeom, Jung, and Song 2007) and those reporting the opposite or equivocal results (Bahr, Pfeiffer, and Oelkers 2008; Bjelakovic, Nikolova, Gluud, Simonetti, and Gluud 2007; Borst 2008; Catley and Anderson 2006; Creagan et al. 1979; Hoffer et al. 2008; Moertel et al. 1979; Stanner, Hughes, Kelly, and Buttress 2004). Lawenda et al. (2008), stating that although concurrent administration of vitamin C with chemotherapy or radiation treatment may reduce treatment-related side effects, conclude that the use of supplemental antioxidants during treatment should be discouraged because of possible tumor proliferation and reduced survival due to lessening the effectiveness of the radiation therapy. Gerber et al. (2006) suggest vitamin C to lessen side effects of radiation, as does Valtuena et al. (2008). Grasad (2004) presents an improved efficacy and lowered toxicity using antioxidants with standard and experimental cancer therapies.

The type of vitamin C, as well as the dose and mode of administration, may be important and needs to be evaluated (Berube et al. 2008; Cameron and Pauling 1976 1978: Hoffer et al. 2008; Padayatty and Levine 2000; Paddayatty et al. 2004). This will be discussed in detail in chapter 4 and chapter 5 since high doses of vitamin C were used by the patient presented.

Green Tea

Green tea contains the V compound (-) epigallocatechin gallate (EGCG) which has been shown to inhibit the growth and cause apoptosis of cancer cells (Fujiki 1999; Zhang, Holman, d'Arcy, Huang, and Xie 2007; Yuan, Koh, Sun, Lee, and Yu 2005). Japanese researchers demonstrate a decreased recurrence in Stage I and Stage II breast cancer in women who drank green tea before and after the clinical onset of cancer (Nakachi 1998). Five or more cups of tea, or a higher dose of polyphenols, give a better prognosis (Yang 1999; Zhang et al. 2007). Usually, this dose of green tea is not achieved in western countries. There may also be some possible effects on the hormone axis and immune system due to the caffeine and phytosterols in the green tea (Hirayama 1990; Ovaskainen et al. 2005; Yang 1999). Sowers et al. (2006) show an effect on estrogen metabolism by measuring levels of hydroxyestrone (a metabolite of estrogen), which is decreased by increased intake of green tea, and hypothesizes this may be the health benefit related to breast cancer. Catechol-containing tea polyphenols are very rapidly O-methylated by human catechol-o-methyltransferase (COMT), and tea catechins appear to reduce breast cancer in the study by Wu, Tseng, Van Den Berg, and Yu (2003) of Asian American women. In this study, the strongest decrease in risk was among patients with a low activity of COMT, suggesting that they were metabolically less efficient in eliminating tea catechins and thus received the most benefit. Besides populations, there may be a difference in age groups that also explains some margin for error in studies comparing different groups (Yuan et al. 2005). Green tea is an antioxidant source used by the patient presented.

Soy/Dairy

There has been considerable research on the use of soy as a substitute for dairy products. Although current information from large reviews and epidemiologic evidence does not support any relationship between dairy products and breast cancer risk (Moorman and Terry 2004; Parodi 2005), an unknown factor is the contamination of dairy products with pesticides, antibiotics, and hormones fed to dairy animals.

Several studies support the relationship of high soy intake and decreased risk of breast cancer (Bernstein and Ross 1993; Lampe et al. 2007; Trock, Hilakivi-Clarke, and Clarke 2006; Yamamoto, Sobue, Kobayashi, Sasaki, and Tsugane 2003). Others show no definite relationship (Shanon et al. 2005; Touillard, Thiebault, Niravong, Boutron-Ruault, and Clavel-Chaperon 2006) and it is pointed out that not only is there little human data showing definite support but phytoestrogens may interfere with the ability of Tamoxifen in the inhibition of breast cancer (Duffy, Perez, and Partridge 2007; Wood, Register, Franke, Anthony, and Cline 2006). Rice and Whitehead (2006) point out that the intake of soy phytoestrogens in eastern countries is greater than 30 mg/day, whereas in the west it is under 10 mg/day. However, they also indicate that the decreased risk of breast cancer in migrants increases with subsequent generations, supporting some dietary component in the causal relationship. Duffy et al. (2007) and Rice and Whitehead (2006) both show that exposure early in life may be protective. Others also demonstrate a beneficial effect and reduced breast cancer risk with high soy intake in childhood and adolescence (Lampe et al. 2007; Wu et al. 2002).

The relationship of soy and sex hormones is complex and not completely understood (Allred et al. 2004; Hilakivi-Clarke, Wang, Kalil, Riggins, and Pestall 2004; Mahady 2005; Maskrinec et al. 2004; Ross 2006). Besides the intricate biochemical picture, Martinez, Thomson, and Smith-Warner (2006) support the difficulty in applying assumptions of meta-analysis due to heterogeneity of genetics and metabolism in different populations. In addition, Atkinson, Frankenfeld, and Lampe (2005) review the various isoflavones in soy products which may be available in varied amounts depending on processing. Metabolism by gut flora affecting absorption may also differ in individuals, and this concept is introduced by Atkinson et al. (2005). Relationship of soy products in hormone modulation will be discussed in greater detail in chapter 4 and chapter 5.

Stress

Two reports are available that provide a link between development of breast cancer and perceived stress and psychological factors (Cooper, Cooper, and Faragher 1989; Hilakivi-Clarke, Rowland, Clarke, and Lippman 1994). A lateral study found no relationship between job stress and breast cancer (Achat, Kawachi, Byrne, Hankinson, and Colditz 2000). Management of stress and spirituality certainly appears to promote positive results in some people as demonstrated in the case study, but this is an area that is difficult to measure objectively.

Women with breast disease fit a stress profile that is consistent with an integrated theory of mammary carcinogenesis that combines a number of the observations previously noted. If women who are constitutionally stressed have a genetic mechanism that promotes secretory activity in breast tissue as a result of endogenous catecholamine stimulation, and if a subset of these women have high-circulating beta-glucuronidase levels that concentrate carcinogens consumed by a diet high in fats, nitrates, and transformed hydrocarbons; it is possible that carcinogenic agents may be transported to breast ducts in unusually high levels (Bammer and Newberry 1981; Horwitz, Maguire, Pearson, and Segaloff 1975; Whittiker and Clark 1971). The excessive catecholamine release by individuals who are sensitive to caffeine may also have the effect of decreasing the normal function of natural killer (NK) cells involved in cancer surveillance (Blazar 1986; Papatestas and Kark 1974; Tonnesen, Brinkley, Schou Oleson, and Christensen 1985). Hrushesky et al. (1988) suggest that circadian rhythm changes in NK cell activity may, in part, be responsible for an intermittent frequency of postsurgical metastatic dissemination of tumor. Lee (1984) looks at delayed cutaneous hypersensitivity and lymphocyte counts in relationship to relapse in the period of five years following mastectomy. Obviously, these observations and hypotheses are very difficult to prove.

Reactions of women to breast cancer range from fear, denial, guilt, anger, and/or grief (Siegel 1986). Women also have major concerns of loss of personal control as well as bodily deformation (Love 2000). Simply being at risk is a major factor. The nature of self-directed visits and options adds to the sense of personal control and leads to a tendency of CAM use by this group. The patient presented has a very strong spirituality as part of her stress management.

Other Factors

The relationship of exercise and cancer appears to be biologically plausible given that physical activity has been associated with changes in endogenous hormones, menstrual patterns, body fat distribution patterns, and alteration of immunologic parameters (American Cancer Society 2003). The strongest support for physical activity as a potential preventive mechanism is derived from a studies of early-onset breast cancers in which a reduction of risk is associated with regular physical activity and found to be independent of body size (Bernstein and Ross 1993; Hu 1997).

Other less commonly mentioned factors include cigarette smoking, mutagenic effects of hair dyes, prenatal exposure to hormones, ionizing irradiation from cell phones, computers, and television, and occupational/environmental exposure to DDT and polychlorinated biphenyls (PCBs) (Brinton et al. 2002; Jackson 2008). Howard (2009) cites the possibility of artificial lighting as a risk factor. This may feed into the circadian rhythm, melatonin, and subsequently HGH and the hormonal axis. These items probably have no significant impact in this particular case.

Many of the biological mechanisms in the etiology of breast cancer are unknown as can be seen by the complexity of hormonal relationships and other factors such as diet and environment (Beral 2003; Pritchard, Hill, Dijkstra, McDermott, and O'Higgins 2003). Only 55% of cancer cases can be explained by certain factors (Bruzzi, Green, Byar, Brinton, and Schairer 1985). The rationale for presenting this data is to lay a background for chapter 4 and chapter 5.

Skin Metastases (Locoregional Recurrence)

In breast cancer relapse, skeletal metastases are the most common, followed by visceral metastases (usually liver), locoregional recurrence (skin metastases), and then pulmonary spread (Donegan and Spratt 2002; Fentiman, Mattews, Davison, Mills, and Hayward 2005; Veronesi et al. 1995). The probability of relapse after mastectomy with chest wall lesions is directly related to both tumor size and the extent of axillary lymph node involvement (Early Breast Cancer Trialists Collaborative Group 1995). This paper will focus more on locoregional recurrence as found in the patient presented in the case summary.

Locally advanced breast cancer with satellite nodules in the skin (cutaneous metastases) has a generally poor prognosis (Crowe et al. 1991; Demarec 1951; Fentiman et al. 2005; Gage et al. 1998; Kurtz et al. 1989; Magno, Bignadi, Micheletti, Bardelli, and Pleban 1987; Pawlias, Dockerty, and Ellis 1958; Recht et al. 1999; Whelan, Clark, Roberts, Levine, and Foster 1994). This is usually related to simultaneous distal dissemination that is found in 17%-60% of patients with locoregional recurrence (Chu, Cope, Russo, and Lew 1984; Crowe et al. 1991; Curcio et al. 1997; Recht et al. 1999). Five-year survival of patients with skin metastases is reported at 20% to 40% by Kennedy and Abeloff (1993) and 23% by Tomin and Donegan (1987), while Willner, Kiricuta, and Kolbl (1997) and Willner, Kircutal, Kolbl, and Ftetje (1999) report 14% alive and free of distal dissemination at ten years. Fentiman et al. (2005) state there is a 10% five-year survival and zero survival at ten years in patients with skin recurrence following mastectomy. Bedwinek, Fineberg, and Ocwieza (1991) find an overall five-year survival of 36% and DFS of 13%. Le, Arriagada, Spielman, Guinebretriere, and Richard (2002) give a moderate prognosis with a ten-year survival of 56% and find an increased survival in premenopausal women following systemic treatment, although this does not hold true for postmenopausal women.

Often, little hope is given for long-term survival of patients with locally advanced or recurrent breast cancer (Curcio et al. 1997; Halverson et al. 1992; Pawlias et al. 1958; Willner et al. 1997 1999). This is primarily related to development of distal metastatic disease. Recht et al. (1999) show 55% of over 2000 patients in four randomized trials conducted by the Eastern Cooperative Oncology Group (ECOG) developed recurrent disease, most with distal metastases. Fisher et al. (1991) report likewise. Kennedy and Abeloff (1993) indicate that local recurrence was a grave prognostic indicator and represents a marker for an increased risk of distal dissemination. Irradiation in their group did not improve survival and they emphasize that most had an exceedingly poor outlook.

Chagpar et al. (2003) report a 5% to 40% incidence of chest wall recurrence after mastectomy for breast cancer and relate that this generally forecasts a grim outcome, often with distant metastases and death. They give a 20% survival for ten years in patients with a low to intermediate risk, and 25% metastatic-free survival at ten years in the same group. However, they cite several studies showing that survival after chest wall recurrence is influenced by many factors (Moran and Haffty 2002; Willner et al. 1999). Although they point out that the length of DFI between mastectomy and chest wall recurrence is the *key* prognostic factor, it is felt that low to intermediate risk for overall and distant metastasic-free survival is based on the features of time to recurrence, negative axillary lymph node metastases at the time of mastectomy, and no prior radiotherapy. Patients at high risk (two or more of the characteristics described by Chagpar et al. (2003) show 0% survival at five years. Tomin and Donegan (1987), reporting a 23% survival in five years, associate a better prognosis with negative lymph node metastases and an ER positive tumor This is supported by Fisher, Redmond, Fisher, and Caplan (1988), Haffty et al. (1996), and Maguire, Horwitz, Pearson, and Segaloff (1997).

However, the multivariate factors that are significant have not been consistently defined. Schmoor, Sauerbrei, Bastert, and Schumacher (2000), reporting from the German Breast Cancer Study Group, emphasize that local recurrence increases the risk of developing distal metastases and that factors predicting DFS were negative nodal status, length of DFI, and ER positivity. Pike, Spicer, Dahmdush, and Press (1993) evaluate PR levels and other criteria and note that these factors should be taken into account with future studies and stratification. Janjan, McNeese, Buzdar, Montague, and Oswald (1986) demonstrate that locoregional control and additional chemotherapy increases DFS in these patients. Others find prognosis is best with a single-nodule primary and a disease-free interval of greater than twenty-four months (Bedwinek et al. 1981; Mora, Singletary, Buzdar, and Johnston 1996).

Although most treatment has been aimed at relieving painful and disabling symptoms (Bartus, Schreiber, and Kurtzman 2004), the ability to control chest wall disease may be associated with a more favorable survival (Ames and Balch 1990; Arriagada, Rutqvist, Mattson, Kramar, and Rotstein 1995; Chu et al. 1984; Cokun, Gunel, Yamal, and Altinova 2001; Halverson et al. 1992; Janjan et al. 1986; Kouloulias et al. 2003; Mora et al. 1996; Schwaibold, Fowble, Solin, Schultz, and Goodman 1991). Further studies using DNA cytometry demonstrate that diploid tumors appear to have a better prognosis

(Hedley et al. 1993) and that the S-phase fraction (SPF) may also be a useful finding to indicate a good prognosis. Another characteristic is the growth rate of cutaneous nodules of breast cancer that recur after mastectomy. The average gross doubling time is reported at forty days by Pearlman (1976) with similar findings by Phillipe and Le Gal (1968). This demonstrates a greater growth rate for skin metastases when compared to the primary tumor. Treatment for locoregional recurrence ranges from local control that includes excision and closure, fulguration, photodynamic therapy, radiotherapy to the chest wall (Ames and Balch 1990; Halverson et al. 1992), and adjuvant therapy that may include chemotherapy, immunotherapy and/or hormonal manipulation (Huinik ten Bokkel and van Leeuwenhoek 1999; Kennedy and Abeloff 1993; Recht et al. 1999).

Reviewing basic epidemiology basically emphasizes that carcinoma of the breast continues to be a common disease in white females in the western civilization and has many possible causative factors. Locoregional recurrence (skin metastases), in general, portends a very poor prognosis and serves as a predictor for visceral metastases. Biologic principles support that breast cancer is a systemic disease and locoregional recurrence merely reflects the high risk of distal dissemination. According to the criteria presented, the patient in the case report falls into the category of moderately increased risk for development of distant metastases.

Treatment

In 1891, Halsted published results of radical mastectomy (removal of the breast, pectoralis major and minor muscles, and axillary contents) as treatment for breast cancer with a 6% local recurrence rate (Cameron 1997). The trend in surgery has changed from radical surgery to local control (Spratt and Donegan 2002), and the current philosophy for treatment of breast cancer is to approach this as a systemic disease (Bando 2007; Benda et al. 2004; Chen et al. 2004; Christante et al. 2008; Fabian and Kimler; 2005; Newman and Washington 2003; Steeg and Theodorescu 2008). Some regional variation in the United States is reported (Sariego 2008). The allopathic methods of medical and surgical treatment of breast cancer in the past thirty-five years include surgical extirpation, external beam irradiation, chemotherapy, and hormonal manipulation. Neoadjuvant (preoperative) and adjuvant (concurrent or subsequent to surgical treatment) chemotherapy, as well as hormonal manipulation (considered a strong component), are currently accepted in the present treatment approach to breast cancer (Baum 1998; Charefare et al. 2005; Chen et al. 2004; Elkin et al. 2004; Kamen, Rubin, and Assiner 2000; Lipton et al. 1987; Mouridsen, Rose, Brodie, and Smith 2003; Newman and Sabel 2003; Saphner et al. 1996; Sariego 2008; Wheler 2005).

There are many factors in the treatment of breast cancer that have created a large group of women at risk for therapy-related complications, local breast cancer recurrence, distal metastases and relapse, or the development of a new primary tumor. Despite improvements in diagnosis and treatment of early stage disease, the general aim of therapy in breast cancer is to improve the quality of life and the length of DFS. There still is not a defined treatment that provides complete cure unless it is in cases of early or minimal (small primary) tumors.

Many of the biological mechanisms targeted by chemotherapy suggest a link to a scientific basis for effectiveness of some CAM therapy. These include angiogenesis (Fox, Generali, and Harris 2007) and apoptosis (Gholam, Chebib, Hauteville, Bralet, and Jasmin 2007). Hormone manipulation or modulation by chemical or natural means also plays a significant part in the health of the patient presented. These topics will be discussed in detail in chapter 4 and chapter 5.

CAM Use

There is no question that there is an increasing trend of CAM use for various health conditions in the United States (Astin 1998; Barnes, Powell, McFann, and Nahin 2002; Eisenberg et al. 1998; National Center for Complementary and Alternative Medicine 2004) as well as an increasing popularity throughout the industrialized world (Bouchayer 1990; Fisher and Ward 1994; Goldbeck-Wood et al. 1996; Greger 2001). Eisenberg et al. (1998) point out in a large national survey that the use of CAM in the United States increased from 34% in 1990 to 42% in 1997. This amounts to eighty-three million people admitting to the use of at least one type of alternative therapy and results in up to 10.3 billion dollars in out-of-pocket expenses annually. In another review, Eisenberg et al. (1993) indicate that CAM is not taught widely in medical schools, nor is it generally available in U.S. hospitals. They further state that it is primarily used for chronic rather than life-threatening conditions. Carlston et al. (1999) further discuss presentation of alternative medicine in medical schools. Astin (1998) identifies chiropractic, lifestyle and diet, exercise and movement, and relaxation as the top four categories of CAM use in the United States, although psychological treatment, self-help groups, exercise, and limited dietary changes have always been part of conventional (allopathic) medicine.

Astin (1998) further finds no ethnic or sex differences in usage and reports that patients using CAM do not necessarily have a negative opinion or experience with allopathic medicine. However, 60%-70% of patients do not tell their medical physician that they use CAM. Astin also points out that CAM use may be underreported in the poor and less-educated population. This is supported by observations from Eisenberg et al. (1993) and Drivdahl and Miser (1998). The fact that up to 70% of the respondents who used unconventional therapy did not inform their medical doctor is not surprising and is likely similar to the dishonesty that is seen when illegal drug use is questioned in the medical interview. This may be related to an anticipated negative response from allopathic medical practitioners (Adler and Foskett 1999).

Dissatisfaction with conventional medicine is not a significant predictor of alternative care use (Astin 1998; Eisenberg et al. 2001; Fogel 2006). Most often, individuals report a desire to keep control in their own hands and look at promoting personal health rather than focusing solely on illness (Hough, Dower, and O'Neil 2001). These reports point out that education may increase the likelihood that people will be exposed to various nontraditional forms of health care through their own reading. Use of the internet further adds to self-education about illnesses and information on the variety of treatment available. There currently seems to be more of a challenge to the authority of conventional practitioners and less unquestionable acceptance of the physician's knowledge and expertise (Astin, Marie, Pelletier, Hansen, and Haskell 1998). In Western cultures, middle-class, white females with a college education and a higher economic status appear to be the most open-minded to CAM use (Astin 1998; Eisenberg et al. 1993 1998). As such, evaluation of CAM use in women with breast cancer is complementary.

Despite the argument that there is no scientific basis for CAM, significant background is available showing use in Eastern medicine and the folk medicine of Latin and American Indian cultures (De Pacheco and Hutti 1998; Ortiz, Shields, Clausen, and Clay 2007; Shiang and Li 1971; Spector 2004). It is interesting to note that in the Hispanic theory of disease, ailments are thought to develop as a result of an imbalance between two humors: hot or cold. This is similar to hot/cold and Yin/Yang of Ayurvedic and Chinese medicine (Harwood 1971; Kaptchuk 2000; Lad 2004; Shiang and Li 1971).

Ortiz et al. (2007) present a meta-analysis of CAM use in the Hispanic population. Higher CAM use in this group compared to the general population is based on ethnic beliefs about the part the moon and natural forces play in health (DePacheco and Hutti 1998; McGoldric, Pearce, and Giordano 1996; Pachter 1994; Spector 2004). In addition, some herbal remedies have been introduced by African slaves in Brazil and the Caribbean. Many illnesses in the Hispanic population are managed outside the formal health-care system. It is at the discretion of the care giver, often a mother or other family member, when a decision for "professional help" is required (McGoldric et al. 1996; Ortiz et al. 2007; Pachter 1994; Yoder 1987).

Eisenberg et al. (2001) and others (Lee, Lin, Wrench, Adler, and Eisenberg 2000; MacKenzie, Taylor, and Blum 2003) report on ethnic CAM use as well as CAM use worldwide. Lee et al. (2000) give information on four ethnic groups in San Francisco: Latin, White, Black, and Chinese. These groups all show a high prevalence of use. A telephone interview with 379 patients was performed in their preferred language and more than one-half of these groups state they use alternative methods. Blacks are more likely to use spiritual healing; Chinese, herbal therapy; Latins, dietary therapy and spiritual healing; while White patients follow dietary measures and use physical methods, such as massage and acupuncture. Only 50% of the patients in this group feel free to inform their medical physician of CAM use. Fujiki (1999) demonstrates a significant use of alternative medicine techniques in post-treatment cancer prevention, showing that Japanese patients with Stage I and II breast cancer who consume five or more cups of green tea a day have a lower recurrence and longer disease-free interval. Abdullah, Lau, and Chow (2003) cite a 27.8% usage of CAM in Chinese breast cancer patients in two centers in Hong Kong. This and the report by Lee et al. (2000) further emphasize that middle-aged females with a higher education were more likely to consider CAM use.

CAM use is also widely accepted in Canada (Hoffer 2003). Ohlen, Balneaves, Bottorf, and Brazier (2006) report that in British Columbia the patient's "significant other" plays a major role in decision-making for CAM. Later, several reports will be cited as far as CAM use by breast cancer patients in Canada. Fisher and Ward (1994) report on prevalence of use in various western European countries.

An observation that comes from reviewing these studies is the widespread acceptance and use of CAM. Bonakdar (2006) attempts an evidence-based update. Dunne Boggs and Mittman (2004) emphasize that naturopathic medicine is forging a path very parallel to, albeit some decades later, the development of allopathic medicine over the last century. An admonition to medical practitioners is for an increased awareness that patients using CAM may be at risk for possible interactions with allopathic treatments (Fogel 2006). This will be discussed in the following sections.

CAM Use/ Little Evidence and Risks

Despite the previous reports demonstrating widespread CAM use, there are also a host of reviews available that disagree with the usefulness of CAM (Atwood 2004; Ernst and Cassileth 1998; Trindle, Davis, Phillips, and Eisenberg 2005). A careful appraisal of CAM use is proposed in other papers (Angell and Kassirer 1998; Cassileth 1999; Hoffer 2003; Oppel 2003). In studying the use of alternative health care by a family practice population, Drivdahl and Miser (1998) find that less than one-half of CAM users are satisfied with their alternative care even though there is increasing interest and use by family practitioners (Astin 1998; Barnes et al. 2002; Dunne Boggs and Mittman 2004). Perkin, Pearcy, and Fraser (1994) demonstrate attitudes and opinions of practitioners of allopathic medicine toward alternative medicine. In their editorial, Angell and Kassirer (1998) argue that there cannot be two kinds of medicine: *conventional* and *alternative*. They further point out that the ideology of alternative medicine largely ignores biological mechanisms and that assertions, speculations, and testimonials do not substitute for evidence.

Cost is identified as a negative aspect of CAM use, particularly when discussing nutritional supplements and vitamins from health food stores (Mills, Ernst, Singh, Grass, and Wilson 2003). Eisenberg et al. (1998) address the over ten billion dollars spent annually for supplements, which are rarely covered by conventional health insurance. The report by Mills et al. (2003) draws attention to the heterogeneity of advice provided by natural health food stores to individuals seeking treatments for breast cancer. They consider this group of patients to be vulnerable and promote regulations to protect them from the significant cost, as well as the safety implications, of some products. Additionally, patients might delay or discontinue orthodox treatment at the advice of a CAM practitioner because the discussion of CAM use with allopathic physicians is limited (Adler and Foskett 1999). In many instances, personnel in the stores do not discuss the potential for adverse effects of products or the possibility of drug interactions (Algner 1998; Gotay and Dimitriu 2000; Heldet 1992; Palmer, Haller, McKinney, and Klein-Schwartz 2003; Stoffer, Szpunar, Coleman, and Mellos 1980; U.S. Food and Drug Administration 1993). The use of CAM with cancer will be discussed in detail in the following section.

There is the question of interactions between herbal medicines and prescribed drugs (Boon and Wong 2004; Cassileth and Deng 2004; Izzo and Ernst 2002). Izzo and Ernst (2002) bring up the point that patients believe natural health products can do little harm since they are natural and therefore, less toxic. In fact, the converse may be true since there is no oversight of these products. Recent reports on adverse effects reveal that some "natural" products thought to be safe may, in fact, be harmful (Izzo and Ernst 2002; Cassileth and Deng 2004). In addition, a comprehensive review of herbal supplements has been introduced as a routine part of the preanesthetic history in patients prior to elective surgery, presenting a safety and medicolegal hurdle in patient care (Ang Lee, Moss, and Yuan 2001; Tessier and Bass 2004). Massage therapy and acupuncture are two of the CAM practices most generally accepted by the medical profession (Astin et al. 1998). Ernst and Cassileth (1998) point out that many CAM remedies are based on folklore and have not yet been scrutinized to the scientific rigor that is required for drug therapies. This is also supported in reviews from the United Kingdom (Cassidy 2003; Holmes 2004).

CAM/Breast Cancer

There is significant interest regarding CAM use in cancer. Cheblowski (2003) comments on advised American Cancer Society guidelines for nutrition and exercise for cancer survivors and congratulates the panel members on a careful and objective analysis. He further adds that this group concludes that many dietary regimens and supplements, suggested as an alternative to the standard of care, have little or no evidence to support their use. However, many oncologists and cancer centers now consider CAM as an option in the overall management for their patients (Antman et al. 2001; Cassileth and Deng 2004; Gansler, Kaw, Cramer, and Smith 2008; Richardson, Sanders, Palmer, Greisinger, and Singletary 2000; Weiger et al. 2002). Boon and Wong (2004) provide a good review of the safety and efficacy of herbal use in cancer. Guidelines from an oncology standpoint are presented by Nahin (2002) and White (2002) in two other reports. Lodovico (2000) presents an evidence-based review in the management of the elderly with cancer.

Given the fact that neither massage nor acupuncture involve taking anything orally, they are likely perceived to have fewer potential adverse effects or interactions with conventional cancer treatments than some other CAM therapies (Boon et al. 2000; Patterson et al. 2002). It is pointed out that there are currently no herbs with significant evidence of efficacy as cancer treatment (Boon, Olatunde, and Zick 2007; Weiger et al. 2002). Matsuyama, Reddy, and Smith (2006) indicate that the perspective of the patient who has metastatic cancer is different from that of a well person, and state that these patients are willing to undergo treatments that have a small benefit with major toxicity when choosing chemotherapy near the end of life. This may also reflect the perspective of some patients who choose CAM in the treatment of cancer. Fogel (2006) brings up the point that the effects of CAM usage were more psychological rather than having any clear-cut evidence for their benefit. This is also mentioned by Moschen et al. (2001) as a primary reason for CAM use. Holmes (2004) emphasizes possible adverse effects of CAM use in cancer, and Wells et al. (2007) note that no literature exists on CAM use and symptom control for women with lung cancer. Weiger et al. (2002) give insight on advising patients seeking CAM outside the conventional treatment for cancer.

In a systematic review of studies published between 1995 and 2005, Gerber et al. (2006) identify the objectives of CAM as being very diverse. These include a reduction of therapy-associated toxicity, improvement of cancer-related symptoms, fostering of the immune system, and even direct anti-cancer effects. Gerber et al. (2006) further indicate that some CAM methods may have adverse effects or reduce the efficacy of conventional treatment and conclude that available data on CAM modalities in the treatment of early-stage breast cancer does not support their application. Thangapazham et al. (2006) found no measurable effects on cell growth or gene expression in vitro in patients using homeopathic remedies for cancer. Chustecka (2007) negates the usefulness of shark cartilage.

Jacobson, Rokman, and Kronenberg (2000) review English-language articles published in the biomedical literature from 1980 to 1997 that report results of clinical research on complementary and alternative medical treatments of interest to patients with breast cancer. They conclude that although many studies have encouraging results, none definitely show that a CAM treatment altered disease progression in these patients. Furthermore, they state that if CAM studies are well founded, well designed, and meticulously conducted in their hypotheses with methods and results reported clearly and candidly, then research in this controversial area should achieve credibility both in the scientific community and among advocates of unconventional medicine. Despite these reports, Gansler et al. (2008) point out the increasing frequency of CAM use in cancer patients. The fact that women are high consumers of alternative or complementary therapies (Astin 1998; Eisenberg et al. 1993 1998) would lead to breast cancer patients being particularly prone to purchasing such remedies (Morris, Johnson, Holmer, and Walts 2000).

In a large survey of cancer survivors across the United States, more than one-half of these patients report using CAM (Gansler et al. 2008). Primary modalities are prayer in 61%, relaxation in 44%, faith/spiritual healing in 42%, nutritional supplements/vitamins in 40%, and meditation in 15%. Females are more likely to use CAM than men and include younger age groups and white females with higher education levels and income. This may indicate the ability to afford CAM modalities that are not covered by health insurance as well as the interest to investigate and provide self-education on the availability of various modalities. Females reported in this survey present with a more advanced stage of breast or ovarian carcinoma at diagnosis. Patterson et al. (2002) report a 70% use of CAM in patients with cancer, most often dietary supplements. They state that patients using CAM tend to have a better income, which may be related to the cost involved with CAM that is not covered by health insurance.

Several large studies are available as far as CAM use and breast cancer. Data from multiethnic samples of early breast cancer patients is available (Alferi, Antoni, Ironson, Kilbourn, and Carver 2001; Ernst and Cassileth 1998; Lee et al. 2000; Lins, Rensch, Adler, and Eisenberg 2000). Boon et al. (2007) provide survey results among breast cancer patients over two time periods: 1998 and 2005. There is an increase in CAM use during these time periods from 67% to 82%. There is also a decrease in radical surgery and the utilization of more chemotherapy and hormonal treatment in the second group (2005). This report refers to several other large studies, including a prior one by Boon et al. (2000), demonstrating the prevalence of CAM use ranging from 16.5 to 84% (Balneaves, Bottorf, and Hislop 2006; Burstein, Gelver, Guadagnolie, and Weeks 1999; Crocetti et al. 1998; Moschen et al. 2001; Rees et al. 2000). According to Boon et al. (2000), less than 50% of patients with breast cancer inform their medical physician of CAM use, and the decision to use CAM is seen in younger, better—educated females with higher income. The apparent rationale for CAM was to take a more active role in their self-care. Boon et al. (2000 2007) question if CAM use may be overestimated somewhat because of the type of survey and response rate, but Adler and Foskett (1999) state that in the United States the incidence of CAM use may actually be underestimated. This is based on the fear of telling the allopathic physician about CAM in anticipation of a negative response. In another paper, Adler (1999) cites that younger women were more likely to consider CAM use, with a danger in delay of conventional treatment. The American Cancer Society provides its guidelines for nutrition and exercise in cancer patients and mentions that increased folic acid and antioxidant intake may counteract some effects of chemotherapy (2003). Morris et al. (2000) present a comparison between CAM use in breast cancer versus other primary sites, while Tagliaferri, Cohen, and Tripathy (2001) show a fairly common pattern of CAM use in early-stage breast cancer. Kaegl (1998) gives information on the Canadian experience with unconventional therapies for cancer, again showing frequent use. Cassidy (2003) and Holmes (2004) present a British view with similar findings.

VandeCreek, Rogers, and Lester (1999) find that breast cancer outpatients involved in conventional treatment are more likely to use a wide range of alternative treatments than the general public. Frequent modalities are exercise and spiritual healing. Nahleh and Tabbara (2003) review a large number of various other studies reporting a range of 48%-70% CAM use in breast cancer patients in the U.S. population. Reasons given in these studies for CAM are to boost the immune system, improve the quality of life, prevent recurrence of the cancer, provide control over their own treatment decisions, treat the breast cancer itself, and ameliorate the side effects of conventional treatment. A survey by Lengacher et al. (2006) finds that the use of CAM is thought to relieve physical and psychological stress in patients with breast cancer. These patients report gaining control over their treatment. Most of them have more than a high school education. Also, patients who have undergone chemotherapy are more likely to use CAM for symptom control (Wells et al. 2007).

DiGianni, Garber, and Winer (2002) indicate that, apart from psychosocial interventions, there is little scientific evidence that exists regarding the efficacy of CAM use for breast cancer patients. Among women with newly diagnosed, early-stage breast cancer who have been treated with standard therapies, initiation of alternative medicine appears to be a marker of greater psychosocial distress and a worse quality of life (Burstein et al. 1999). In this review, the mental health scores of these women are worse after three months and associated with depression, fear of recurrence of the cancer, lower scores for mental health and sexual satisfaction, and they tend to have more physical symptoms as well as symptoms of greater intensity. Sered and Agigiani (2008) present this in terms of "holistic sickening" where patients tend to speak about breast cancer as a symptom of problems that exceed the cancer itself, at times suggesting that women themselves are responsible to some extent for their own breast cancer. Siegel (1986) explores this further with examples that the development of cancer in some cases seems to provide an escape from an irresolvable situation.

Damkier, Paludan-Muller, and Knoop (2007) present Danish patients with breast cancer and one-third report using CAM in their treatment program. Primary reasons given for CAM use were to increase quality of life and alleviate symptoms. van der Weg and Streulie (2003) give information on oncology outpatients in rural Switzerland. 50% of the group interviewed suffers from breast cancer and their motivation for CAM use is not based on distrust. Instead, with a goal of maintaining hope, they prefer to take an active role in self-care. In this study, 79% of patients discuss CAM use with their medical doctor. Feedback, in general, is that medical physicians in Switzerland encourage CAM use.

There is a prevalent use of CAM with cancer, and in particular, breast cancer. The purpose of this information is not only to demonstrate the increased use of CAM in women with breast cancer, but to provide a background to explore specific CAM modalities used in the case presentation. It also shows the importance of seeking information about CAM use from patients. It may be difficult for the allopathic practitioner to make recommendations about CAM, especially in conjunction with chemotherapy, radiotherapy, and hormone treatments, due to lack of concrete studies on specific CAM use. This data should encourage well-organized research into these areas, as well as promote allopathic practitioners to become better informed about what modalities patients may be considering.

Purpose of the Study

Although there has been some improvement in survival rate due to earlier diagnosis of breast cancer, patients with metastases are reported in the literature with DFI and DFS as goals in treatment. However, the use of the term "cure" is not used. Patients with skin metastases (locoregional recurrence) have a particularly poor prognosis. The trend of increasing CAM use is widely supported in the literature, including large groups of females with breast cancer. A focus on specific CAM methods used by the patient presented will lay a foundation for areas to be discussed.

Looking at the epidemiology, risk factors, and biological principles involved with breast cancer (Merlot, Pepper, Reid, and Maley 2007), certain aspects will be analyzed in depth. Antioxidant use (vitamin C and green tea) is a specific area to be developed. Areas targeted by chemotherapy, such as angiogenesis (Baidas et al. 2000; Fox et al. 2007) and apoptosis of cancer cells (Gholam et al. 2007; Harley 2008; Lewis, Osipo, Meeke, and Jordan 2005), suggest mechanisms for effectiveness of CAM use. In addition, IGF may be an important area (Yu and Berkel 1999).

Hormonal manipulation is currently a significant area found to be beneficial in the treatment of breast cancer. There are many environmental, including dietary, factors that may naturally affect hormone levels (Jensen 2005; Sicat and Brokaw 2004). The use of soy will be covered, and its place in natural hormone modulation can provide one of the strongest supports for a scientific basis for CAM use in the case presented.

A more difficult area to develop is spiritual healing, which may be related to energy fields, but also plays a part in the effect of stress on the hormonal axis and IGF. The importance for the particular patient presented pertains to the major role spirituality plays in her health.

Review of evidence-based medicine (EBM) points out the weakness of many "scientific" studies and also ignores observation and experience as a basis for CAM (Glickman-Simon 2005). A plea will be made for members of the scientific community to consider allopathic as well as CAM modalities in the treatment of breast cancer.

Significance of the Study

The allopathic approach to breast cancer in the past has focused on the part affected. This is supported by the long-standing use of the modified or radical mastectomy. However, there is now widespread acceptance that breast cancer needs to be treated as a systemic disease. Adjuvant chemotherapy and/or hormone manipulation have been developed as a major part of the treatment regimen. The biologic principles of these treatments can be linked to some of the mechanisms of CAM. This argument can be based on current biological factors implicated in the development of breast cancer, as well as biologic mechanisms targeted by chemotherapy. Natural hormone balance can also be linked to regulation of hormonal levels using diet and nutrition.

One of the main arguments against the use of CAM has been the lack of evidence-based studies. There are many weaknesses of EBM pointed out in the allopathic literature (Loewy 2007). In addition, the scientific principles of "curiosity, observation, and experience" support an open-minded approach to consider CAM in the overall treatment regimen. Although it is noted that there is an increased need for further studies of alternative methods and their place in treatment, it is difficult to provide evidence-based studies for their support. However, the presence of multiple uncontrollable variables can also be used in the criticism of conclusions of current evidence-based medicine.

Observations from this interesting case as well as linkage to scientific and theoretical literature will, hopefully, increase awareness for the benefits of CAM in the treatment of breast cancer. The same thought process could be expanded to the treatment of other cancers and chronic diseases. With observation of the frequent use of CAM by patients, third-party payers should consider implementation of some of these methods, not only to improve the health of the population but also as a cost-effective measure in treating cancer and other chronic diseases.

Research Question

What role does CAM play in the treatment of breast cancer?

It is well documented that there is increasing acceptance and use of CAM. To determine the clinical significance, the researcher can find studies supporting beneficial outcomes and also review biologic mechanisms involved in the etiology of breast cancer as well as pathways targeted by current chemotherapy. Hormonal manipulation can also support a scientific basis for some CAM methods. Vitamin C as an antioxidant and soy products for natural hormone balance are two areas that are specifically studied since these are primary methods used by the patient presented.

Can support for a scientific basis of CAM be made?

Reviewing biological pathways gives insight to potential mechanisms for the effectiveness of CAM. Antioxidant use and hormone modulation are two specific areas. The weaknesses resulting from uncontrollable variables in evidence-based or case-controlled studies present an obstacle in scientific studies supporting CAM. The basic clinician/student uses curiosity and observation to remain open-minded when dealing with patients and disease. This represents a strong point in favor of learning by experience, as well as supporting the scientific method. Biologic feasibility of CAM can be observed, and hopefully, further scientific support for its use can be developed.

Scope, Delimitations, and Limitations

Significant literature exists that supports the increasing use and acceptance of CAM. No evidence-based studies or case-controlled clinical trials are available, but there are several reviews that provide meta-analysis of CAM use in Western society. Abundant literature is available supporting the use of CAM in a specific population (middle-aged women with breast cancer). These reviews include not only populations from various regions in the United States, but also Europe and Southeast Asia.

Biological and physiological pathways, not only in the development of breast cancer but also those targeted in treatment by current chemotherapy, are reviewed and suggest a scientific basis for certain CAM methods. Research has defined some biological mechanisms and pathways. This includes studies on vitamin C and other antioxidants that affect DNA repair and apoptosis. An interesting aspect is the IGF pathway. However, such understanding on a cellular or molecular level is limited (Gholam et al. 2007) and represents one of the most significant limitations (Bigelow and Cardelli 2006). Amounts of vitamin C and green tea are not well controlled in the literature reviewed. There is always the question that results of animal studies are not completely transferable to humans.

A strong point involves the use of diet and nutritional supplements to bolster normal physiologic cell repair and healing. In addition, natural hormone regulation using nutrition fits with the well-accepted hormonal treatment of breast cancer. On the cellular level, the mechanics of hormone regulation is incompletely understood and quite complex. In addition, there is no consistent control of nutritional methods, such as type of soy products, processing, and amount; or the amount of fresh fruit and vegetable intake. Certain other factors, such as lifestyle and premenopausal exposure to environmental toxins are difficult to control and compare between populations. Differences in genetics and metabolism between populations pose another variable. Many times, enough variables are present to make it difficult to compare population-based studies and find a definite basis for an individual method.

The patient presented has a very strong spirituality. Stress and psychological factors affecting health have no concrete system for evaluation. Possible mechanisms include effects on the hormonal axis and IGF. Energy fields (Bruyere 1987) are described in the realm of CAM and may present a potential link here, but obviously, can only be presented in an abstract and hypothetical sense.

EBM is the current trend to accept treatment methods in modern health care (Freedman 1987; Lie 2006). No case-controlled studies or comparison clinical trials are available to support CAM. Arguments are found in the allopathic literature which criticize methods and point out weaknesses in the development of evidence-based medicine (Peterson, Woodard, Urech, Daw, and Sookanan 2006; Ramana 2008; Sa Couta 2003). Halsted and Osler (Aequanimitas; Cameron 1997; Lyons and Petrucelli 1978; Halsted and Osler biographies) both made significant contributions in the development of the modern practice of allopathic medicine and surgery. Halsted and Osler emphasize the characteristics of curiosity and observation in the role of the clinician/scientist. If continued observations support CAM in the treatment of breast cancer, this can be expanded to the current practice of medicine with increased awareness of the usefulness of CAM with other diseases or conditions.

Definition of Terms

The term *patient*, instead of *client*, will be used since the woman interviewed is part of an allopathic medical/surgical practice. General, acceptable medical terminology will be used, with the exception of lay terms as utilized during the patient interview. Scientific terminology will also be used pertaining to the literature review. This includes biological and experimental terminology, such as reactive oxygen species (ROS) and catechol-O-methyltransferase (COMT). In addition, ER (estrogen receptor), PR (progesterone receptor), and biological terms such as *epidermal growth factor* (EGF), *insulin-like growth factor* (IGF-1), and other terms will be identified as they occur throughout the paper. Common biological terms, such as *DNA* and accepted scientific units of measurement, will not be specifically identified.

CAM (complementary and alternative methods) and *EBM* (evidence-based medicine) will be abbreviations commonly used throughout the paper. Others may be cited in the text one time, but otherwise will be listed in the abbreviation list in the table of contents.

There are multiple research groups that will be identified, such as National Surgical Adjuvant Breast and Bowel Project (NSABP), as referenced in the literature.

Summary

This paper reviews the course of a woman diagnosed with breast cancer sixteen years ago, who subsequently developed skin metastases (locoregional recurrence) within a year of her mastectomy. Refusing conventional treatment (radiotherapy, chemotherapy, or hormonal manipulation), she follows a strict diet and uses other types of CAM. She did not receive any local treatment for the skin metastases, and photographs (see appendix A) demonstrate progression and regression of these lesions through her post-diagnosis course. The patient uses the changes in these skin lesions as a guideline to alter her personal regimen. She has had a remarkable ability to cope with her disease and maintains a high quality of life with no systemic metastases noted over sixteen years.

A review of the strong points of her lifestyle changes and personal use of diet and nutritional supplements raises speculation on a possible scientific basis for these methods. Attention will be paid to antioxidant use since she uses green tea and high doses of vitamin C. In addition, natural hormonal manipulation may be a strong point of her cancer management. Spirituality is another aspect of her lifestyle that will be analyzed.

Biology of breast cancer, biological pathways targeted by chemotherapy, and basic physiology in diet and nutritional supplements provide support for the scientific basis for some CAM. Natural hormone modulation using diet and soy, along with the use of high doses of vitamin C and green tea as antioxidants are strong points of the case presented. Using a review of current biological pathways described in the literature, an attempt will be made to link scientific and theoretical literature that may support CAM use in the treatment of breast cancer.

Although there are criticisms to the lack of EBM for CAM use, some allopathic literature provides arguments against the current methods used to develop guidelines for EBM (Gupta 2003). In addition, the scientific principles of curiosity, observation, and experience cannot be ignored and provide support for an open-minded approach to CAM in the current practice of medicine (Fitzgerald 1999).

Chapter Two

Review of Related Literature and Research

Introduction

After the initial patient interview, a descriptive review of the current literature was performed to present contemporary breast cancer statistics. Included in this review is a summary of available literature on locoregional recurrence with an emphasis on its significance as an indicator for distant metastases and poor prognosis. Current, accepted treatment for breast cancer is outlined and includes a trend toward minimal surgery along with the use of adjuvant chemotherapy and hormonal manipulation. Various risk factors are included to introduce possible links to a scientific basis for CAM. The review introduces the possible relationship of hormone modulation using diet and soy. Nutrition with fruits and vegetables, soy, nutritional supplements, and vitamins are evaluated with a possible relationship to breast cancer. An emphasis on vitamin C as an antioxidant will be developed since high doses are one of the principle methods used in the patient presented.

Next, a general review of CAM demonstrates increased worldwide acceptance and use, including North America. Many meta-analyses are available in this area and the most commonly used CAM modalities are presented. Middle-class white females with a college education are identified as the most frequent North American population group for CAM usage. Many reports are seen in favor as well as many against CAM. The use of CAM by cancer patients is selectively reviewed, then narrowed to CAM use in women with breast cancer.

Research Literature Review

The performance of a descriptive literature review began with current allopathic medical and surgical textbooks and journals to establish a background of current breast cancer epidemiologic statistics and accepted treatments. Known and presumed risk factors for development of breast cancer were reviewed. These were also used to introduce some biological and physiological pathways involved in the development (etiology) and treatment of breast cancer. Major sources of information were textbooks on breast cancer (Spratt and Donegan 2002; Schwartz 2005), as well as oncology textbooks (DeVita, Hellman, and Rosenberg 2003). Environmental and nutritional factors related to the hormonal axis were also reviewed (Williams 2003). In addition, journal references from chapters in the textbooks were used to assist in a general literature search. Textbooks on various aspects of natural health were also reviewed (Hough 2001; Kirchfield and Boyle 1994; Page 2002; Williams 2003). A list of lay sources used by the patient in the case study is included at the end of the case presentation.

The next part of the literature review involved the Internet. This began with the Boolean operators of "breast cancer and CAM" and led to recovery of reports of use in the United States as well as worldwide, and was further subdivided into use by specific populations. Literature supporting CAM use was encountered and balanced with reports questioning its effectiveness. An attempt was made to keep the literature search current by focusing on the past ten years. Information was then gathered for CAM use in cancer, and subsequently narrowed to CAM in females with breast cancer.

Further Internet searches were performed for the various subtopics that developed as information was collected. Again, use in the United States as well as worldwide was reviewed and included clinical, as well as experimental studies. Specific biological pathways targeted by current chemotherapy were studied and include angiogenesis, apoptosis, alterations in DNA, and DNA mutations. Specific CAM use and its potential effect on these pathways were explored. Animal studies were avoided with isolated exceptions since it is difficult to transfer this information to humans.

Hormonal manipulation is a widely accepted modality in the treatment of breast cancer. Articles were encountered covering the controversy regarding hormone use in adolescence, premenopausal, and postmenopausal females, and the relationship to breast cancer. Some evidence was found that included estrogen as a genotoxic agent. The use of isoflavones as a phytoestrogen and its possible effect on the hormonal axis was evaluated, noting the complexity of hormonal pathways related to estrogen as well as other hormones. This led to the hormonal effect on glucose metabolism and IGF, with reviews on the part these play in carcinogenesis, as well as the metabolic syndrome. Key in the progression of cancer is underlying inflammation, with this process affected by antioxidants, as well as modulation of the hormone axis, and will be developed in chapter 4 and chapter 5.

The importance of isoflavones in hormonal pathways was evaluated, not only in clinical studies, but also with regard to cell biology. Controversial literature was found both in support and against the part that soy plays in prevention and treatment of breast cancer. An important factor seen in the literature search was the lack of accurate measurement of the amount, as well as the particular type of isoflavone used, and the genetic difference affecting metabolism found in populations. This presents a particularly difficult control measure when attempting to compare studies and results. In addition to soy, red clover, which also contains isoflavones, was used by the patient presented.

Since diet/nutrition support a holistic approach using the organism's natural biological mechanisms for repair and immune function, the literature was pared to focus on two important aspects in this particular patient's presentation. These include antioxidants (vitamin C and green tea) and other nutritional factors, including soy, which could potentially affect her hormonal status. Natural aspects of diet and nutrition, particularly consumption of fresh fruits and vegetables, were reviewed in comparison to nutritional supplements. Whole foods or natural sources contain molecularly similar compounds which may work synergistically with the targeted agent (such as vitamin C) with improved benefit.

Abundant literature regarding vitamin C metabolism and use was encountered, and information from authors with several publications was gathered since they serve as potential experts in this field. Literature was also found related to vitamin C and IGF, which will be covered in chapter 4 and chapter 5. As far as clinical treatment of cancer, controversial articles, both in support and against the use of vitamin C, were reviewed. In addition, it was found that the dose and route of administration of vitamin C (oral versus intravenous) present an interesting aspect that adds to the controversy to the use of vitamin C in cancer treatment. The patient in the case study uses a regimen with high doses of vitamin C.

Finally, no specific case-controlled studies were found that definitely prove CAM is beneficial in the treatment of cancer. This is narrowed to CAM use and its effectiveness in the treatment of breast cancer. With many decisions for current practice emanating from evidence-based medicine (EBM), which form the basis of current standard of care decisions in modern medicine, allopathic literature was found criticizing the methods used to formulate these evidence-based principles. In addition, uncontrollable variables present an obstacle in many studies. There may also be a conflict of interest between patients, third-party payers, and health-care organizations. Literature was reviewed from allopathic pioneers (Halsted and Osler biographies) who emphasized the basic qualities of "curiosity, observation, and experience" in the student/scientist/clinician. Several arguments in allopathic literature were found encouraging the study of CAM in the future.

The patient presented has a very strong spiritual life. Supporting the scientific basis of spirituality is quite abstract and complicated. Reviews in this area involved theoretical and observational textbooks (Hampshire 1989; Love 200; Siegel 1986).

Various allopathic professionals were used for their insight on current practice and options for breast cancer treatment. These include a general oncologist, a general surgeon, a surgeon who is a breast specialist, an oncologist specializing in the treatment of breast cancer, and a gynecologic oncologist who has a special interest in natural medicine. A standard questionnaire was developed (see appendix B) to gain feedback from their personal experience in the use of CAM by their patients. These professionals were also used to help validate some of the articles reviewed in the literature search with specific attention to areas addressed in this research paper. In addition, they were able to guide the search to other sources. One of the practitioners has personal experience with the use of vitamin C in cancer patients.

Contemporary Theoretical Perspectives

Many etiologies have been presented as far as causal or aggravating factors in the development of breast cancer. Only a small proportion of females with breast cancer have an underlying genetic tendency. Hormonal factors in the adolescent, premenopausal, and postmenopausal groups have been implicated. Other environmental factors, such as smoking and radiation exposure, have been shown to be significant. Nutritional aspects are felt to be important, but despite abundant literature in this area, specific data is lacking. Stress has also been identified as an aggravating factor with possible effects on the hormonal axis.

The treatment of breast cancer is currently expressed in terms of disease-free interval (DFI) and disease-free survival (DFS) rather than complete cure. Locoregional recurrence (skin metastases) is associated with a very poor prognosis and, in general, portends the development of visceral or systemic metastases. The trend in surgery is for minimal surgery accompanied by local irradiation. The current approach to treatment is consideration of breast cancer as a systemic disease with adjuvant chemotherapy and hormonal manipulation commonly used in addition to the initial surgical treatment and irradiation.

There is increasing acceptance and widespread use of CAM demonstrated, not only worldwide, but in North America. Upper middle class, well-educated, white females appear to be among those who more widely accept and use CAM. As such, CAM use in patients with breast cancer is increasing. There has been no specific CAM method identified as a "magic bullet." Some methods, such as shark cartilage, have been shown to be ineffective.

The oncology literature is rich in studies of many of the biological pathways that have been identified in the development of cancer, as well as breast cancer specifically. Information about mechanisms on a cellular basis can be found. These include angiogenesis, apoptosis, and DNA mutations, all of which have been targeted by specific chemotherapy. General dietary methods, such as increased vegetable and fruit intake, may affect antioxidant levels, which then interact through the mechanisms of angiogenesis and apoptosis on a cellular level. Certain nutritional supplements may also affect DNA metabolism and mutations.

Vitamin C administration in the prevention or treatment of cancer is controversial. However, abundant literature is available with studies supporting and just as many refuting the importance of vitamin C. Much of this relates to serum levels achieved by oral or intravenous dosing. There is clear evidence of its effect as an antioxidant, but interesting information was found regarding vitamin C, glucose metabolism, and IGF. The patient presented uses high doses of vitamin C and this area will be explored in detail.

Chemical hormonal manipulation is also a strong point in current breast cancer treatment. Endogenous or exogenous hormones may play a part in cell proliferation as it relates to breast cancer development. Natural hormonal manipulation, by use of soy products (isoflavones) and other dietary measures, can be supported in the current literature. The hormone axis is complex, and effects probably include HGH (human growth hormone) and IGF.

An attempt is made by modern allopathic medicine to present evidence as far as case-controlled studies and meta-analysis, and then formulate these into EBM. Despite this, there are many variables present that are difficult to control, such as comparison of population-based studies, where genetic differences in metabolism and personal lifestyles may exist. Not only does this threaten external validity for implementation of evidence-based studies to general medical practice, but is also a consistent flaw in studies that attempt to provide supporting evidence for or against CAM.

Relationship of Current Literature to Present Study

Although there is much yet unknown at the cellular and molecular level regarding breast cancer development and mechanisms currently used in its treatment, certain biological pathways can be linked to support why some CAM methods are useful in the treatment of breast cancer. Breast cancer is currently approached as a systemic disease with a trend of less aggressive local treatment (less aggressive surgery). This supports a holistic approach using general diet and nutritional principles to promote host defense mechanisms in the treatment of breast cancer. Antioxidant use, which is promoted in many chronic and degenerative diseases, as well as those that evolve from general inflammation, such as atherosclerosis and arthritis, can be boosted by diet changes and nutritional supplements. In addition, current mechanisms targeted by chemotherapy, such as angiogenesis, apoptosis, and DNA mutations, can also be supported by antioxidants and supplements, as well as other aspects of general nutrition.

Hormonal manipulation is a mainstay of current breast cancer treatment. However, hormonal interrelationships are quite complex. Attention has been focused on the use of isoflavones (soy products) as phytoestrogens that provides natural hormone protection. The explanation may very well be more complicated, likely involving other hormones, such as IGF and HGH. It is very difficult to isolate one single factor when these interrelationships are so complex. Natural hormonal manipulation appears to be a major factor in the case of the patient presented.

This patient also has a very strong spirituality. It is quite difficult to find any evidence-based studies in support of spirituality. Ayurvedic and Chinese medicine rely on energy fields for the health of the organism as a whole. Stress has also been shown to play a part in general health and may be related to the immune system and the effect of stress on the hormone axis. In the patient presented, regression and progression of her skin lesions may sometimes be explained on this basis alone. There is no solid research available in this area, but observation and experience should not be ignored

Although modern medicine would like to base treatment protocols on EBM, there are certainly many arguments, both pro and con. Control over one modality is attempted in evidence-based medicine or case-controlled studies, but there are still many variables when dealing with the complex human organism. These include genetics (metabolism of drugs or utilization of nutritional regimens), environmental factors, such as diet or radiation exposure, smoking, stress, and even the non-uniform control of substances used (such as processing, concentrations, or types of soy products). Subsequently, it is difficult to find solid studies to definitely support or condemn the use of CAM. Observation supports a biologic plausibility of CAM in women with breast cancer.

Summary

The current allopathic approach to breast cancer as a systemic disease supports holistic principles. There is no question of the increasing acceptance and use of CAM, not only worldwide, but also in North America. CAM encompasses a large area and variety of modalities. As such, it is difficult to focus on any specific CAM method or support any particular method as a "magic bullet." CAM use may be a reflection of an attitude encouraging general lifestyle changes. No definite scientific studies are available proving the effectiveness of CAM. However, if patients did not feel a benefit, there would not be increased use demonstrated in the world literature.

Reviewing biological mechanisms in the development of cancer, chronic inflammation, also seen in other degenerative and chronic diseases, plays a part. In addition, environmental toxins and conditions, such as diet and nutrition, can be seen in the background of cancer. Scientific support for CAM methods is suggested by focusing on some of these biological mechanisms on a cellular level. Antioxidants, for example, are used for conditions with chronic inflammation.

The primary barrier to critiquing the literature reviewed in this study is that there are no case-controlled studies or meta-analytic reviews available which definitely prove the effectiveness of CAM. Although there are studies available attempting to demonstrate the benefit of a single agent or method of CAM, usually there were a combination of factors or variables that make it very difficult to identify the effect of a single agent. For example, review of studies of vitamin C show variance in the dose and the methods of administration (oral versus parenteral).

The use of isoflavones (soy products) may fit into the pathway of hormone manipulation. However, consistent flaws found in research studies include genetic differences in populations that may affect metabolism, the type of soy consumed (processing), and inconsistencies in dose or amount ingested. This results in many uncontrolled variables. There is no FDA (United States Food and Drug Administration) regulation of soy or nutritional products.

Hormonal manipulation is a commonly accepted modality in the current allopathic treatment of breast cancer. The hormone axis is quite complicated and not completely explained in the current literature. Furthermore, hormone interrelationships may involve mechanisms which include glucose levels, IGF, and HGH. Studies are available that demonstrate estrogen by itself can be a genotoxic agent. The use of isoflavones (soy products) and other dietary measures may affect natural hormone modulation and was explored in clinical as well as research literature.

More detail will be focused on specific CAM methods used by the patient presented. These include vitamin C, linking its role as an antioxidant and known biological pathways. In explaining some of the controversy of vitamin C use in cancer, dose, and route of administration (oral versus parenteral) was explored. In addition, glucose metabolism and the role of IGF and HGH are suggested as a major pathway for CAM use in cancer treatment, and information is available on the effect of vitamin C in these areas.

Spirituality, stress, and energy fields are more complex with no black-and-white evidence to support this as an effective CAM method. Spirituality is an aspect that is very difficult to measure even though it has been demonstrated that stress itself can alter hormone levels. However, the patient presented has a very strong spirituality and objective progression and regression of the skin metastases can be directly correlated to stress levels and her spirituality. It will be difficult to form any concrete conclusions in this area, but observations of the patient's clinical response will be emphasized.

Additional concerns in general involve the difficulty in controlling all aspects of an individual's lifestyle and environment. Reported cases of spontaneous tumor regression make it sometimes difficult to provide a biologically plausible explanation. Another unknown is the patient's innate immune system. Other concerns involve drawing conclusions from individual case studies. The National Cancer Institute has a "best case series" that attempts to present case studies. These do not present any definite useful conclusions but provide thought for further exploration in these areas. Finally, the complex interrelationship of the hormone system is strongly emphasized since it presents a barrier in drawing conclusions based on one particular hormone or its manipulation.

A final concern has to do with forming clinical guidelines based on EBM. Even in the allopathic literature, arguments are made regarding the inaccuracy involved in case-controlled studies, as mentioned in the preceding paragraphs. The scientific principles of "curiosity, observation, and experience" encourage continued exploration of CAM use in breast cancer.

The widespread patient acceptance and use of CAM should lead to increasing physician awareness and open-mindedness for the potential usefulness of CAM in the treatment, not only of cancer, but also other chronic diseases. Future studies that are designed should take into account the holistic approach and realize that no specific modality can be used as a "magic bullet." Finally, consideration by third-party payers for the acceptance of CAM coverage in patients may be a measure to improve overall health and help control health-care costs.

Chapter Three

Design of the Study

Introduction

The case study was developed during an office-based interview that included a review of the chart in the patient's presence accompanied by a narration of the history in her own words. Interval photographs of the chest wall and mastectomy site showing progression and regression of the skin metastases are enclosed (see appendix A). A theoretical study was chosen since there are no clinical trials or evidence-based studies available for the research topic chosen and included a descriptive literature review. The initial review utilized allopathic textbooks and journals, which included surgical and oncology texts for a general review of breast cancer and its current treatment. This was then narrowed to literature specifically related to locoregional recurrence (skin metastases). The review started with texts, moved to references cited in the texts, and then an Internet search was initiated. The general review looked at epidemiology and factors implicated in the development of breast cancer. This was narrowed to cellular biology and physiology associated with these factors, and then focused on biological mechanisms targeted by chemotherapy in an attempt to identify a link with CAM.

The initial Internet search started with Medscape.com using the Boolean operators "breast cancer and CAM." Articles were reviewed to see if there were any ethnic or regional differences worldwide, and then focused on North America. Although attempts were made to limit literature to the past ten years, some review articles compared population groups outside this time period. In addition, some of the basic background information regarding skin metastases and breast cancer (locoregional recurrence) were outside the ten-year time period. Meta-analyses were quite helpful in developing a broad base of information regarding CAM use.

The review then focused on specific aspects of CAM. Since the patient presented used high doses of vitamin C, green tea, and soy products, the search was concentrated and systematically performed in these areas. This also included a general review of nutritional and detoxification textbooks, and nutritional articles from the internet. In addition, biological mechanisms of angiogenesis and apoptosis were reviewed, in an attempt to discover a possible link with the aforementioned pathways, since these are areas targeted by chemotherapy. The hormone review was a little more difficult because the interrelationship between hormones is quite complex, but this is an important aspect since hormonal manipulation plays a major role in the current approach to treatment for breast cancer.

The search generally included a variety of worldwide clinical and research journals. However, when pertinent information was found, lay literature and news articles were also reviewed. In addition, the initial reference sources used by the patient interviewed led to several lay sources dealing with CAM (see case presentation). Natural medicine textbooks were utilized, attempting to link natural methods with scientific principles by comparing mechanisms outlined in the scientific literature (Hough et al. 2001; Kirchfield and Boyle 1994; Page 2002; Williams 2003). Most of the links were related to nutritional pathways, and included a focus on antioxidants (vitamin C) and isoflavones (soy).

The patient interviewed has a very strong spirituality, and books she uses include Love (2000) and Siegel (1986). These sources could also be used to link spirituality with energy fields (Bruyere 1989), although this remains somewhat abstract since there is no concrete scientific research literature related to spirituality.

The personal interviews with allopathic professionals were initiated using a questionnaire (see appendix B). Several specialties were chosen so that both medical and surgical aspects could be reviewed. Besides asking the practitioners regarding their own personal experience with patients' use of CAM, feedback was also received regarding the literature and references used in this study. In addition, one of the professionals has experience with vitamin C in the treatment of cancer.

Methodology

The most recent editions of allopathic textbooks for a general review of epidemiology, biology, and pathophysiology involved in breast cancer were used to present the most up-to-date statistics as well as a scientific background in these areas (DeVita et al. 2003; Spratt and Donegan 2003; Schwartz 2005). Recent editions of nutritional and detoxification textbooks were also reviewed (Haas and Levin 2002; Page 2002). All of these are standard, basic, well respected, and widely used sources.

The practical screen for the Internet review started with the Boolean operators, as mentioned. Subsections included operators of the specific CAM used by the patient interviewed. Baseline information included the following:

a) The study had to have an English equivalent, although articles from throughout the world were reviewed to prevent a North American prejudice.

b) Worldwide review allowed collection of information from various ethnic groups and populations.

c) Information found in lay literature, periodicals, and newspapers was also screened. This included references presented by the patient interviewed (see case presentation).

d) Although articles in the last ten years were preferred, older articles were accepted when they presented statistical or other information pertinent to this study.

e) There are no case-controlled studies of CAM and the majority of the articles were retrospective in nature. Large review series (meta-analyses) were helpful, and articles were found that compared CAM use in the same population groups over two separate time periods.

f) Scientific literature for up-to-date information on biological pathways was reviewed. This included literature related to breast cancer as well as specific areas, such as vitamin C, soy, angiogenesis, apoptosis, and IGF. Animal studies were not emphasized since this presents another variable when attempting to establish a scientific link with CAM.

g) The relationship of hormones and hormone manipulation in breast cancer was reviewed in texts as well as scientific periodicals.

h) When several articles by the same author on a specific topic were encountered, these served to identify potential experts in the field.

a.) A standard questionnaire was used to perform the personal interviews (see appendix B) and was expanded during the interview depending on the responses and the experience level of the practitioner determined during the interview. These professional contacts were also used as content experts for review of the information collected in this study.

When the literature reviewed was observational rather than experimental, the quality screen was a little more complicated. However, support for a scientific basis for biological mechanisms and physiology was based on experimental studies and observation. Positive information and pertinent negative findings were reviewed. The quality screen could also be affected by internal validity, which will be mentioned in the subsequent paragraph. No case-controlled studies could be found comparing CAM with traditional allopathic treatment. A scientific basis for some CAM methods was suggested by linking biological mechanisms in CAM with those described in the allopathic literature for mechanisms targeted by chemotherapy. Although the hormonal axis is complicated and not completely understood, literature in this area was sought since hormone manipulation is a strong point of current breast cancer treatment and appears to play a major role in the health of the patient presented.

Internal validity was attempted by selecting a specific population (breast cancer in females and CAM use). Several published studies by the same author indicated a researcher with experience in the field. Pertinent negative information or discrepancies were reviewed to improve the credibility of the study. Internal validity was potentially threatened when results of different studies came from separate populations, where genetics and metabolism may be difficult to compare.

Although there is some evidence of external validity in this review since information gained could be expanded to other cancers or other types of chronic diseases, no conclusions are made to expand this to the other areas. General arguments in favor, as well as those opposing the use of CAM, are presented to allow a general overview. Emphasis is on open-mindedness rather than making any definite conclusions. It would appear that results could be generalized to several subpopulation groups, with the exception that strict control over environment and diet is not possible. In addition, differences in genetics may affect metabolism, leading to another area making comparison of results difficult. A link between natural methods and scientific support for their use is strongly suggested when looking at specific biological mechanisms, but no case-controlled scientific studies are available.

Finally, a combination of allopathic as well as naturopathic literature was used to minimize bias. The lack of evidence-based studies supporting CAM is balanced by allopathic literature providing arguments that contradict the development of EBM in current medical practice. No conclusions were made to expand any findings to areas other than breast cancer. A plea is made to maintain an open-minded approach, supporting the scientific principles of curiosity, observation, and experience. Peer comments and feedback about the articles and texts used in the study were obtained from allopathic professionals who served as content experts.

Summary

A qualitative and descriptive literature review was chosen for this theoretical study since it is difficult to find any case-controlled studies with CAM. A diversified search to provide a diffuse background of CAM utilized textbooks, both allopathic as well as naturopathic, journals, lay literature, and medical professionals. The research topic is introduced by reviewing use of CAM and the personal experience in a middle-aged woman with breast cancer. The physiologic mechanisms outlined in the biology of breast cancer, as well as areas targeted for chemotherapy and hormonal treatment, were reviewed in an attempt to narrow the study to specific types of CAM used by this patient with an attempt to link this to a scientific basis. Another strong point to the development of a link will be the plea for an open-minded approach and support of the scientific principles of curiosity, observation, and experience. Appropriate literature from the history of medicine, as well as information regarding EBM and its potential weaknesses were reviewed.

Chapter Four

Results and Findings

Introduction

The initial purpose of this study was an attempt to identify a specific CAM modality and establish a scientific link for its effectiveness in the treatment of breast cancer. However, progressing through the literature review, the focus changed. Findings led to a comprehensive review of pathways in basic cell physiology and the relationship with the development and treatment of cancer. Looking at the same pathways, specific CAM modalities used by the patient presented were then studied to see if a scientific link could be established. The resulting information fails to identify a "magic bullet." This study is not meant to be a complete scientific review of breast cancer, but attempts to present basic findings to support a natural approach using the body's innate mechanisms in a holistic fashion.

Discussion and Evaluation of Research

The information presented in chapter 1 demonstrates that breast cancer is a significant disease in Western society. In addition, locoregional recurrence (skin metastases) presents a very poor prognosis. The epidemiology review identifies various risk factors. Questionable factors relate to hormone exposure and use, dietary factors, such as fruit and vegetable intake, nutritional supplements and vitamins, dairy products that may be tainted with hormones, the use of exogenous hormones such as those found in soy, and stress. Factors with an unquestionable relationship are genetics, a high intake of saturated fats and animal protein, and ingestion of moderate to high amounts of alcohol. The use of saturated fats and animal protein, junk food, and psychological factors (stress) are among those that appear to be related to the case presented.

Various biological principles lend a better understanding to mechanisms and cell physiology in the development of cancer, as well as the usefulness of certain CAM modalities. These will be presented as far as cancer in general with specific references to any differences related to breast cancer.

Cancer—A Dynamic Process

Hanahan and Weinberg (2000) point out that cancer is a dynamic process with multiple steps. Tumors are complex tissues with a redundancy of components and substances and not simply cells gone wild. Merlo, Pepper, Reid, and Maley (2006) make the further point that neoplasms are microcosms of evolution and Nowell (1976) presents cancer as a disease of clonal evolution within the body. Somewhere there is a breakdown of natural defenses. The p53 tumor suppressor protein, otherwise known as a genomic caretaker, is frequently involved (Weinstein and Ciszek 2002). This affects the DNA damage signaling pathway that is lost in most human cancers.

The purpose of the normal human genome is to maintain a multicellular organism. Neoplastic cells are different. TK-based genetic instability is involved in many of these processes. TK is also a signaling system that can be affected by various CAM modalities (Hanahan and Weinberg 2000; Merlo et al. 2006). Changes in methylation can alter expression of genes, such as p53, at a rate faster than the mutation rate of a cancerous growth (Hanahan and Weinberg 2000; Merlo et al. 2006; Ziyaie et al. 2000). Genetic variability within the cell lines may allow for selection of more aggressive sublines of tumor. Crespi and Summers (2005) and Heppner and Miller (1997) present such results in a somatic evolution of cell lines. Metastases cause 90% of human cancer deaths (Steeg and Theodorescu 2008).

Telomerase Activity

There is a fine balance between telomerase activity involved in normal aging and what occurs in cancer, as well as other diseases and degenerative conditions. Progressive telomere shortening has been demonstrated in programmed cell death and aging, and shortening of telomeres in humans contributes to mortality in many age-related diseases (Bryan, Englecou, Gupta, Bacchetti, and Redell 1995; Cawthorn, Smith, O'Brien, Sivatchenko, and Kerver 2003; Oshimura and Varrett 1997). Replicative senescence may have evolved to curtail tumorigenesis and thus serves as a powerful tumor suppressive mechanism (Campsi 1997). Without detectible telomerase activity, telomere elongation has been found within immortal human cells (Bryan and Redde 1997). However, there is a balance between senescence and tumorigenesis that is not entirely clear (Holt, Wright, and Shay 1997; Weinsein and Ciszak 2002). Telomere activation for degenerative diseases may actually reduce, rather than increase, the frequency of age-related tumorigenesis (Harley 2002) even though increased telomerase activity has been detected in cancerous cells (Shay and Baddhetti 1997).

Tumor cells can be considered in terms of acquisition of capabilities that enable cancer growth. One such property involves the ability to go through countless cycles of chromosome replication followed by cell division (Hanahan 2000). This may serve as a checkpoint that influences the mutational spectrum of tumors and has been demonstrated in breast and thyroid cancer (Wynford-Thomas 1997). Attempts at anti-aging therapy and administration of exogenous HGH may increase cancer risk based on the mechanism of telomere maintenance, as will be demonstrated in the hormone section of this chapter. This relationship is complex and may also involve serum activity of IGFBPs.

Growth Factor/ Apoptosis/ Angiogenesis

There are many GFs involved in normal development of cell lines. Activity of these GFs has also been studied as far as their relationship to cancer with attempts to manipulate GF activity as a form of cancer therapy. These growth signals may work to evade programmed cell-death (apoptosis), inducing a limitless replicative potential depending on sensitivity or insensitivity to growth-inhibitory signals. Self-sufficiency may be stimulated by the well-recognized growth factors PDGF, HIF, FGF, EGF, and VEGF, as well as IGF itself. Integrin also has growth factor properties (Giancotti 1999).

GFs may also up or downregulate genes, which is postulated as part of the mechanism involving p53. In addition, these growth factors may play a part in angiogenesis and tumor invasion in metastases as they affect fibroblasts and endothelial cells.

Genetic mutations, tumor invasion by breakdown of the extracellular matrix, and angiogenesis from new blood vessel growth are similar to effects that have been demonstrated by these various aforementioned growth factors (Steeg and Theodorescu 2008). Invasion or metastases occur by exceedingly complex processes that are incompletely understood.

Thirty-eight years ago Folkman (1975) demonstrates that tumors secrete substances which induce neovessel formation from preexisting neighboring blood vessels. This neovascularization is basic for tumor growth. Benign breast lesions associated with a high vascular density are shown to correlate with an increased risk for developing breast cancer (Fox et al. 2008). In this manner, neoplasia represents uncontrolled angiogenesis (D'arcangelo, Facchiano, and Barlucchi 2000).

There are many factors that have been identified as potential activators of neovascularization. The GF system exerts multiple physiologic effects on the vasculature through endocrine, as well as autocrine (self) and paracrine (neighboring) mechanisms (Delafontaine, Song, and Li 2004). Delafontaine et al. (2004) report that GFs affect cell growth through gene expression. Fox et al. (2008) discuss various substances that have been identified in this process, such as HER-1, VEGF, FGF, placenta growth factor, and pleiotrophin. In addition, Fox et al. (2008) point out that tamoxifen inhibits angiogenesis. Some chemotherapy also targets this mechanism. Examples are bevacizumab and paxil, targeting the TK portion of VEGF. Papetti and Herman (2002) demonstrate the same affects with TNF and other factors, and Nicosia, Nicosia, and Smith (1994) report on IGF-1. McMahon (2000) introduces the concept that inhibition of the TK portion of EGF is effective in blocking neovascularization. In addition, Fox et al. (2008) point out that oncogenes and tumor suppression genes are frequently associated with cellular transformation and appear to be important in activating the angiogenic switch.

The extracellular environment is important in this mechanism. Hypoxia and decreased pH stimulate angiogenesis in tumors (D'arcangelo et al. 2000). Ferrara and Davis-Smith (1997) demonstrate that HIF can encourage an aggressive phenotype in the tumor, contributing to its resistance to both chemotherapy and radiotherapy. In addition, Fox et al. (2008) point out that tumors recruit inflammatory cells (macrophages and mast cells) and activate platelets. All of these cells are rich in angiogenic factors, and Fox et al. (2008) refer to other studies demonstrating that increased levels of tumor-associated macrophages can be a marker of poor prognosis in tumors.

Folkman (1989) presents studies showing that tumors are angiogenesis dependent. Gimbrone, Leapman, Cotran, and Folkman (1972) point out neovascularization as a necessary condition for malignant growth of a solid tumor. Without an adequate vascular supply, tumors become necrotic or apoptotic (Hanahan and Folkman 1986). Feldman and Libutti (2000) discuss studies dealing with the inhibition of angiogenesis as a promising strategy for antitumor therapy. Weidner, Semple, Welch, and Folkman (1991) show that neovascularization may serve some prognostic relevance, although Freidman, Humblet, Ponjean, and Boniver (2000) demonstrate no correlation. Furthermore, Ingehom et al. (1999) point out a need for standardization of techniques to reduce inter- and intra-observer variation, while Prehn (1993) presents the concept of variable levels of GF activity leading to competing influences. One such example is what occurs in the local environment versus effects from systemic circulatory inhibitors and stimulants produced by normal tissue and tumors. D'arcangelo et al. (2000) show that short-term hypoxia upregulates VEGF expression while long-standing hypoxemia involves increasing VEGF activity to influence tumor growth. Fidler (2003) emphasizes the importance of angiogenesis for the establishment of metastases in terms of a favorable microenvironment for implantation of tumor cells, his so-called "seed and soil hypothesis." The fact that tumors may actually be the body's response to a toxic environment with an attempt for survival (Moritz 2008) is a controversial topic and will be discussed in chapter 5.

Nutritional Modulation of the Cell Cycle

Hilakivi-Clarke et al. (2004) present an extensive discussion on nutritional modulation of the cell cycle as related to breast cancer. This involves hormone signaling and cell function, as well as nutritional aspects that serve as checkpoints in the mammalian cell cycle. TK cell membrane receptors are a common denominator in many metabolic pathways. The discussion of this paper is important as far as dietary prevention and intervention in human breast cancer.

Hilakivi-Clarke et al. (2004) point out PDGF and FGF promote entry of the cell into the G 1 phase of mitosis. IGF-1 and EGF have similar actions. Over expression of cyclin D-1 correlates with a poor prognosis in tumors and appears to convert the usually good prognosis of ER positive tumors to a worse status. Cell proliferation may be induced by estrogen, particularly during fetal, prepubertal, and pregnancy time periods. Pointed out in the previous section to be a common factor in promoting angiogenesis, the mechanism appears to be through membrane TK receptors. There also appears to be a subset of breast cancer that is sensitive to the proliferative effects of androgens. DHEA stimulates growth of the skin metastases in the case presented.

Hilakivi Clarke et al. (2004) state that diet contributes to the etiology of 30%-50% of diagnosed breast cancer. This is not precise since most studies report dietary intakes at the time of the diagnosis. As cancer development is a multistep process there may be a time lapse, making it difficult to identify the contributing components (Welsch 1987). Not only this, but there are multiple pathways involved with nutritional aspects. As presented in chapter 1, the strongest evidence for a link between nutrition and breast cancer is a high intake of alcohol and also polysaturated fats and animal protein (Cho et al. 2006; Djuric et al. 1998; Howe et al. 1990; Katsouyanni et al. 1994; Longnecker et al. 1995).

Phytoestrogens have been extensively studied as far as their relationship to endocrine-related cancers. Isoflavones are in this class and many types are found in soy products, red clover, and berries. Genisitein is one of the more commonly used isoflavones. At a low dose, isoflavones have been shown to have a cell-proliferative effect. In higher doses, an inhibitory effect on TK activity is seen, which may inhibit angiogenesis and induce apoptosis. Cabanes et al. (2004) point out that prepubertal exposure to genisitein upregulates BRCA-1 mRNA, providing an explanation for improved DNA repair capacity.

Finstad et al. (1984) and Rudolph, Kelley, Clasing, and Erickson (2001) show that n-3 and n-6 fatty acids impact cell proliferation and differentiation. n-6 PUFA consumption may directly enhance aromatization (Richards and Brugemeier 2003). Adipose tissues may also serve to aromatize DHEA into increased amounts of estrogen (Lipton et al. 1987). Again, timing of the exposure and a clear definition of pathways is difficult to identify (Welsch 1987). Premenopausal females that are overweight may have higher circulating estrogens derived from adipose tissue. This likely affects the pituitary-gonadal axis secondary to the additional estrogen produced by fatty tissue. Obesity has also been shown to affect insulin sensitivity. This brings IGF and its place in the hormonal axis into the picture, which will be discussed later in chapter 4.

Caloric restriction appears to have a protective effect on the development and progression of cancer (Kritchesky 1992). Insulin resistance brings serum glucose levels into play as far as stimulation of IGF, which then feeds into the stress axis via ACTH. G1 cell arrest may occur secondary to adrenocorticoid secretion (Zhu, Jiang, and Thomson 2002; Jiang, Zhu, and Thomson 2003). Kadowaki et al. (2003) make a case that adenopectin is related to the mechanism of insulin resistance in obesity. They also discuss the concept that energy restriction may reduce oxidative damage and free radical generation, affect the hormone axis, and reduce tumor cell proliferation via reduced gene expression and G 1 cell cycle arrest. Hilakivi-Clarke et al. (2004) point out the extensive literature available that links IGF-1 to breast cancer through interaction with GH and the hormonal axis in general.

Retinoid receptors are members of the nuclear steroid/thyroid hormone receptor family which control cell growth and differentiation. Activation of retinoid receptors are shown to be growth inhibitory by downregulation of p53, affecting the G 1 phase (Amos and Lotan 1990; Seewaldt et al. 1997; Seewaldt, Dietz, Johnson, Collins, and Parker 1999; Weinstein and Ciszak 2002). The difference between an effect from vitamin A or other carotenoids seems to be more pronounced using whole foods and vegetables rather than supplements (Cheung et al. 2003; Fairfield and Fletcher 2002; Howe et al. 1990). This suggests a synergistic action from structurally similar molecules that may occur in whole foods versus a specific, solitary chemical formulation from manufactured supplements.

Chemotherapy Mechanisms

Many chemotherapy regimens are based on interference with the ability of DNA to replicate in tumor cells. Looking at differentiated patterns of expression of ninety-two genes to tailor treatment based on gene expression of the patient, Charfare et al. (2005) present gene profiling and proteomics to predict tumor response, sensitivity to chemotherapy, and patient prognosis. p 53 downregulation allows aggressive tumor growth by decreasing levels of apoptosis (Symonds et al. 1994). As will be discussed later, antioxidants, such as vitamin C and green tea, repair DNA damage and assist in DNA signaling. This, hopefully, promotes healthy DNA function in noncancerous cells. Other pathways are via antiangiogenic and pro-apoptic mechanisms.

Chemotherapy regimens work in various manners. Older agents include the antibiotics doxorubicin and mitomycin-C, which affect mRNA signaling and DNA synthesis (Stewart and Ratain 1997; Dahl, Weiss, and Issel 1985), and antimetabolites, such as 5-flourouracil (replaces pyrimidine) and methrotrexate (a folic acid analog), interrupting metabolic pathways in DNA synthesis (Stewart and Ratain 1997). Alkylating agents (Berger 1993) and the platinum-based compounds, cisplatin and carboplatin, break or otherwise affect DNA cross-links (Sledge, Loeher, Roth, and Einhorn 1988). The drugs bevacizumab and trastuzumab inhibit specific gene receptors of VEGF (Wheler 2005) and HEGF (Kim, Lobocki, Dubay, and Mittal 1997), again noting the mechanism via cell membrane TK inhibition (Hennipman et al. 1989). Trastuzumab amplifies HER-2/neu signaling to focus on programmed cell death, angiogenesis, and cellular signaling (Green 2003; Moshin, Weiss, and Gutierrez 2005)

Vinca alkaloids inhibit microtubule synthesis in mitosis (Stewart and Ratain 1997). The drug GRN 163 L causes specific telomere dysfunction and is found to increase radiation sensitivity in breast cancer cells (Gellert, Dikman, Wright, Gryaznov, and Shay 2006; Gomez-Millan, Goldblatt, Gryaznov, Mendonca, and Hebert 2007). Taxanes (paxlitaxel and docetexel) affect cells by preventing the formation of a normal mitotic spindle resulting in G2/M phase (mitosis) blockade (Belotti et al. 1996; Lee et al. 2001) and are among the most active agents in treatment of breast cancer (Chakravarthy and Pietenpol 2003). Telomerase-based therapies are of interest in that tumors may be less likely to develop resistance than other targets of cancer therapy since telomerase acts as a mitotic clock of replicative aging, conferring normal cells a finite capacity for division (Chakravarthy 2003; Kim 1997; Lee et al. 2001).

HGH and IGF are hormones implicated in telomerase activity (Harley 2008; Rosen and Conover 1997; Yu and Rohan 2000). This shows a factor in common when treating cancer or providing treatment for age-related and degenerative disease. Melatonin further demonstrates some crossover effect with the hormonal axis (Harley 2008), probably related to HGH. This may be important in developing therapies based on circadian rhythm and cell-division cycle.

A local environment of acidosis and hypoxia may affect angiogenesis, but also plays a significant part in apoptosis. Resveratrol inhibits both processes by direct local effects as an antioxidant, as well as inducing basic FGF and VEGF expression (D'arcangelo et al. 2000; Garvin, Ollinger, and Dabrosin 2006; Gimbrone et al. 1972). Vaccines have an antiangiogenic effect through inhibition of epithelial proliferation (Belotti et al. 1996; Lam 1998), further pointing to a crossover effect by more than one mechanism. Biphosphonates have been used to strengthen bone in patients with metastases, and it has been shown that they may also have an antitumor effect by inhibiting the anti-apoptotic effects of growth factors, such as eliminating the stimulation of FGF by IGF (Clemons and Rea 2004; DeBuis et al. 2001; Fromigue, Kheddoumi, and Body 2003; Hillner et al. 2003; Mincey 2000; Nevill-Webbe, Holen, and Coleman 2002).

Scheduling of chemotherapy regimens can also be used to improve efficacy (Kamen et al. 2000). Metronomic dosing is another novel approach, which uses smaller dosing at constant intervals without rest periods, eliciting repeated waves of apoptosis of tumor and epithelial cells (Hanahan, Burgers, and Bergsland 2000). Melatonin and circadian rhythm may be involved, suggesting effects on the hormonal axis via GH. Cyclophosphamide, used in this fashion, affects both apoptosis and angiogenesis in resistant tumors (Browder et al. 2000). Slaton, Perrotte, Inoue, Dinney, and Fidler (1999) show that maximal antiangiogenic therapy typically requires prolonged exposure to low drug concentrations, which is exactly counter to the maximum tolerated doses administered when tumor cell kill is the goal.

Shark cartilage was purported in the 1990s as an anticancer agent on the basis of inhibiting angiogenesis since the extract comes from an avascular tissue. However, no definite benefit is shown (Chustecka 2007; Miller, Anderson, Stark, Granick, and Richardson 1998), and no improvement was noted in the case presented. Thalidomide and sulindac demonstrate equivocal results in the inhibition of angiogenesis (Baidas et al. 2000; Minchinton, Fryer, Wendt, Clow, and Hayes 1996; Verheul, Panigrahy, Yuan, and D'Amato 1999), although Verheul et al. (1999) report an animal study.

Immunotherapy is another target area for cancer treatment (Early Breast Cancer Trialists Collaborative Group 1992; Hudsen, Humphrey, Mantz, and Morse 1974; Lennox 1985; McGuire, Carbone, and Vollmer 1975; Mueller and Ammers 1978; Slamon et al. 2001; Slaton et al. 1999), with an emphasis on lymphocyte function (Lee 1984; Meyer 1970; Papatestas 1977; Papatestas and Kark 1974; Whittiker and Clark 1971). MGN-3 is a modified arabinoxyline from rice bran that presumably serves as an antiviral and immunomodulator by increasing TNF, NK cells, and B and T lymphocytes (PDRHealth.com). IP-6 facilitates signal transmission between the cytoplasm and nucleus to regulate cell growth (Inositol Hexaphosphate; PDRHealth.com). Although there are no good human studies, it may affect induction of cell division (mitosis) and inhibit vascular and epithelial GF by means of IGFBP-3 (Jariwalla 1999; Memorial Sloan-Kettering Cancer Center 2004; Singh, Agarwal, and Agarwal 2003). Certain synthetic drugs are potentially useful as immune response modifiers by exerting biological effects through induction of IFN (an antiviral agent) polynucleotides (LaCour 1982). Nonspecific passive immunotherapy with bacterial endotoxin has also been used to stimulate the cytokine TNF (Old 1985).

Hormonal Manipulation

There is much controversy in the literature on the implication of hormone exposure and hormone replacement on the development of breast cancer (Beral 2003; Cauley et al. 1999; Chewbloski et al. 2003; DeBuis et al. 2001; Early Breast Cancer Trial Collaboration Group 1995; Genezani and Gambacciniani 1999; Grabric et al. 2000;

Hankinson 1997; Kabuto, Akiba, Stevens, Meriishi, and Land 2000; Kelsey 1993; McGuire et al. 1975; Phillips et al. 2004; Pike et al. 1993; Sener et al. 2009; Thomas, Reeves, and Key 1997). Spratt (1993) demonstrates that hormone exposure results in the development of a more biologically favorable cancer than to non-users. Age-specific breast cancer incidence rates show decline in the rate of increase after menopause, leaving the question whether key carcinogenic events occur before rather than after menopause (Pike et al. 1993). Retrospective studies may be problematic and reliability questioned since specific data on hormone levels is not consistently available. In addition, other factors, such as environmental and nutritional aspects, present as uncontrollable variables. Progesterone, prolactin, androgens, and other steroid hormones may play a part but have not been sufficiently studied. Exactly how hormones increase cancer risk is not completely understood, including which of the specific hormones, estradiol or estrogen, is the most significant (Bernstein and Ross 1993; Falk, Dorgan, Potischman, and Loncope 1997: Falk et al. 1999; Hankinson et al. 1995 1999; Migliaccio et al. 1996).

Hilakivi-Clarke et al. (2004) discuss hormonal control of the cell cycle. Estrogen is a potent mammary mitogen which stimulates cell cycle progression, particularly in the G1 phase (McCarty 1989). Piao et al. (2008) show this G1 effect occurs by TK receptors inhibition in the cell membrane. Besides the ovary, estrogen is also synthesized in other areas, such as the adrenal gland, adipose tissue, and by mammary tumors themselves. Lyons, Li, and Johnson (1958) show that estrogen stimulation of breast development is ineffective in the absence of anterior pituitary hormones. Estrogen increases GH secretion and inhibits prolactin. Not only is estrogen a major factor in mammary gland growth, but it also plays a part in somatogenesis and angiogenesis in breast tissue in a process involving estrogen itself, as well as other hormones and multiple growth factors (Davis et al. 1994; Eddy et al. 1996; Johns, Freay, Fraser, Korach, and Rubanyi 1996; Korach et al. 1996).

Estrogens are synthesized by aromatization of androgens via the enzyme aromatase. This serves as a rate-limiting step in estrogen production and increased aromatase activity can be found in classic endocrine tissues in the ovary, adrenal, and hypothalamus, as well as adipose tissue, fibroblasts, small amounts of muscle tissue, and even cancerous tissue itself (Lipton et al. 1987). Hall (1974) proposes that estrogens can flood the system, causing tumors to mature, differentiate, and stop proliferation. Androgens can induce proliferation of ER positive cells (Hilakivi-Clarke et al. 2004), with the TK receptor on cell membranes as the common denominator (Yeager 2000).

Estrogen has also been shown to be an endogenous genotoxic agent, increasing the risk of uterine and mammary cancer (Cavalieri, Frenkel, Liehr, Rogan, and Roy 2000). Cavalieri et al. (2000) present evidence that high levels of circulating estrogen act as a carcinogen, resulting in cancer by mutating critical regulatory genes and causing abnormal cell proliferation (Weinberg 1996). This may be related to an effect combined with ingestion of saturated fat, discussed in the following paragraph. Fluctuation of hormones leading to NK cell cytotoxicity favors the periovulatory period as the most favorable prognostic time for surgery (Hrushesky 1988; Ratajczak, Sothern, and Hrushesky 1988; Spratt 1993).

PAH are investigated as model carcinogenic compounds by Cavalieri and Rohan (1992), who describe the route by which catechol estrogens, the major metabolites of estradiol and estrone (the natural hormones in the estrogen family), may be oxidized to catechol estrogen quinones (CE-Q). These subsequently may react with DNA to form depurinating adducts, leading to mutations that give rise to breast, prostate, as well as other cancers. Occurring through mutagenic oxygen radicals produced by estradiol-induced lipid peroxidation, particularly in the presence of reduced transition metal ions (Fe^{2+}, Cu^+), an inflammatory pathway is suggested. Cavalieri et al. (2000) propose that this is the rationale of the increased cancer risk seen with saturated fat and animal protein intake, demonstrating another action involving the hormone axis. Understanding the origin of these mutations opens the door to strategies for controlling and preventing cancer.

The use of tamoxifen is unchallenged as a first-line agent in the hormonal treatment of breast cancer (Early Breast Cancer Trialists Collaborative Group 1998; Fisher et al. 1999; Veronesi et al. 2005). It has antiangiogenic properties, in addition to its ability to block the action of estrogen on tumor cells by inhibiting the synthesis of estrogen while blocking its binding to estrogen receptor sites (Baum 1998; Jensen 2005). Tamoxifen appears to interfere with mitosis in the early G1 phase (Osborne, Boldt, Clark, and Trent 1983). Aromatase inhibitors, such as Femara, have also been used to affect this pathway (Mouridsen et al. 2003). Side effects seen with these agents include an increase in osteoporosis, fractures, myocardial infarction, thromboembolic events, and an increased incidence of endometrial cancer and other secondary malignancies (Hulley et al. 1998; Rossouw et al. 2002). This suggests a systemic effect on multiple physiological pathways in the human organism.

More than thirty years ago, PR expression is presented as a better indicator of responsiveness to endocrine treatment then ER alone in advanced breast cancer (Horwitz et al. 1975; McGuire, Horwitz, Pearson, and Segaloff 1977), although clinical indications are not entirely clear and continue to be controversial (Gasparini 1992; Huseby, Ownby, Brooks, and Russo 1997; Stierer et al. 1995). Progestin is considered a second-line hormonal agent of choice with the dominant activity being antiestrogenic through progesterone receptors (Chewbloski et al. 2003; Shi 1994). Allegra and Kiefer (1985), Pike et al. (1993), and Rochefort (1984) show a direct cytotoxic effect by progestin on human breast cancer cells. Side effects include mild glucocorticoid activity and weight gain (Ingle et al. 1999). Progesterone antagonists are also used in hormonal manipulation of breast cancer (Michna, Nishino, Neef, McGuire, and Schneider 1992), suggesting more than one mechanism of action.

Older therapies, not used nearly as frequently since the development of the aforementioned agents, include adrenalectomy and oophorectomy, to remove the hormonal influence from the secretion of estrogen by these organs (Ferrara, Raiches, and Minton 2006; Ingall 1984; Rush 1982; Spratt and Donegan 2002). In addition, alternative methods, such as isoflavones (discussed in the soy section of this chapter) (Mahady 2005), dong quai (Lau, Hoi, Chan, and Kim 2005), and other substances (Sicat and Brokaw 2004) are purported to affect the hormonal axis.

Local effects present another aspect which demonstrates the complexity of hormonal axis balance. Estrogen has a synergistic effect on PDGF and fibroblast-related GF in angiogenesis and the development of mammary stromal tissue by means of somatostatin receptors (Hilakivi-Clarke et al. 2004; Lyons et al. 1958). Somatostatin can inhibit GH release, prolactin secretion, insulin and glucagon release, and pentagastrin-induced gastric secretion. Somatostatin receptors have been demonstrated to facilitate a direct inhibitory effect on cell growth (Karashima and Schally 1987; Schally 1986).

Next to estrogen, prolactin is the most important hormone involved in breast function and development and is a potent mitogen for breast tissue (Shiu and Friesen 1980). Higher plasma levels of prolactin are associated with an increased risk of breast cancer in postmenopausal females (Hankinson et al. 1999). Diets rich in saturated fats increase prolactin levels (Ingram et al. 1990) and is presented as a possible explanation of breast cancer risk. This also leads to pituitary feedback affecting estrogen and GH, demonstrating the complexity of events that can occur from the action of a single hormone.

Interesting information was encountered regarding HGH and IGF-I (Li et al. 1998; Yu and Rohan 2000). HGH levels will be presented as IGF-I in the discussion since serum levels of this hormone represent the best marker reflecting a mean level overall of HGH (Biller et al. 2002; Boquete et al. 2003; Brabant et al. 2003; de Boer et al. 1996; Pandian and Nakamoto 2004; Stasburger 2001; Yu and Berkel 1999). Somatostatin and tamoxifen, acting by inhibition of IGF-1, should be synergistic, but this is not definitely proven (Ingle et al. 1999). This is a starting point for linking IGF with sex hormones in the overall hormone axis.

Hormonal Axis/HGH/IGF

GH/IGF has been studied in aging populations as far as frailty, chronic illness, and degenerative conditions (Balducci 2000; Carroll et al. 1998; Drake, Howell, Monsoon, and Shalet 2001; Frost et al. 1996; Juul et al. 1997; LeRoith 1997; Poehlman and Copeland 1990; Roizen and Oz 2008; Rosen and Conover 1997) and involves an elusive pathway (Baserga 1997; Firth and Baxter 2002; Rajaram, Baylink, and Mohan 1997; Rosenfeld et al. 1999; White and Khan 1994) from a multifunctional protein family (Cohen 2006). IGF is important for normal physiologic function in virtually every tissue (Khandwala, McCutcheon, Flyvberg, and Friend 2000). IGF-I plasma concentrations are reported to decline with advancing age and may be reflected in growth and maintenance of connective tissue, muscle, and bone during the aging process (Donahue, Hunter, Sherbolm, and Rosen 1990; Yu and Rohan 2000). Just as other aspects of the hormonal axis, the IGF family is characterized by a complex interrelationship within the group of factors themselves, as well as effects on other portions of the hormonal axis in general.

The IGF family consists of multiple growth factor ligands, receptor proteins, and binding proteins (Wu et al. 1999). IGF-I has both immediate and long-term effects on various cellular activities, and these effects are mediated mainly through IGFRP-I (Wu et al. 1999). IGF-I exerts an anabolic action on protein and carbohydrate metabolism by increasing cellular uptake of amino acids and glucose, thereby stimulating glycogen and protein synthesis (Jones and Clemmons 1995). The IGFRPs are glycoproteins located on the cell membrane primarily triggering a cascade of reactions by means of the TK receptor on the cell membrane (LeRoith, Werner, Beitner-Johnson, and Roberts 1995; Stewart, Johnson, May, and Westley 1990). The various IGFBPs have multiple and complex functions and can either be IGF dependent or independent (Collett-Solberg and Zohen 1996; Kelley et al. 1996). IGFBPs have an inhibitory, as well as potentiating, effect which is independent of IGF actions (Elgin, Busby, and Clemmons 1987; Firth and Baxter 2002; Mohan, Daylink, and Pettis 1996; Rajaram et al. 1997; Sepp-Lorenzino 1998; Weinzimer et al. 2001). The difference in structure and function among the components of the IGF system show the complex relationship of this axis, sometimes with a suppressing function, sometimes stimulatory, and even opposing functions at the same time. As an example, Vadgama, Wu, Datta, Khan, and Chillar (1999) show that tamoxifen decreases IGF-I levels significantly.

Cancer is a disease associated with aging, with the highest cancer incidence seen in later life when GH and IGF-I levels are low. This is evaluated in many research studies in an attempt to establish a relationship between GH and cancer risk. The trend seen in the literature reviewed shows that increased levels of IGF-I are associated with an increased cancer risk, only if IGFBP-3 is low, presumably seen since elevated levels of IGFBP-3 decrease the amount of IGF-I available (Yu and Rohan 2000). The complexity of this relationship can be seen in multiple published series. Information is available attempting to identify which of the factors (IGFs, IGFRPs, or IGFBPs) serve as the most important marker. This is somewhat controversial and indicates that elevated or low levels of one factor must be considered with changes in others rather than the measurement of one component alone (Bonneterre, Peyrat, Beuscart, and Demaille 1990; Hankinson et al. 1998; Ohmuller, Pham, and Rosenfield 1993). Data found in the literature is still not completely clear regarding a direct or inverse correlation with individual factors in this family, or whether this involves a combination of factors (Bohlke, Cramer, Trichopoulos, and Manzoros 1998; Chen et al. 1994; Rocha et al. 1997; Sheikh et al. 1992). Although several decades of basic and clinical research have demonstrated an association between members of the IGF family and neoplasia, this is still not completely understood.

Since expression of the IGF-I gene is regulated primarily by GH, Hankinson et al. (1998) report that measurement of plasma IGF-I concentrations may be useful in the identification of women at high risk for breast cancer. IGFRP-I is also implicated in breast cancer (Surmz, Gukakova, Nolaw, Nicosia, and Scirra 1998). Although receptor proteins have an effect through TK receptors on the cell membrane (Piao et al. 2008), inhibition of breast cancer cell growth and apoptosis also occurs by affecting the FGF family and the beta transforming GF family (Colomer et al. 1997; Nass 1996; Yiangou 1997). Information is available regarding which of the factors of binding protein serve as the most important markers (Cohen 2006; Jones and Clemmons 1995; Rosenfeld et al. 1999). Many other studies demonstrate changes in physiologic levels of a combination of various factors in the family, as well as IGFBPs, may be related to an increase in cancer risk and development, among these breast cancer (Bohlke et al. 1998; Bruning et al. 1995; Hankinson et al. 1998; Krywicki and Yee 1992; LeRoith et al. 1997; LeRoith, Vaserga, Hellman, and Roberts 1995; McCauley 1992; Pekonen, Partanen, Makinen, and Rutanen 1988; Pekonen, Nyman, Ilvesmaki, and Partanen 1992; Yu et al. 1998). Lee, Hilgenbeck, and Yee, (1998) find over-expression of IGFRP-I is associated with a longer disease-free survival and better overall survival in breast cancer. These relationships of the IGF family and breast cancer risk also holds true for other ethnic groups (Agurs-Collins, Adams-Campbell, Kim, and Cullen 2000; Vadgama et al. 1999; Yu et al. 2002).

In looking at the various aspects of HGH, IGF-I is described as similar to, but distinct from, the insulin receptor and may cause stimulation of DNA synthesis (Chen et al. 1994). Aberrant activity may lead to expression of oncogenes (Berns, Klijn, van Stavern, Portengen, and Fockens 1992; Papa et al. 1993). One of the target genes for IGFBP-3 is p53, which, when downregulated, leads to deregulation of the cell cycle and DNA replication (Buckbinder, Talbott, Seizinger, and Kley 1994; Buckbinder et al. 1995; Kelley et al. 1996).

Antimitogenic and apoptotic suppression has also been identified in the IGF axis (Yu and Rohan 2000). IGFs are mitogens that play a pivotal role in regulating self-proliferation, differentiation, and apoptosis (Baserga 1997; Butt, Fraley, Firth, and Baxter 2002; Cohen 2006; Sepp-Lorenzino 1998; Tomolo et al. 2000; White and Khan 1994; Yu and Rohan 2000). This is also demonstrated with IGFRP-I (Resnicoff et al. 1995; Stewart and Rotwein 1996). Furthermore, IGFBPs have mitogenic and apoptotic properties independent of the ability to modulate bioavailability of the individual IGF protein fractions (Butt, Firth, and Baxter 1999; Tonner 2000; Yee, Favoni, Lippman, and Powell 1991). Wetterau, Francis, Ma, and Cohen (2003) show stimulation of telomerase activity by IGF-I in prostate cancer cells. A novel approach uses the inhibition of IGF-I action as an adjunct to cytotoxic chemotherapy in breast cancer (Gooch, Van Den berg, and Yee 1999).

Another interesting aspect of HGH has to do with glucose metabolism, glycemic status, and the metabolic syndrome. Baxter (1994) describes the actions and bio-availability of the IGFs with insulin in counter-regulation, blocking "free" insulin activity during fasting or hypoglycemia. Steele-Perkins et al. (1988) present IGF-I stimulation of glucose uptake, glycogen synthesis, and DNA synthesis, whereas others go a step further linking these mechanisms to affecting GH, leading to insulin resistance and the metabolic syndrome (Forouhi, Luan, Cooper, Boucher, and Wareham 2005; Kadowaki et al. 2003). Insulin pathways and Type II diabetes are implicated with an increased risk of breast cancer (LaJous et al. 2008; Wolf, Sadetski, Catane, Karsik, and Kaufman 2005; Wu, Yu, Theng, Stanczyk, and Pike 2007).

Finally, links to sex hormones and the overall hormone axis continue to show the complexity of these systems. IGF-I, acting through an endocrine pathway by interacting with estrogen and progesterone receptors, may stimulate tumor growth (Owens et al. 1993; Pekonen et al. 1988; Peyrat, Bonneterre, Beuscart, Dijane, and Demaille 1988; Stewart et al. 1990). Favoni et al. (1995) show that patients with higher estradiol and progesterone do not present different IGF-I concentrations compared to patients with lower serum sex hormone levels, and values of IGF-I do not depend on estrogen receptor status.

The components IGF-I or IGFBPs may be secreted differently depending on the ER status (positive or negative) of the patient (Clemmons, Camacho-Hubner, Coronado, and Osborne 1990). This brings up the point whether autocrine production of IGFBP by breast cancer cells may be more important than IGF-I levels in predicting breast cancer risk and prognosis (Figueroa, Jackson, McGuire, Krywicki, and Yee 1983; Foekens et al. 1989). Induction of mRNA by IGF fractions are shown to cause proliferative effects in breast cancer, particularly the MCF-7 cell line (Stewart et al. 1990), and may explain one of the mechanisms for the mitogenic effect (Diorio, Brisson, Berube, and Pollack 2008; Ruan, Catanese, Weizzorek, Feldman, and Kleinberg 1995). This may be on an autocrine (Huynh, Yang, and Pollack 1996; Thorsen, Lahoot, Hrasmussen, and Aakvaag 1992) or paracrine (Clarke, Howell, and Anderson 1997) basis in addition to the endocrine effects. Dependent on the presence of a combination of prolactin, hydrocortisone, GH, and insulin, stimulation by estrogen from the ovaries is shown to cause arborization of the ductal system in breast development (Farrar and Walker 2000; Tonner 2000). There is an independent effect by certain IGF components as well (Tonner 2000). Barni et al. (1994), Rajaram et al., (1997), and Shiu and Friesen (1980) present data on the IGF-I effect on another hormone, prolactin. Used in breast cancer hormonal manipulative therapy, part of the antitumor effect of tamoxifen may be from reducing IGF-I levels (Khandwala et al. 2000; Vadgama et al. 1999).

Finally, further complexity of the effects and actions of the IGF family is noted related to nutrition (Yu and Rohan 2008). Nutritional status and dietary energy intake are critical regulators of IGF-I levels (Thissen, Ketersleger, and Underwood 1994). This is seen in both overnutrition (Forbes, Brown, Welle, and Underwood 1989), as well as caloric restriction (Smith, Underwood, and Clemmons 1995). Yu and Rohan (2008) present a review of studies looking at other aspects, such as physical activity, body mass, alcohol consumption, and cigarette smoking, with conflicting results and are unable to present any solid relationship with serum levels of the IGF family.

Antioxidants

In discussing the case presented, antioxidants are utilized and represent one of the common agents of CAM (Arrigoni and de Tullio 2002; Assouline and Miller 2006; Li and Schellhorn 2007; White 2002), usually in the form of ascorbic acid (vitamin C) or green tea. In general, antioxidants serve as potent reducing agents of free radicals produced by normal metabolic respiration (Paddayatatty et al. 2003), and Halliwell (1992) hypothesizes a possible role of ROS in the pathogenesis of many chronic diseases while stating that they may also be a consequence of a pathological condition. Controlling free-radicals may prevent DNA mutations (Lutsenko, Carcamo, and Golde 2002; Pflaum-Kielbassa, Garmyn, and Epe 1998) and repair oxidized amino acids to maintain protein integrity (Barja et al. 1994; Cadenas, Rojas, and Varga 1998; Hoey and Butler 1984), thus modulating gene expression (Allen and Trisini 2000; Arrigoni and de Tullio 2002). Affecting signal transduction and gene expression is shown to attenuate cell proliferation, arresting the cell cycle and inducing apoptosis (Simon, Haj, Ehia, and Levi-Schaffer 2000). Salginak (2001) introduces the concept of screening tests for ROS in populations to try to identify an increased cancer risk.

Vitamin C

Ascorbic acid has been shown to serve several functions. Besides the aforementioned antioxidant effects, others include synthesis of carnitine from lysine, stimulation of cytochrome p450 activity, increased cholesterol metabolism, and detoxification of exogenous compounds such as nitrates (Gonzales 2005; Li and Schellhorn 2007). In addition, ascorbic acid functions in neurotransmitter synthesis, converting dopamine to norepinephrine, suggesting a link to the stress hormone axis (Arrigoni and de Tullio 2002). It is involved as a cosubstrate in multiple enzyme systems (Arrigoni and de Tullio 2002). Gene expression is shown to occur via p73, inducing apoptosis (Catani et al. 2002), or through p53 (Ikawa, Nakagawara, and Ikawa 1999; Reddy, Khanna, and Singh 2001), providing a mechanism to restore healthy cell checkpoints. Attenuation of cell proliferation, by inducing apoptosis via the IGF system and reduced expression of IGFRPs, is shown by Naidu et al. (2001) and Naidu,

Karl, Naidu, and Coppola (2003). Zou et al. (2006) defines another pathway in the IGF system with the same effect. Chen et al. (2005 2007) and Simon et al. (2001) report on the pharmacologic pathway of ascorbate serving as a pro-oxidant to generate hydrogen peroxide in the extracellular space which then leads to cytotoxicity of tumor cells. In addition to antioxidant properties, Arrigoni and de Tullio (2002) cite other examples of ascorbic acid functions that are often underestimated or ignored. Downregulation of VEGF, which may affect angiogenesis, is also reported (Nespeira et al. 2003; Rodriguez, Nespeira, Perez-Ilzarbe, Eguinda, and Paramo 2005).

Transport and mechanisms are reviewed extensively by Li and Schellhorn (2007), Gonzales (2005), and Wilson (2005). Genetically, humans do not have the ability to synthesize vitamin C as do other mammalian systems due to an evolutionary inactivating mutation of the involved gene (Li and Schellhorn 2007). Absorption occurs by two pathways, facilitated diffusion and active transport, but not by simple diffusion. This determines the maximum serum concentration that can be achieved by the oral route (Brubacher, Moser, and Jordan 2000; Hoffer et al. 2008; Padayatty et al. 2006). Ascorbic acid may serve as an anti- or pro-oxidant depending on the environment. Three factors are involved: the redox potential of the environment, the local concentration of ascorbate, and the presence or absence of free transition metals (Fe^{+2}, Cu^{+1}), which can frequently be released in the presence of cancer cells.

Vitamin C status has been related to mortality in U.S. adults (Asplund 2002; Bjelakovic et al. 2007; Khaw et al. 2001; Loria et al. 2000), with the most significant correlation seen with low levels of the vitamin and increased cardiovascular deaths. Epidemiological studies for decreased cancer risk with vitamin C use are controversial (Cui, Shikany, Liu, Shagufta, and Rohan 2008). Block, Patterson, and Subar (1992), looking at more than two hundred studies, find a protective effect of increased fruit/vegetable intake in 128/156 well-designed reports in their large meta-analysis. Steinmetz and Hunter (1996), looking at 206 human epidemiological studies and twenty-two animal studies, and Gandini et al. (2000), using meta-analysis of twenty-six published studies, report similar findings. The difficult aspect of these studies is that a standard serving size is not well defined. Bjelakovic et al. (2007) make the interesting comment that elimination of free radicals from the body may actually interfere with some essential defense mechanisms like apoptosis, phagocytosis, and detoxification. This supports the complexity and multiplicity of the pathways involved.

Stanner et al. (2004) state that although scientific rationale and observational studies are convincing, randomized primary and secondary studies fail to show consistent benefit from the use of antioxidant supplements to reduce cancer risk. They present arguments that there are many trials attempt to isolate high doses of one agent, that appropriate doses or combination of agents is unknown, that doses of single agents, such as vitamin C, are not at consistent levels in various studies, and that whole food and plant sources may provide a variety of similar structural molecules that work synergistically and are more effective than a manufactured single molecule supplement. Asplund (2002) argues that an uncontrolled variable is that the use of supplements may actually be only one element of overall healthy behavior.

Nutrition and vitamins are generally accepted as an aid in treatment of cancer (Block et al. 1992; Gandini et al. 2000; Salganik 2001; Steinmetz and Hunter 1996), not only as an overall benefit, but also to enhance efficacy and decrease the toxicity of standard treatment (Block et al. 1992; Li and Schellhorn 2007; Prasad 2004; Stanner et al. 2004). Others report possible adverse consequences of the use of vitamin C with chemotherapy and radiation treatment through various mechanisms (Catley and Anderson 2006; Drisko, Chapman, and Hunter 2003; Lawenda et al. 2008; Zou et al. 2006). Moss (2006) argues that a blanket rejection of vitamin C is not justified, instead seeking a balance between toxicity and the nutritional advantages of vitamin C use. Yeom et al. (2007) emphasize that an improvement in the "quality of life" associated with vitamin C use may be as important as a cure.

Cameron and Pauling (1976; 1978) cause controversy in their reports that vitamin C increases the quality of life, as well as survival in patients with cancer. In the 1976 paper, they report that in one hundred terminal cancer patients, the mean survival was 4.2 times greater in subjects receiving ascorbate and state that vitamin C has a definite value in terminal cancer. Cameron and Campbell (1974) and Cameron, Campbell, and Jack (1975) have earlier publications regarding the use of high doses of ascorbic acid. The dose in these studies is 10 g/day given orally, although in their later paper Cameron and Pauling (1978) use vitamin C as a continuous intravenous infusion.

Recalling the limitation for the maximum concentration that can be achieved by the oral route, intravenous and/or oral dosing is a major point when discussing the use of vitamin C for therapeutic purposes (Borst 2008; Duconge et al. 2008). Padayattay et al. (2004) emphasizes that optimal dosing is critical to interventional studies using vitamin C and that adequate serum levels for cytotoxicity of cancer cells can only be achieved by the intravenous route. The major difference in reports regarding inefficacy of vitamin C use in cancer in the controlled study by Creagan et al. (1979) and "blind comparison" by Moertel et al. (1985) is the use of a dose of 10 g/day given orally with no intravenous infusion. Assouline and Miller (2006) define numerous pitfalls in these studies, including determination of the most biologically active dose, which tumor types might be the most sensitive, and the potentially confounding role of additional concomitant complementary and alternative modalities used. Hoffer et al. (2008) reports that ascorbic acid is selectively cytotoxic to many cancer cell lines. Using intravenous administration at higher doses than Cameron (1991), Hoffer et al. (2008) find that in patients with previously treated advanced malignancy, vitamin C fails to demonstrate anticancer activity and propose that prior treatment may have affected the cellular biology and selected for resistant cell types.

In looking at vitamin C use in cancer, it is necessary to remember the metabolic pathways. Padayatty and Levine (2001) emphasize that the maximum plasma level of ascorbic acid by oral administration is limited by renal excretion. Contraindications to high dose vitamin C are glucose 6-phosphate dehydrogenase deficiency and renal insufficiency (Padayatty et al. 2006). Padayatty et al. (2004) present evidence that the maximum tolerated dose of oral vitamin C is 18 g/day and produces peak plasma concentrations of about 200 mg/dl. Normal vitamin C plasma levels are 0.6mg/dl to 2 mg/dl, which are achieved by the nutritional guidelines of 250 mg of vitamin C per day (Haas and Levin 2006). Brubacher et al. (2000) state that in the general population the assumed optimal plasma concentration of vitamin C can be achieved by the intake of approximately 100 mg/day. By intravenous infusion, ascorbic acid serves as a pro-oxidant which is then oxidized to dehydroascorbic acid, considered the most potent antioxidant in extracellular fluid. This leads to generation of hydrogen peroxide with subsequent diffusion into the intracellular cytoplasm. This presumed mechanism for the cytotoxicity of cancer cells does not appear to affect normal cells and furthermore, antioxidant activity may be enhanced by lipoic acid, coenzyme Q 10, B complex vitamins, vitamin K3, and magnesium (Bahlis et al. 2002; Chen et al. 2005; 2007). Chen et al. (2005 2007), Paddayatty et al. (2004; 2006), and Bahlis et al. (2002) show that 30 g given intravenously achieves a serum concentration greater than 200 mg/dl, the level which was shown to cause in vitro cytotoxicity. Gonzales (2005) reports that an intravenous infusion of 60 g over sixty minutes, followed by an additional 20 g over sixty minutes, achieves serum levels of greater than 400mg/dl for four hours. Much of the controversy in reports regarding the efficacy of vitamin C use in cancer may be related to the fact that oral dosing cannot reach these pharmacologically effective plasma levels (Padayatty and Levine 2000).

Finally, other interesting aspects in the physiology of vitamin C were found. Padayatti et al. (2007) look at paracrine secretion from the adrenal gland and report finding that adrenal vein vitamin C release preceded that of adrenal vein cortisol. This suggests a link to a hormone-regulated vitamin C paracrine secretion that occurs as a part of the stress response. Bahr et al. (2008) also describe the release of vitamin C release from the adrenals in response to ACTH, although this is an animal study. Other studies attempt to link vitamin C and the IGF family with a possible role in insulin resistance and type II diabetes (Chen et al. 2005; Naidu et al. 2001 2003). Baynes (1991) and Chen, Jia, Qiu, and Ding (2005) show that changes in serum glucose levels affect the bioavailability of vitamin C and attenuate its actions, proposing that some of the secondary pathology found in diabetes may be vitamin C related.

Green Tea

Polyphenols in green tea are described in the literature for their antioxidant ability and chemoprotective role, as presented in chapter 1. Ovaskainen et al. (2008) present information supporting additional benefits of polyphenols when taken in natural form, including berries and coffee, rather than supplement form. This may relate to a combination of molecularly similar agents providing synergism of action and increased efficacy in the natural form. Other mechanisms of a beneficial effect include growth inhibition and apoptosis (Fujiki 1999), inhibition of hepatic growth factor signaling to potentially block invasive cancer growth (Bigelow and Cardelli 2006), and other relationships supporting tea consumption with a decreased risk of breast cancer (Zhang et al. 2007), including the folate pathway (Inoue et al. 2008). Variables consistently found in the literature include dosing, such as number of cups per day, which is definitely higher in Southeast Asia (>750 g/year) than Western society (Zhang et al. 2007). Zhang et al. (2007) and Yuan et al. (2005) discuss the inconsistency found in literature reports that may be explained epidemiologically by genetic differences in metabolism of the catechol-containing polyphenols.

Yuan et al. (2005) discuss the angiotensin-converting enzyme (ACE) genotype, and find that women with a low-activity ACE genotype have a reduced risk of breast cancer compared to those possessing a high-activity ACE genotype. Green tea polyphenols inhibit angiotensin II ROS production, and Yuan et al. (2005) propose that breast cancer protection occurs by this mechanism since ACE is involved in polyphenol metabolism and women with a low activity genotype have a lower ROS production.

Another mechanism producing an effect on ROS is shown by Wu et al. (2003) when they review the methylation of polyphenols by catechol-o-methyl transferase (COMT), and state that Asian Americans with the lowest risk of breast cancer have a low activity level of COMT, making them less efficient in eliminating tea catechins and thus receiving the most antioxidant benefit. Sun, Yuan, Koh, and Yu (2006) demonstrate that green tea decreases breast cancer risk, whereas black tea does not.

Isoflavones

Soy

In the case presented, soy products are used as part of the nutritional regimen. The relationship between soy intake and the risk of breast cancer is extensively studied in the literature. Soybeans are a dietary source uniquely rich in isoflavone phytoestrogens (Beecher 2003; Hilakivi-Clarke et al. 2004; Messina, McMaskill-Stevens, and Lampe 2006; Powles 2004; Setchell, Boriello, Hulme, Kirk, and

Axelson 1984). The types of isoflavones most often discussed are genistein and daidzen in soy (Messina et al. 2006) and quercitin, a red clover extract (Powles 2004). Soy is highly processed in the West as compared to Asian countries, and Allred et al. (2004) points out that natural soy, containing a complex mixture of bioactive compounds, is affected by processing by providing a more constant amount of genistein, thereby increasing estrogenicity. Missing from our knowledge-base is the systematic identification of the cellular and biochemical targets of isoflavones and the mechanism by which they produce their influence (Barnes 2004). Most of the effect of soy is thought to be in the competitive binding of estrogen receptors, or so-called "selective estrogen receptor modulator (SERM)" (Fabian and Kimler 2005; Setchell 2001).

Breast tissue is shown to concentrate isoflavones (Fabian, Kimler, Mayo, and Khan 2005; Hilakivi-Clarke et al. 2004; Medina 2005; Messina 1999; Setchell 2001; Wood et al. 2006), further pointing to their importance in breast cancer. Soy has no progesterone effect and may actually decrease serum progesterone levels (Messina 1999). Rice and Whitehead (2006) point out that it is not known whether phytoestrogens accumulate in tissues and whether they accumulate in conjugated forms (as they are mostly found in children) or in their free active form. Thus, the risk of developing breast cancer may be related to exposure early in life as seen in the decreased breast cancer risk in Southeast Asian migrants, with an increased risk occurring in subsequent generations (Rice and Whitehead 2006; Sowers et al. 2006).

Many studies demonstrate a benefit from soy in decreasing breast cancer risk, and emphasize the difference between Southeast Asian and Western populations (Barnes, Grubbs, Setchell, and Carlson 1990; Lampe et al. 2007; Maskarinec et al. 2004; Sarkar and Li 2003; Shanon et al. 2005; Trock et al. 2006). However, contradictory evidence is also presented (Daniells 2009; Martinez et al. 2006; Maskarinec et al. 2007; Messina 1999; Potischman et al. 1998; Touillard, Thiebault, Niravong, Boutron-Ruault, and Clavel-Chapelon 2006; Wu et al. 2007). In addition, information regarding timing of exposure during lifetime is discussed. Concentration of genistein in breast tissue from soy consumption during the neonatal and prepubertal time periods favors a protective role (Duffy, Perez, and Partridge 2007; Lamartiniere et al. 1995; Rice and Whitehead 2006; Ross 2006; Wu et al. 2002), and a protective aspect is shown with lifelong intake (Messina et al. 2006). This may be an important factor when comparing the difference in risk between Southeast Asian with Western populations (Wu et al. 2002 2007; Yamamoto, Sobue, Kobayashi, Sasaki, and Tsugane 2003), including an increased risk in Asian Americans in the second generation (Rice and Whitehead 2006), although even this can be controversial (Potischman 1998). Martinez et al. (2006) state that many variables make it difficult to apply assumptions to meta-analyses because of the heterogeneity in populations, genetics, metabolic differences, dose, and timing of intake during lifetime. Furthermore, Martinez et al. (2006) postulate that the potential increased risk of breast cancer is also related to other factors that predispose the woman to this disease. Wu et al. (2005) present data about decreased breast cancer risk with soy use, but this is a study related to short term intake (two months).

Maskarinec et al. (2009) find no change in mammographic density from soy consumption, while Atkinson et al. (2004) present the same for red clover. Aldercreutz et al. (1992) show data from in vitro and in vivo studies of phytoestrogens and the relationship to breast cancer risk. Setchell (2001) emphasizes the possibility that phytoestrogens may be a double-edged sword, beneficial to some groups while creating risks to others (effect may be estrogen or antiestrogen), and may be a dose-dependent response.

The above discussion primarily involves the interaction of phytosterols with estrogen. Maskarinec et al. (2004) postulate that the preventive effects of soy on breast cancer in premenopausal females may not be mediated by circulating sex hormones and encourage investigation of a different mechanism. Martinez et al. (2006), Rice and Whitehead (2006) and Sowers et al. (2006) point out other lifestyle factors that may be involved. Medina (2005) emphasizes research that has moved from the biological to the molecular level. Genistein, acting via inhibition of the TK pathway, may inhibit EGF activity promoting apoptosis (Akiyama et al. 1987; Akiyama and Ogawara 1991; Dampier et al. 2001; Dave et al. 2005; Ferry et al. 1996; Kim, Peterson, and Barnes 1998; Migliaccio et al. 1996; Peterson and Barnes 1991; Wang, Higuchi, and Zhang 1997), leading to inhibition of tumorigenesis. Cabanes et al. (2004) find prepubertal exposure to soy (genistein) or a low fat n-3 PUFA diet upregulates

BRCA-1 and other genes that may then lead to an increased ability to repair DNA.

Other mechanisms are seen. Su et al. (2005) discuss the antiangiogenic activity of genistein. Soy consumption lowers serum markers of inflammation, which is pertinent to cancer development (Willett 2007). Effects may also be mediated through the hormonal axis with insulin resistance and the metabolic syndrome playing a part (Azadbakht et al. 2007). Cooke, Selvaraj, and Yellayi (2006) and Jiang et al. (2008) introduce the concept and evidence for soy affecting the function of cells in the immune system.

Significant variables recognized in the use of soy, which may be generalized as far as vitamin C and other aspects of CAM (or allopathic pharmacotherapy for that matter), include the amount ingested, differences in metabolic utilization based on genetics, absorption, and the effect of gut flora.

Dosing itself has multiple variables. First of all, the amount of soy intake in Southeast Asian populations is much greater than in Western societies (Alderkreutz and Mazur 1997; de Kleijn et al. 2001; Messina et al. 2006). Rice and Whitehead (2006) point out that Eastern intake of soy amounts to the equivalent of 30 mg/day of genistein, whereas Western intake is less than 10 mg/day. There is no standardization in the processing of soy products, which then leads to the variable of intake being estimated rather than directly analyzed (Allred et al. 2004; Chen, Lin, and Hu 2007; Erdman, Badger, Lampe, Setchell, and Messina 2004; Setchell et al. 2003). Furthermore, processing removes molecularly similar substances that may work synergistically in the actions of soy. There may be difficulty in comparing the amount of isoflavones in various soy products, such as tofu, tempeh, or soyburgers. Even supplements may have different isoflavone concentrations (Manach, Scalber, Morand, Remsey, and Jimenez 2004; Setchell et al. 2003). Intermittent intake versus one large serving daily may also lead to different levels of serum activity (Manach et al. 2004; Setchell et al. 2003).

Genetic differences in populations where soy has been a basic foodstuff for centuries may play a part in the pharmacokinetics/ utilization/metabolism (Setchell 2001; Setchell et al. 1984). There can be genetic differences in a mixed population itself. In addition, absorption can affect bioavailability (Kano, Takayanagi, Harada,

Sawada, and Ishkawa 2006; Setcell et al. 2003), which brings up the question of intestinal function.

Availability and utilization of soy may be affected by intestinal flora. This includes absorption (Setchell et al. 2002), recycling (Chen et al. 2003), and conversion to more active metabolic forms (Atkinson, Frankenfeld, and Lampe 2005; Decross, Eekhaut, Possemieres, and Verstraete 2006). Although Nattleton et al. (2005) did not find that soy consumption and probiotics increased equol production. Another aspect of probiotics and prebiotics in general nutrition, besides their immune system effect, can be seen. Furthermore, it presents a variable between populations and even in the same population group when looking at results of a relationship between soy use and breast cancer.

The length of time of soy intake used in the studies reviewed is a further variable (Maskrinec et al. 2004; Nattleton et al. 2005; Wu et al. 2002). Timing of exposure during lifetime with regard to risk of breast cancer has been discussed previously (DeCroos et al. 2006; Duffy et al. 2007; Lamartiniere et al. 1995; Rice and Whitehead 2006; Ross 2006; Wu et al. 2002). Wu et al. (2005) present a study with only a two-month intake of soy, which ignores the potential importance of soy exposure early in life with long-term accumulation in tissues.

Red Clover

Red clover (trifolium pretense) contains various flavonoids, among these genistein and daidzen, as well as coumarin, a commonly used blood thinner (Atkinson et al. 2004). A common brand name for a red clover nutritional supplement is Promensil. Additional isoflavones found in red clover are demethylated in the liver to genistein and daidzen, felt to be the biologically most active forms (Atkinson et al. 2004). Red clover has primarily been used as an alternative method for treating menopausal symptoms, particularly hot flashes (Coon, Vittler, and Ernst 2007; Lathaby et al. 2007; Lukaczer, Darland, and Tripp 2005; van de Weijer and Barnsten 2002). One argument favoring natural sources, such as a tea infusion prepared from the plant, relates to the molecular variety of isoflavones available, again promoting improved utilization and function from natural sources that may provide an ideal spectrum of isoflavones compared to an isolated, chemically fabricated form (Powles 2004). Tsumoda, Pomeroy, and Nestel (2002) demonstrate that absorption is similar to soy. Related assimilation and metabolism also appears to be the same (Atkinson et al. 2004).

Sugar

Hyperglycemia is commonly manifest in cancer patients (Krone 2005) and high intakes of sugar and refined carbohydrates with subsequent elevation of blood sugar is strongly associated with an increased risk of cancer and possible decreased survival after cancer diagnosis (Talamini et al. 1997; Weindruch 1992; Wolf et al. 2005; Wu et al. 2007). Krone (2005) points out that hyperglycemia may affect the actions of ascorbic acid and the promotion of proper intracellular antioxidant function via the hexose monophosphate shunt. Many studies provide data that there is also an effect which influences sex hormone levels via insulin pathways, insulin resistance, and the metabolic syndrome (Forbes, Brown, Well, and Underwood 1989; Forouhi et al. 2005; Talamini et al. 1997; Wu et al. 2005 2007). Hyperglycemia also increases plasma markers of inflammation (Azerbakht et al. 2007). Del Giudice et al. (1998) link this to the hormonal axis via increased IGFBP-3 levels, again emphasizing metabolic pathways that are interrelated with effects in more than one aspect of the hormonal axis.

Other CAM

Other less studied CAM were reviewed. Brassica vegetables (Haas and Levin 2006) are shown to have an anti-proliferative effect that decreases breast cancer risk (Ambrosone 2004 2006; Brandi et al. 2005; Fowke et al. 2000 2003; Lampe and Peterson 2002; Smith-Warner et al. 2001). Alteration of hormone metabolism is presented with the use of cruciferous vegetables in this family (Auborn et al. 2003; Fowke et al. 2000 2003; Greenlee, Atkinson, Stanzyk, and Lampe 2007). Flaxseed, which has an ability to alter estrogen metabolism, is shown by Brooks et al. (2004) to have very similar actions compared with soy and is also used by the patient presented. Interval high-intensity exercise is shown to affect estrogen metabolism, likely on the basis of an increase in GH secretion that occurs with such exercise (Atkinson et al. 2004). This type of exercise regimen is promoted in hormone modulation programs in an attempt to stimulate GH levels naturally (personal communication with Cenegenics Medical Institute, Las Vegas).

The patient presented added IP-6 later in her course. Although there are no substantial clinical trials regarding IP-6 and the treatment of breast cancer, evidence is available on its use in prostate cancer (Singh et al. 2003). The mechanism is purported to be the ability of IP-6 to relay messages to the cell nucleus for gene transcription. This may block certain abnormal signals in cancer cells, leading to apoptosis and also possibly inhibit angiogenesis (Jariwalla 1999; Memorial Sloan-Kettering Cancer Center 2004; PDRHealth.com; Bucenik 2003). MGN-III appears to work on the immune system by bolstering activity of NK cells, TNF, and B and T lymphocytes (www.PDRHealth.com). These two agents, although considered investigational, demonstrate the pathways shared by general nutrition and pharmocotherapeutic agents.

Spirituality

The next area researched is one where there are no clear conclusions available, but one that appears to play a major role in the health of the patient presented. Integration of spirituality into the practice of medicine is elusive at best (Braverman 1987). There is no clear definition of the measurement of spirituality despite having been used for thousands of years. In addition, energy fields, so important in Ayurvedic and Chinese medicine, are abstract in Western thinking (Bruyere 1989). As demonstrated in chapter 1, prayer and meditation are among the modalities frequently used as CAM. Nevertheless, there is a relative lack of literature linking spirituality and health.

Religion is the man-made or developed system attempting to improve general health and well-being by teaching spirituality. Spirituality itself represents the capacity to change (Burke 1993; Dossey 1996; O'Hara 2002). Clarification of what is meant in this area includes five terms commonly used in nursing interventions: prayer, scripture, presence, listening, and referral (Emblen and Halstead 1993). Professional caregivers themselves have different experiences and attitudes (Kay and Robinson 1994; King, Sobil, Haggerty, Dent, and Patton 1992; Koeig, Bearon, and Dayringer

1989; Maugans and Wadland 1991). The healing significance of prayer has been used as far back as recorded history, and involves populations throughout the world and religious groups in the United States (al'Krenawi, Graham, and Maoz 1996; Berkel and de Waard 1983; Braverman 1987; Ellison 1995; Kaptchuk 2000; Kirchfield and Boyle 1994; Lad 2004; Spector 2004), each of which may have differing values.

When used in medicine, prayer is usually combined with other treatment modalities. Isolated cases accompanied with healing or cure by means of a "miracle" using religion/spirituality alone are frequently associated with skepticism (Abbot 2000; Astin, Harkness, and Ernst 2000; Levin and Banderpool 1987; Levin and Schiller 1987; O'Hara 2002). O'Hara (2002), Larson, Pattison, and Blazer (1986), and Orr and Isaac (1992) discuss the lack of literature regarding the power of prayer and health. Many reviews of medical, psychological, and social science literature affirm the positive link between spiritual motivation and well-being with improved general health (Burke 1993; Byrd 1988; Collipp 1969; Dossey 1993; Duckro and Magaletta 1994; Emblen and Halstead 1993; Kay and Robinson 1994), and increased life expectancy (Berkel and de Waard 1983; Hummer, Rogers, Nam, and Ellison 1999; Jarvis and Northcott 1987). Hilakivi-Clarke et al. (1994) discuss lifestyle aspects, including prayer, related to development and progression of breast cancer. Not all literature is conclusive as far as benefits (Bergin 1983; Glik 1999; Levin and Banderpool 1987; Levin and Schiller 1987; Propst, Ostrom, and Watkins 1992). Sered and Agigiani (2008) present the concept of holistic sickening, whereas Galantar (1997) states that reliance on prayer may prevent seeking complementary traditional medical treatment and promote harmful regimens.

Variables that exist in the literature include the significant heterogeneity among fifty-nine randomized clinical trials as reported by Abbot (2000), as well as heterogeneity and methodological limitations precluding a formal meta-analysis of twenty-three trials (Astin et al. 2000), making it difficult to draw definite conclusions about these studies. Orr and Isaac (1992) discuss the difficulty not only in defining the quality and quantity of prayer, but also how to assess and measure the same. Frequency of prayer as a qualitative measure of spirituality is presented by Walker and Anderson (1999). They state that the failure of clinical investigators to report on religious variables of their subjects may miss important factors related to their overall treatment. Assessment of quality requires a proper environment, which is difficult to control (O'Hara 2002). Furthermore, quality may have an individual variance (Poloma and Pendleton 1991). In the patient presented, an attitude of "Thy will be done" is certainly different then specific requests of God.

A combination of prayer with other treatment modalities (Ellison 1991) and population differences (al'Krenawi et al. 1996; Berkel and de Waard 1983; Ellison 1995) present additional variables. In fact, Berkel and de Waard (1983) point out that the prudent diet and prohibition of smoking in Seventh-Day Adventists may play a significant part in the health benefits seen in this group. Braverman (1987) describes the difficulty and potential inability to diagnose the spirituality of the individual patient from differences in interview techniques used by health-care professionals. Ellison (1991) states that it may be difficult to maintain religiosity as a constant variable throughout a study. The ability of a patient to use spiritual aspects can also affect social support and environmental variables, as well as determine an attitude toward related decisions and treatment overall (Jarvis and Northcott 1987). When patients are told, "there is no more to be done," Siegel (1986) states that a hug, hand-holding, or listening may still provide a positive benefit. The pertinence of methods used in the literature regarding spirituality suggests that a qualitative design research protocol may be the best method to evaluate spirituality as well as other elements of CAM (Kiene and von Schon-Angeror 1998; Walker and Anderson 1999).

A link with biological mechanisms can be postulated from some of the aforementioned discussion on cell physiology. Potential effects of prayer on biology of the human organism are presented by Cmich (1984), who emphasizes spirituality on a holistic basis. Measuring 8-hydroxydeoxyguanosine level in female subjects, perceived stress appears to be related to the pathogenesis of cancer via oxidative DNA damage (Irie, Asami, Nagata, Miyata, and Kasai 2001; Irie, Asami, Ikeda, and Kasai 2003). Additionally, the impact of stress on health by modulating the rate of cellular aging through the mechanism of accelerated telomere shortening is presented by Epel et al. (2004). These studies introduce the aspect of biological mechanisms, but do not identify a specific pathway. However the stress-linked hormonal response through the adrenal is well-known to be detrimental to health, presenting a complex link between spirituality and the hormonal axis.

EBM

Loewy (2007) points out that medical treatment consists of much more then prescribing drugs or operating on people. There is an art, as well as the science of medicine. Modern medicine currently follows a trend to develop the best available methods for objectively comparing and pooling results among multiple studies to determine the efficacy of an intervention or predictive power of an assessment technique (Gray 2008). Thus, it is important to review the relevance of evidence-based medicine (EBM) in terms of the effectiveness of CAM in the care of patients overall.

The term EBM can be traced to McMaster University in Canada in the 1980s (Rosenberg and Donald 1995) and was first published in 1992 (Evidence-Based Medicine Working Group). The term is now common in the medical work place, lay literature (Bavley 2009; Groopman and Hartzband 2009; Zimmerman 2009), and is spreading internationally (Ramana 2008). It has expanded to support the standard of care on a medical-legal basis, serves as a report card for physicians, and may form a basis to deny services by third party payers (Bavley 2009; Feldman, Novack, and Gracely 1998; Grace 2009; Groopman and Hartzband 2009; Iglehart 2009). Isaacs (1999) jokingly refers to other alternatives, among them "eminence-based medicine," "eloquence-medicine," and "nervousness-based medicine." Indeed, Loewy (2007) emphasizes the danger of detention of the thought process that could occur with EBM.

Although EBM is intended to solidify the science of medicine, Gupta (2003) also appraises it from a "state of the art" prospective. Prospective, randomized, meta-analysis and case-control studies are frequently used to present scientific support to a concept (Gillenwater and Gray 2003; Hicks 1995; Hughes 1996; McManus, Wilson, and Delaney 1998). Loewy (2007) further points out the weakness of double-blind studies. Other approaches may need to be used when dealing with populations and multiple risk factors for cancer (Bruzzi et al. 1985), including what Balducci (2000) describes as level IV-common sense. Interpretive bias is frequently involved in the evaluative process (Kaptchuk 2003).

Many uncontrolled variables exist in attempting an EBM evaluation of CAM (Antman et al. 2001; Loewy 2007; Weiger et al. 2002; White and Ernst 2002). Hoffer (2003) defines many of the barriers to practical testing of CAM, making it onerous to provide black-and-white evidence for the effectiveness of CAM. The difficulty in the scientific study of spirituality was covered previously. Many of the same variables exist in EBM studies of conventional allopathic treatments. Among these are age, ethnicity and genetics, metabolism, lifestyle habits including cultural and economic factors, patient beliefs and spirituality, environment, and the personal responsibility necessary for discipline in following certain regimens. Variables involved with the processing of nutritional supplements have been discussed in the sections on Vitamin C and soy (see chapter 4) as well in the section on nutrition (see chapter 1).

There may be a place for the best-case series published in the *Journal of the National Cancer Institute* (Nahin 2002; Vanchieri 2000), since patients may refuse randomization but still need to be treated. Many evidence-based protocols present results of a large statistical group of people which cannot simply be mindlessly applied to the individual patient (Loewy 2007). Alternatives to conventional means in research studies include uncontrolled clinical trials (White and Ernst 2001), randomized studies with patients having a choice to receive alternate therapies (Zelen 1979), single-case causality assessment (Kiene and von Schon-Angeror 1998), and using guidelines with scientific rigor in qualitative research when evaluating CAM within a research protocol (Bunne 1999; Hamberg, Johansson, Lindgren, and Westman 1994; Mallenrude 1993; Walker and Anderson 1999).

Hoffer (2003) also presents many valuable arguments regarding manners in which information is gathered to support the biologic and clinical plausibility for CAM. He points out that some CAM therapies, such as glucosamine or St.-John's-wort, can be easily tested using the design of randomized control trials (RCT) because they are simple drugs or druglike products with standard clinical indications. Many other CAM modalities are more difficult because of their complexity or nature of the alternative medicine philosophies from which they are derived. The most difficult point is performing a rigid RCT when dealing with the complex interrelationships that may involve metabolic pathways or the hormonal axis where it is nearly impossible to isolate one aspect when looking at its holistic response. Hoffer (2003) states that while the barriers to practical testing of CAM are real, they are not insurmountable, and suggests that the plausibility of several case studies evaluated with intellectual rigor (n-of-1 experiments) may be useful.

Much of what was accepted as EBM ten years ago has now changed since guidelines are based on the current existing evidence. Loewey (2007) proclaims that merely following an EBM protocol can be destructive to thinking and leads to inappropriate use. Medical professionals have years of training to develop experience. To be criticized by conventional medicine for using a "hunch" (experience is such a sixth sense) versus "hard facts" as being unscientific is discussed by Loewey (2007) and Hampshire (1989). They present this "hunch" as no less scientific then numbers or x-rays, but it certainly does not lend itself to EBM. Experience and judgment are necessary as well as hard scientific data in making good clinical decisions. Kiene and von Schon-Angeror (1998) support this concept when using CAM in patient care. Atwood (2004) presents many of the arguments between allopathic medicine and naturopathy, describing attitudes from both sides as far as pseudoscience, myths, fallacies, and truth. He emphasizes that validity of health claims may be influenced by political institutions, popularity, history, catch phrases ("emerging profession"), or other irrelevant means.

The trend in healthcare is the development of an "industry," (Rowe 2006; Sanderson 2006) with financial incentives for treatment (Loewy 2007; Peterson, Woodard, Urech, Daw, and Sookanan 2006; Sage and Kalyn 2006; Yong and Conrad 2007) and a preoccupation with profit (Rowe 2006; Sanderson 2006). Creeping into the picture, Pay-for-performance (P4P) may serve as a barrier to physician-patient relationships (Feldman et al. 1998; Sage and Kalyn 2006; val Krishnan, Dugan, Camacho, and Hall 2003; Yong and Conrad 2007). EMB may be used by payers to deny services (Grace 2009) and may lead to a conflict of interest among various providers in the system. For instance, the patient desires the best, most modern techniques for evaluation and treatment, while the physician is being evaluated by insurance carriers, hospitals, and attorneys as far as the utilization of resources, results, and costs. Financial incentives may be provided, such as from pharmaceutical companies to hospital formularies. Loewy (2007) argues that to be ethically valid, EBM must be aimed at the patients' best interests and not the financial interests of others.

If EBM suppresses curiosity and imagination, it gets in the way of the sort of speculation necessary for scientific progress (Loewy 1998). Loewy (1998) emphasizes that merely following an EBM is destructive to thinking. Loewy (2007) and Fitzgerald (1999) question if progress can be made without challenging the status quo and current habits. Halsted (www.Answers.com 2008; Cameron 1997; Lyons and Petrucelli 1978) and Osler (www.Answers.com 2008; Aequanimitas; Lyons and Petrucelli 1978) were pioneers in modern medicine and essential in developing the current system used in the United States for training physicians and surgeons. Both considered clinical wards as classrooms of the highest order with the concept of the physician as a clinician-scientist. Curiosity was encouraged to further investigation, and observations were accumulated to provide experience. Financial incentives in research provided by parties with a motive for cost-cutting and profit-gaining are adversaries of these attributes encouraged by Halsted and Osler. Fitzgerald (1999) believes that it is curiosity that converts strangers (the objects of analysis) into people with whom can be empathized. The overwhelming bulk of information available to the current practitioner and EBM may suppress the expression of curiosity and thought processes (the "art") (Fitzgerald 1999) by which advancement can be made in the "science" of medicine (Cushing 1919)

Summary

Biological pathways related to cell physiology, cancer development and treatment, and the hormonal axis are quite complex and interrelated. A review of similar mechanisms utilized by specific CAM modalities in the case presented attempts to establish a scientific link to CAM use in breast cancer. The incomplete understanding and inability to apply concrete proof is very difficult relying on current studies due to uncontrollable variables. These same variables also apply to EBM. Curiosity, observation, and experience continue to play in integral role for the clinician/scientist

Chapter Five

Conclusions

Introduction

The original purpose of this research study was to identify elements of CAM that may be useful in breast cancer. The focus changed into a more detailed review of cell physiology and the development of cancer with an attempt to link a scientific or biological basis to explain the effectiveness of CAM. This study is not meant to be comprehensive in these areas, but instead demonstrates that knowledge at this point is incomplete.

There is an increasing acceptance and use of CAM in breast cancer and other diseases. It is difficult to use EBM to support CAM with solid scientific evidence. Due to inherent flaws and many uncontrollable variables, EBM protocols cannot be accepted without question. In addition, blindly following EBM hinders curiosity and ignores experience gained from serial observation, resulting in a detriment to the advancement of science. Certain aspects of a qualitative review design are probably the most beneficial means in identifying the effectiveness of CAM. The information presented supports a holistic approach to health with the overall organism regulating internal mechanisms if given the proper support.

Conclusions and Implications

CAM

Despite reports negating its usefulness, there is no question of an increasing awareness and use of CAM worldwide. Middle-age white females with a college education and higher economic status appear to form the principle group accepting CAM. This economic level may allow affordability of a CAM modality when not covered by insurance, but an increased interest in self-education and improvement is also seen. A pervasive feeling of hopelessness, sadness, fear, and anxiety associated with a diagnosis of breast cancer enables those with discipline and personal responsibility to find CAM helpful in assuming control of their own health. Disease cure may be one goal, but symptom control and an increased "quality of life" are important considerations.

However, no "magic bullet" is identified despite attempts to thoroughly research literature on CAM modalities used by the patient presented. To be fair, the same applies to many allopathic treatments. As far as the scientific basis for CAM, this study focuses on modalities used in the case presentation. Effectiveness of CAM also appears to be a reflection of a basic mind-set of those using CAM, simply portraying healthy behaviors undertaken by these individuals. Those taking supplements tend to look at general lifestyle changes overall and maintain a personal responsibility that accompanies spirituality. This supports a holistic approach.

Antioxidants

Vitamin C is one of the more commonly used and extensively studied CAM modalities. The antioxidant protective effect on DNA from vitamin C and green tea is well accepted. With vitamin C, the mechanism of cytotoxicity in cancer cells occurs via pro-oxidants and the generation of hydrogen peroxide in the extracellular space. The gray area using antioxidants as an effective modality in breast cancer pertains to dosing. Clinical studies in the literature achieve effective plasma concentrations of ascorbate by using an intravenous infusion. Oral dosing is limited in reaching the serum levels needed for cytotoxicity of cancer cells. However, other benefits of vitamin C may still be attained.

An important variable when attempting to compare studies regarding the effectiveness of polyphenols in green tea involves the number of cups of tea ingested daily to be useful. No standard amount is established. In addition, there may be a difference between natural and manufactured sources of antioxidants. Molecularly similar structures to ascorbate found in fruits and vegetables or other polyphenols that are present in a prepared natural green tea infusion lead to the possibility that multiple substances in natural or whole foods, working synergistically, may lead to a greater benefit. Finally, a relationship between antioxidants and IGF with effects on the hormonal axis likely plays a part in their effectiveness.

Soy

Since hormonal manipulation is a well-accepted method in the treatment of breast cancer, it was initially felt that soy and red clover use may be the beneficial CAM in the case presented. The most biologically active agent in soy that produces a pharmacologic response is genistein. Red clover provides an isoflavone that serves as a precursor to genistein. Small amounts of genistein have an antiestrogen effect, whereas a higher dose demonstrates more estrogenlike qualities.

Again, several variables are identified related to the use of these substances. First of all, the timing of exposure, emphasizing that during prepubertal and neonatal years soy is protective, may be more important than later soy use, such as in the postmenopausal female, or after a cancer has been diagnosed. Second, variation in the amount ingested includes several factors. Differences exist in amounts of soy used by Southeast Asian compared to Western populations. There is no good control as far as the amount of genistein found in different soy products. Processing is more common in the West and may affect the amount of isoflavones available. Thus, pharmacologically different responses can be expected. There can also be a difference related to a large single dose compared to ingesting soy throughout the day. Third, there is the genetic variable, which may affect metabolism, when attempting to compare two separate groups or even individuals within the same population. Additionally, Southeast Asian women generally have early-age exposure more commonly than those in the United States. Finally, intestinal flora affects absorption and metabolism, which can differ even among individuals of the same population. This introduces the concept of probiotics playing another role besides immune system enhancement.

Basic Nutrition

Basic nutrition serves to provide an energy source as well as building blocks for the "human machine." At present, the human organism itself appears to be the most effective means to balance metabolic processes and to manufacture what is needed if provided with proper substrates. Complicated pathways exist and interact with a complex hormonal axis. The use of antioxidants as built-in free radical scavengers protect DNA and normal gene signaling with resulting apoptosis of worn out or improperly functioning cells. Probiotics affect metabolism in soy intake and also promote a healthy immune system overall. These concepts further support a holistic approach.

Spirituality

Spirituality was another area researched since it appears to be a strong point in the recovery of the patient presented. Representing a nontangible CAM modality, prayer is frequently practiced but is difficult to quantify and also to identify quality. One of the strongest links of spirituality to a scientific basis may be its relationship to the stress/hormonal axis.

An interesting concept is one explored by Siegel (1986). Stating that when patients profess their disease is not stressful, he attempts to learn if this is performance or the truth. According to Siegel, cancer and death may not be stressful if "it's a solution to life's problems" (p. 80). There is much lacking in the understanding how attitudes can affect the immune system. Spirituality displays personal responsibility, a basic concept of natural medicine.

Hormonal axis

The hormonal axis is complex and incompletely understood. Multiple interrelationships make control of one hormone without eliciting a response in another portion of the axis virtually impossible. Besides pharmacologic manipulation, the hormonal axis can be affected by diet, blood glucose, exercise, and stress. There are endocrine (systemic) effects as well as autocrine (self) and paracrine (neighboring) effects from endogenous hormones or hormonelike substances secreted by normal or tumor cells. These, in turn, may further lead to subsequent changes in the hormonal axis and also explain paraneoplastic syndromes that are seen with various tumors. Hormones have different effects depending on serum levels. Estrogen itself, in certain situations, is shown to have cytotoxic properties.

Hormonal manipulation, one of the principle therapies currently used in breast cancer, targets sex hormones and cell membrane hormone receptors. Potential effects involving the IGF family and the hormonal axis are presented. Controversy surrounds the role of GH and IGFs on cancer risk, and there appears to be a fine balance between levels of GH aimed at prevention of degenerative conditions and those levels that may lead to the development of cancer. Controversy also exists on what serum levels of various factors in the IGF family—IGF-I, IGF-II, IGFRPs, and IGFBPs—are significant. IGFBP seems to be a reliable marker of cancer risk, but a concomitant relationship with other factors in the IGF family needs to be considered. Again, the fine balance and complex interrelationship that exists within the hormonal axis is evident.

IGF is well documented as far as an effect on telomeres and apoptosis. Mechanisms of chemotherapy attempt to target angiogenesis and apoptosis via biological pathways involving various GFs. Similar pathways are shared by members of the IGF family. Thus, targeting areas such as angiogenesis by one mechanism can, in this manner, subsequently affect the hormonal axis by feedback. Melatonin influences GH secretion and brings up the possibility of a circadian rhythm relationship to cell function and may provide one reason the novel approach of metronomic dosing in chemotherapy is useful.

Holistic Approach

Cell Biology/Physiology

The literature search repeatedly portrays the extreme complexity and interrelationships in the physiological pathways involved in the development of breast cancer as well as its treatment. Within the hormonal axis, attempts to affect one hormone in a pathway may have uncontrollable consequences in another area. When looking at the breadth of the material presented in this study, a lack of complete understanding of these pathways can be seen. In addition, absence of a biologically plausible explanation for the so-called "spontaneous regression" seen in some cancer patients supports a contention that the practice of medicine today is 20% science and 80% experience and judgment. Regarding cell physiology and complex pathways, such as the hormonal axis, a fundamental question remains. Science may have identified a certain mechanism, but leaves unanswered, "What actually tells a specific cell to function as it does?"

Cancer

The concept that cancer is a disease of clonal evolution is introduced by Nowell (1976). Hanahan et al. (2000) describe cancer as a dynamic process, and Merlo et al (2007) call it a microcosm of evolution. Moritz (2008) presents a unique perspective describing cancer as a survival mechanism of the body rather than a disease. He asserts that cancer is the final attempt of the human organism to live by altering cells to survive in a toxic environment. Without dealing with the underlying cause for the development of cancer cells, treatments that attempt to eliminate these very cells, which have mutated for survival, represent an incomplete approach. Detoxification, as well as proper nutrition, should be considered jointly in cancer care and treatment. A balance between allopathic treatment and natural medicine is encouraged.

The philosophy of natural medicine supports the contention that symptoms of disease result from the body's response in an attempt to heal itself. Disease and treatment should be approached in a holistic fashion, not just focusing on symptoms. In his Nobel prize acceptance speech, Albert Szent-Gyorgi uses such a philosophy:

> The medical profession itself took a very narrow and very wrong view. Lack of ascorbic acid caused scurvy, so if there was no scurvy there was no lack of ascorbic acid. Nothing could be clearer than this. The only trouble is that scurvy is not the first symptom of that lack but a final collapse, a

premortal syndrome and there is a very wide gap between scurvy and full health (Li and Schellhorn 2007).

Cancer itself should be approached as a systemic disease, and this concept is emphasized in allopathic medicine by the frequent use of adjuvant therapies with various tumors.

Proper nutrition shares similar pathways utilized by some chemotherapy and immunotherapy, generally supporting the overall function of the organism; again, the holistic approach. Chemobrain, a degree of cognitive impairment frequently seen in patients receiving chemotherapy (Wefel et al. 2004), further demonstrate one of the systemic effects of cancer treatment. This condition is approached through attempts to restore cerebral health and function by supplying nutrients utilized specifically by nerve cells.

Curiosity, Observation, and Experience

Evaluation of CAM is difficult using case-controlled or randomized studies. Too many variables are present. Among population studies, differences in genetics and metabolism, lifestyle aspects, including diet and exercise, and environmental exposure are some of the principle variables noted. Varying attitudes and "faith in God" are apparent in spirituality. The effectiveness of CAM also seems to be a reflection of a basic mind-set of those using these modalities and simply portray healthy behaviors undertaken by these individuals. Personal responsibility accompanies spirituality. The attitude of those taking supplements frequently leads to lifestyle changes overall, supporting the holistic approach.

There is no regulation of type or amount of substances present in nutritional supplements, vitamins, or other natural products including foodstuffs. The so-called pharmaceutical grade is lacking. Based on processing and amount used, the variability in products prevents reproducibility and comparison in some studies. Furthermore, it may be difficult to specifically define which active ingredients are present that produce the desired effect. A healthy diet consists of a combination of substances, which may elicit a varied response between manufactured and whole food sources. Using a combination of foods or supplements may produce a different and greater response compared to a single agent. Furthermore, a variety of very similar molecular compounds in whole foods or natural sources that work synergistically could produce an entirely different response than that of a chemically pure supplement.

EBM attempts to provide the best scientific evidence to support treatment protocols. Methods used in EBM are not ideal for studies of CAM. Walker and Anderson (1999) and Kiene and von Schon-Ageror (1998) discuss development of research protocols using a qualitative research design in the study of spirituality. The pertinence of this method could be expanded to evaluation of other areas of CAM. The National Cancer Institute best-case series are not scientifically proven cases, as in the patient presented in this research project, but demonstrate that observations of biologic plausibility play a role and warrant further exploration. An attempt to use EBM methods to explain the efficacy of CAM is flawed by the multiple variables discussed previously with the individual modalities. Current treatment protocols developed through EBM for allopathic practice can also be criticized using these same variables.

In their teaching, Halsted and Osler emphasized observation on the hospital wards, which they highly encouraged in their clinician-scientist students. An example of an observation by this researcher is the following:

> Occasionally, some postsurgical patients will complain that they have lost their sense of taste. Zinc deficiency is a subtle condition with no overt signs, but a restoration of taste and even improvement in healing of chronic wounds is seen with the administration of a zinc supplement. Most wound-care centers routinely provide zinc in the nutritional regimen for their patients.

Earlier in chapter 1, discussing the role of *Brassica* (cruciferous) vegetables in hormone modulation, Fowke et al. (2000) and Gaudet et al. (2004) point out that isothiocyanates found in these food sources may impart a bitter taste in patients with cancer. Although there is no clear-cut explanation, a relationship to the observation with zinc suggests something similar. Although there is room for speculation as to the cause and its significance, consideration of general nutritional support in treatment follows a holistic approach.

Taking the principle of observation a step further, Huggins received the Nobel Prize in 1966 for his work showing that testosterone stimulated the growth of prostate cancer (Huggins 1941). Since then, the medical profession has considered testosterone as a risk factor for developing prostate cancer, and many believe that testosterone replacement therapy is dangerous and increases the risk of developing prostate cancer. Morgentaler (1996) reports findings that did not fit this pattern. At a national meeting of the American Urologic Association, he was strongly criticized by experts in the field, and responds to them during the initial presentation of his 1996 paper:

> These are the results we obtained We present them here because they do fly in the face of conventional wisdom, which is why we believe they may be of interest to this audience. (Morgentaler 2008)

Subsequently, Rhoden and Morgentaler (2004) and others referenced in this same 2004 paper point out that not a single study in human patients exists to suggest that raising testosterone levels increases the risk of prostate cancer. So, raising deficient testosterone levels does not appear to be "food for a hungry tumor" (Morgentaler 2008, p. 51). In 2004, the Institute of Medicine, a branch of the National Academy of Sciences, summarizes that the influence of testosterone on prostate carcinogenesis and other prostate outcomes remains poorly defined (Morgentaler 2008). However, there is still reluctance in conventional medicine to even consider testosterone replacement for fear of causing prostate cancer.

Morgentaler (2008) further describes his detailed analysis of Huggins's original paper, and finds that Huggins's assertion that higher testosterone caused greater growth of prostate cancer, reported for so long and accepted as gospel, was based on almost nothing at all. This observation by Morgentaler is subsequently supported by further reports in the field and has led to some practitioners providing testosterone replacement in deficient patients for the cardiovascular and metabolic benefits without the fear which arose with Huggins's report. This would not have occurred blindly following an EBM or conventional wisdom policy based on the Huggins's information and discounting an observation that obviously ran counter to current philosophy. Experience gained from observations leads to the advancement of knowledge.

Based on curiosity as a characteristic of the true scientific mind, a series of observations leads to experience. Experience leads to judgment in attempting to individualize treatment for a specific patient. EBM can be used as a guide, but should not be accepted without question. Observation and experience cannot be ignored. There is no "magic bullet." At this point it appears the human machine, when provided with the necessary substrates and following a disciplined routine, has the best mechanism to heal itself.

George W. Hogeboom (1894), in his president's address to the Kansas Medical Society in 1894:

> Every learned profession is subject to popular prejudice. The skill and learning of individuals vary, differences of theory inevitably arise in every profession calling for judgment and opinion. The extreme view would hold every theologian to be a hypocrite, every lawyer to be a rogue, and every doctor to be a quack, because, forsooth, theology is founded upon faith, the lawyer occasionally defends a rascal in court and sustains a losing cause, and doctors are often unable to agree as to what ails a sick man . . . . The medical profession is empirical only in the sense that all scientific pursuit is empirical, but it is the true empiricism—starting from the basis of absolute knowledge and trying all things and holding fast to that which is good. Whatever reproach may have rested upon the medical science in the past for a stubborn adherence to mere tradition and ideas and theories, there can be no doubt of its recent rapid advancement, and this advancement is strictly upon scientific lines. If any criticism can now be entertained, it is not that we are going ahead too slowly, but that enraptured with new ideas, stimulated by new and pregnant suggestions and discoveries, we may not be conservative enough.

Although this address was given over one hundred years ago, there is much that is still pertinent.

Implications for Future Research

CAM should be approached in an open-minded fashion. There is no question that alternative methods are being explored by more and more patients. Allopathic medical practitioners should be aware of this increased acceptance and use of CAM, considering its potential usefulness in the treatment armamentarium with an emphasis on nutrition and detoxification. Many patients appear to be seeking a "magic bullet" out of desperation, and with no regulating agency for "natural" products, studies promoting intelligent and safe choices need to be developed. It is not clear whether this would be better served by a government agency, such as the FDA, or private institutions that do not have a financial interest invested in products. Whichever route is used, outside influence from parties with financial gain from current treatment methods must be avoided. Nonetheless, increased acceptance and use is a factor that cannot be ignored.

This study demonstrates the biologic plausibility of CAM in the treatment of breast cancer. This can be expanded to other cancers as well as chronic and degenerative conditions. Focusing on mechanisms of host resistance, using agents to bolster natural defenses is a reasonable goal. This emphasis should be a "holistic" approach, with nutrition and detoxification being primary areas that can be investigated. Further study is needed into biological and physiologic pathways supporting the effectiveness of CAM. How this can be developed into a research protocol is not entirely clear. The number of uncontrollable variables presents an almost overwhelming obstacle in standard research protocols, but a qualitative research design appears to be the most appropriate. An example is the effect of sugar in the diet that may feed into the hormone axis via IGF-1, realizing that changing one variable may have uncontrollable effects in other areas.

Looking at the molecular profile that distinguishes cancer cells from "normal" tissue, a research goal should be to continue to develop ways to manipulate the cancer cells or organism itself to improve the prognosis of patients (Steeg and Theodorescu 2008). In addition, the proposal of cancer development as a survival mechanism (Moritz 2008) could change attitudes and lead to alternate areas in the study of cancer and its treatment. This is not to say that current treatment methods should be abandoned, but a plea is made to expand research to incorporate strong nutritional and detoxification programs into the overall treatment plan.

EBM has been integrated into the current health-care "industry." Insurance company executives looking for a profitable program and government agencies attempting to control costs promote EBM protocols as gospel in today's healthcare. Some EBM accepted as such twenty years ago has changed to other guidelines now accepted as "standard of care." Thinking outside the box is part of the scientific mind which utilizes curiosity, observation, and experience to develop innovative practices. In addition, when developing or trying new methods, practitioners should have their patient's health and well-being at the forefront, avoiding financial incentives that might be gained from selling products. Although the "snake oil" reputation of many traveling practitioners or salesmen one hundred years ago is remembered, it should be pointed out that the omega-3 oils found in that particular product may have had an unrecognized scientific-based benefit. However, many other products were pushed on unwary customers with unsupported or placebo effects only. Curiosity, observation, and experience support a qualitative research design as a potential method for further studies related to CAM. Nevertheless, further exploration of CAM is scientifically pertinent to present-day care of patients.

Third-party payer coverage should also be on the forefront. Patients are accepting CAM and more allopathic health professionals are taking an open-minded approach to CAM. There is a stream of continued and updated information available on the internet. Overall methods that have a holistic aspect, such as nutrition and detoxification, can be more easily accepted than trying to consider coverage for supplements taken as a "magic bullet." Some supplements, such as CoQ10, are simply extensions of a good nutritional program. However, there still needs to be financial incentive available, not only for the patient but also the insurance company, to be able to advance the use of CAM. It would be interesting to see the effect of CoQ10, magnesium, and potassium supplementation on patients with congestive heart failure, which is the diagnosis related to the largest number of patients hospitalized annually. CoQ10 is not extremely expensive, particularly when looking at the cost of drugs used to treat congestive heart failure, but is out of reach of older patients on a fixed income, particularly if they have to pay for some of their other medications. Also, for patients to be able to take a responsibility in personal health-care decisions, appropriate options need to be available

Summary

Referring to CAM as well as conventional allopathic treatments, there is no "magic bullet." Much information is yet to be discovered in understanding cellular and physiological processes involved in supporting a healthy organism. The weakness of this study is the obvious lack of concrete proof for the effectiveness of CAM in controlled studies. Until researchers are able to develop specific protocols that precisely control all variables, there will continue to be controversy regarding the effectiveness of CAM. Among the strengths is the non bias of the researcher, who has a strong allopathic background. The breadth of the material presented and the increasing acceptance of CAM leads to the observation of biologic plausibility of some modalities. At the present time, a holistic approach using the God-given mechanisms of the human organism is the best chance for health. With the widespread acceptance and use of CAM, an open-minded approach by allopathic medical professionals and third-party payers is justified. Finally, the true wonder of the "human machine" cannot be negated.

References

Abbot, N. C. (2000). Healing as a therapy for human disease: A systematic review. *Journal of Alternative and Complimentary Medicine,* 6, 159-169.

Abdullah, A. S., Lau, Y., and Chow, L. W. (2003). Pattern of alternative medicine usage among the Chinese breast cancer patients: Implication for service integration. *American Journal of Chinese Medicine,* 31, 649-658.

Achat, H., Kawachi, I., Byrne, C., Hankinson, S., and Colditz, G. (2000). A prospective study of job strain and risk of breast cancer. *International Journal of Epidemiology,* 29, 622-628.

Adler, S. R. (1999). Complementary and alternative medicine use among women with breast cancer. *Medical Anthropology Questions,* 13, 214-222.

Adler, S. R., and Fosket, J. R. (1999). Disclosing complementary and alternative medicine use in the medical encounter: A qualitative study in women with breast cancer. *Journal of Family Practice,* 48, 453-458.

Aequanimitas. Celebrating the contributions of William Osler. Retrieved September 15 2008, from *http://www.medicalarchives.jhmi.edu/osler/arquessay.htm*

Agudo, A., Cabrera, L., Amiano, P., Ardanaz, E., Barricarte, A., Berenguer, T., et al. (2007). Fruit and vegetable intakes, dietary antioxidant nutrients, and total mortality in Spanish adults: Findings from the Spanish cohorts of the European Prospective Investigation into Cancer and Nutrition (EPIC) in Spain. *American Journal of Clinical Nutrition*, 85, 1634-1642.

Agurs-Collins, T., Adams-Campbell, L. L., Kim, K. S., and Cullen, K. J. (2000). Insulin-growth factor-I and breast cancer risk in post menopausal Africa-American women. *Cancer Detection and Prevention*, 24, 199-206.

Akiyama, T., Ishida, J., Nakagawa, S., Ogawara, H., Watanabe, S., Itoh, N., et al. (1987). Genistein, a specific inhibitor of tyrosine-specific protein kinases. *Journal of Biological Chemistry*, 262, 5592-5595

Akiyama, T., and Ogawara, H. (1991). Use and specificity of genistein as inhibitor of protein-tyrosine kinases. *Methods in Enzymology* 201, 362-370.

al-Krenawi, A., Graham, J. R., and Maoz, B. (1996). The healing significance of NEGEV's BEDOUIN DERVISH. *Social Science in Medicine*, 43, 13-21.

Albanes, D. (1987). Calorie intake, body weight and cancer: A review. *Nutrition and Cancer*, 9, 199-204.

Aldercreutz, H., Mousavi, Y., Clark, J., Hockerstadt, K., Hamalainen, E., Walhala, K. et al. (1992). Dietary phytoestrogens and cancer: in vitro and in vivo studies. *Journal of Steroid Biochemistry and Molecular Biology*, 41, 331-337.

Aldercreutz, H., and Mazur, W. (1997). Phyto-estrogens and Western diseases. *Annals of Internal Medicine*, 29, 95-120.

Alferi, S. M., Antoni, M. H., Ironson, G., Kilbourn, K. M., and Carver, C. S. (2001). Factors predicting the use of complementary therapies in a multi-ethnic sample of early breast cancer patients. *Journal of the American Medical Womens Association*, 56, 20-123.

Algner, C. (1998). Advice in health food stores. *Nutrition Forum*, 5, 1-4.

Allain, D., Gilligan, M. A., and Redlich, P. N. (2002). Chapter 14: Genetics and genetic counseling for breast cancer. In Donegan, W. L., and Spratt, J. S. (Eds.), *Cancer of the breast*, (5th ed.). Philadelphia: Saunders.

Allen, R. G., and Tresini, M. (2000). Oxidative stress and gene regulation. *Free Radicals in Biology and Medicine*, 28, 463-499.

Allegra, J. C. and Kiefer, J. M. (1985). Mechanism of action of progestational agents. *Seminars in Oncology*, 12 (71), 3-9.

Allred, C. D., Allred, K. F., Ju, Y. H., Goeppinger, T. S., Doerge, D. R., and Helferich, W. G. (2004). Soy processing influences growth of estrogen-dependent breast cancer tumors. *Carcinogenesis*, 25, 1649-1657.

Ambrosone, C. B. (2004). Breast cancer risk in pre menopausal women is inversely associated with consumption of broccoli, a source of isothiocyanate, but is not modified by GST genotype. *Journal of Nutrition*, 134, 1134-1138.

Ambrosone, C. B. (2006). Epidmiological evidence for chemo protective effects of cruciferous vegetables on cancer risk. *American Association of Clinical Research Meeting Abstract*, April 1 2006 (1), 1365.

American Cancer Society. (2002). *Cancer facts and figures*. Atlanta, Ga: American Cancer Society.

American Cancer Society. (2003). Revised ACS guidelines for nutrition, exercise for cancer survivors. *CA: A Cancer Journal for Clinicians*, 53, 268-291.

American Institute for Cancer Research. (1997). *Food, nutrition and the prevention of cancer: A global perspective*. Washington, D.C.: The Institute.

Ames, F. C. and Balch, C. M. (1990). Management of local and regional recurrence after mastectomy or breast-conserving treatment. *Surgical Clinics of North America*, 70, 1115-1124.

Amos, B. and Lotan, R. (1990). Retinoid-sensitive cells and cell lines. *Methods in Enzymology*, 190, 217-225.

Andre, F., Slimane, K., Bachelot, T., Dunant, A., Namer, M., Barrelier, A., et al. (2004). Breast cancer with synchronous metastases: Trends and survival during a 14-year period. *Journal of Clinical Oncology*, 22, 3302-3308.

Ang Lee, M. K.; Moss, J., and Yuan, C. S. (2001). Herbal medicines in peri-operative Care. *Journal of the American Medical Association*, 286, 208-216.

Angell, M., and Kassirer, J. P. (1998). Alternative medicine—the risks of untested and unregulated remedies. *New England Journal of Medicine*, 339, 839-841.

Antman, K., Benson, M. C., Chabot, J., Cobrenik, D., Grann, V. R., Jacobson, J. S., et al. (2001). Complementary and Alternative Medicine: The Role of the Cancer Center. *Journal of Clinical Oncology* 19 (supplement), 55s-60s.

Armstrong, B., and Doll, R. (1975). Environmental factors in cancer incidents and mortality and different countries, with special reference to dietary practices. *International Journal of Cancer*, 15, 617-631.

Armstrong, B. (1976). Recent trend in breast cancer incidence and mortality in relation to changes in possible risk factors. *International Journal of Cancer*, 17, 204-211.

Arriagada, R., Rutqvist, L. E., Mattsson, A., Kramar, A., and Rotstein, S. (1995). Adequate locoregional treatment for early breast cancer may prevent secondary dissemination. *Journal of Clinical Oncology*, 13, 2869-2878.

Arrigoni, O., and de Tullio, M. C. (2002). Ascorbic acid: Much more than just an antioxidant. *Biochimica Biophysica Acta,* 1569, 1-9.

Asplund, K. (2002). Antioxidant vitamins and the prevention of cardiovascular disease: A systematic review. *Journal of Internal Medicine,* 251, 372-392.

Assouline, S., and Miller, W. H. (2006). High-dose vitamin C therapy: Renewed hope or a false promise? *Canadian Medical Association Journal,* 174, 1503-1507.

Astin, J. A. (1998). Why patients use alternative medicines: Results of a national study. *Journal of the American Medical Association,* 279, 1548-1553.

Astin, J. A., Harkness, A. E., and Ernst, E. (2000). The efficacy of "distant healing": A systematic review of randomized studies. *Annals of Internal Medicine,* 132, 903-910.

Astin, J. A., Marie, A., Pelletier, A. R., Hansen, E., and Haskell, W. L. (1998). A review of the incorporation of complementary and alternative medicine by mainstream physicians. *Archives of Internal Medicine,* 158, 2303-2310.

Atkinson, C., Lampe, J. W., Tworoger, S. S., Ulrich, C. M., Bowen, D., Irwin, M. G., et al (2004). Effects of a moderate intensity exercise intervention on estrogen metabolism in postmenopausal women. *Cancer Epidemiology Biomarkers and Prevention,* 13, 868-874.

Atkinson, C., Frankenfeld, C. L., and Lampe, J. W. (2005). Gut bacterial metabolism of the soy isoflavone daidzein: Exploring the relevance to human health. *Experimental Biology and Medicine,* 230, 155-170.

Atkinson, C., Warren, R. M. L., Sala, E., Dowsett, M., Dunning, A. M., Healey, C. S., et al. (2004). Red clover-derived isoflavones and mammographic breast density: A double-blind, randomized, placebo-controlled trial [ISRCTN4294065]. *British Cancer Research,* 6, R170-R179.

Atwood, A. C. (2004). Naturopathy, pseudoscience, and medicine: myths and fallacies vs. truth. Posted March 25 2004 on *Medscape /General medicine,* 6: e53. Retrieved October 3 2008 from http.//www.medscape.com/viewarticle/471156

Auborn, K. J., Fan, S., Rosen, E. M., Goodwin, L., Chandrasken, A., Williams, D., et al. (2003). Indole-3-carbinol is a negative regulator of estrogen. *Journal of Nutrition,* 133, 2470S-2475S.

Azadbakht, L., Kimiager, M., Mehrabi, Y., Esmaillzadeh, A., Hu, F, D., and Willett, W. C. (2007). Soy consumption, markers of inflammation, and endothelia function. *Diabetes Care,* 30, 967-973.

Baer, H. J., Schnitt, S. J., Connolly, J. L., Byrne, C., Cho, E., Willett, W. C., et al. (2003). Adolescent diet and instance of proliferative benign breast disease. *Cancer Epidemiology Biomarkers and Prevention,* 12, 1159-1167.

Bahlis, M.J., McCafferty-Grady, J., Jordan-McMurry, I., Neil, J., Reis, I., Kharfan-Debaja, M., et al. (2002). Feasibility and correlates of arsenic trioxide combined with ascorbic acid-mediated depletion of intracellular glutathione for the treatment of relapsed/refractory multiple myeloma. *Clinical Cancer Research,* 8, 3658-68.

Bahr, V., Pfeiffer, A. F., and Oelkers, W. (2008). Is there a need for vitamin C supplementation of the normal diet? Effects of in vivo ascorbate depletion on adrenal function. *American Journal of Clinical Nutrition,* 87,191-195.

Baidas, S. M., Winer, E. P., Fleming, G. F., Harris, L., Pluda, J. M., Crawford, J. G., et al. (2000). Phase II evaluation of thalidomide in patients with metastatic breast cancer. *Journal of Clinical Oncology,* 18, 2710-2717.

Balducci, L. (2000). Evidence-based management of cancer in the elderly. *Cancer Controls,* 7, 368-376.

Balneaves, L. G., Bottorff, J. L., and Hislop, T. G. (2006). Level of commitment: exploring complementary therapy use by women with breast cancer. *Journal of Alternative and Complementary Medicine,* 12, 459-466.

Bammer, K., and Newberry, B. H. (Eds). (1981). *Stress and cancer.* Toronto: C. J. Hogrefe.

Bando, H. (2007). The treatment of primary breast cancer: Surgical approach. *Gan To Kagaku Ryoho,* 34, 849-852.

Baral, E., Larson, L. E., and Mattsson, B. (1977). Breast cancer following irradiation of the breast. *Cancer,* 40, 2905-2910.

Barja, G., Lopez-Torres, M., Peree-Camdo, R., Rojas, C., Cadenas, S., Prat, J., et al. (1994). Dietary vitamin C decreases endogenous protein oxidative damage, malondialdehyde, and lipid peroxidation and maintains fatty acid saturation in guinea pig liver. *Free Radicals in Biology and Medicine,* 17, 105-115.

Barnes, P., Powell Griner, E., McFann, K., and Nahin,R. (2002). Complementary and alternative medicine use among adults: United States. *Advanced Data,* 343, 1-19.

Barnes, S. (2004). Soy isoflavones-phytoestrogens and what health? *Journal of Nutrition,* 134, 1225S-1228S.

Barnes, S., Grubbs, C., Setchell, K., and Carlson, J. (1990). Soybeans inhibited mammary tumors in models of breast cancer. *Progress in Clinical Biologic Research,* 347, 239-253.

Barni, S., Lissoni, P., Vrivio, F., Fumagalli, L., Nerlini, D., Cataldo, M., et al. (1994). Serum levels of insulin-like growth factor-I in operable breast cancer in relation to the main prognostic variables and their perioperative changes in relation to those of prolactin. *Tumorigenesis*, 80, 212-215.

Bartus, C. M., Schreiber, J. S. and Kurtzman, S. H. (2004). Palliative approaches to the patient with breast cancer. *Surgical Clinics of North America*, 13, 517-530.

Baserga, R. (1997). Editorial: the path less traveled by. *Endocrinology*, 138, 2217-2218.

Baum, M. (1998). Tamoxifen—the treatment of choice. Why look for alternatives? *British Journal of Cancer*, 78 (Supplement 4), 1-4.

Bavley, A. (2009). That surgery may not be best for you. *The Kansas City Star*, March 22 2009, A-1.

Baynes, J. W. (1991). Role of additive stress in development of complications in diabetes. *Diabetes*, 40, 405-412.

Baxter, R. C. (1994). Insulin-like glucose factor binding proteins in the human circulation: A review. *Hormone Research*, 42, 140-144.

BEIR V Report.(1990). Health effects of exposure to ionizing irradiation of the breast. Division of Medical Sciences National Research Council. Washington, D.C.: National Academy of Science Press.

Bedwinek, J. M., Lee, J., Fineberg, B., and Ocwieza, M.(1981). Prognostic indicators in patients with isolated local-regional recurrence of breast cancer. *Cancer*, 47, 2232-2235.

Beecher, G. R. (2003). Overview of dietary flavenoids: Nomenclature, occurrence, and intake. *Journal of Nutrition*, 133, 3248S-3254S.

Belotti, D., Bergani, V., Drudis, T., Eorsoth, E., Ditelli, M. R., Viale, G., et al. (1996). Micro tubule-affecting drug paclitaxel as antiangiogenic activity. *Clinical Cancer Research*, 2, 1843-1849.

Benda, R. K., Mendenhall, N. P., Lind, D. S. Cendan, J. C., Shea, B. F., Richardson, L.C., et al. (2004) Breast-conserving therapy

(BCT) for early-stage breast cancer. *Journal of Surgical Oncology*, 85, 14-27.

Bennett, L. M. (1999). Breast cancer: genetic predisposition and exposure to radiation. *Molecular Carcinogenesis*, 26,143-149.

Beral, V. (2003). Breast cancer and hormone-replacement therapy in the million women study. *The Lancet*, 362, 419-427.

Berger, N. (1993). Alkalating agents. In DeVita, V., Hellman, S., Rosenberg, S., (Eds.), *Cancer, principles, and practice of oncology*, Philadelphia: J. D. Lipencott.

Bergin, A. E. (1983). Religiosity and mental health: A critical re-evaluation in meta-analysis. *Professional Psychology Research and Practice*, 14, 170-184.

Berkel, J., and de Waard, F. (1983). Mortality patterns and life expectancy of Seventh Day Adventist in the Netherlands. *International Journal of Epidemiology*, 12, 455-459.

Berns, E. M. J. J., Klijn, J. G. M., van Stavern, I. L., Portengen, H., and Fockens, J. A. (1992). Sporadic amplification of the insulin-like growth factor 1 receptor gene in human breast cancer. *Cancer Research*, 52, 1036-1039.

Bernstein, L. and Ross, R. K. (1993). Endogenous hormones and breast cancer risk. *Epidemiologic Reviews*, 15, 48-65.

Berube, S., Diorio, C., and Brisson, J. (2008). Multivitamin-multimineral supplement use in mammographic breast density. *American Journal of Clinical Nutrition*, 87, 1400-1404.

Bigelow, R. L., and Cardelli, J. A. (2006). Green tea catechins, (-)-epigallocatechin-3-gallate(EGCG) and (-)-epiccatechin-3-gallate (ECG), inhibit HGF/Met signaling in immortalized and tumorigenic breast epithelial cells. *Oncogene*, 25, 1922-1930.

Biller, M. K., Samuels, M. H., Zagar, A., Cook, D. M., Arafah, V. M., Bonert, V., et al. (2002). Sensitivity and specificity of 6 tests for the diagnosis of adult growth hormone deficiency. *Journal of Clinical Endocrinology and Metabolism*, 87, 2067-2079.

Bjelakovic, G., Nikolova, D., Gluud, L. L., Simonetti, R. G., and Gluud, C. (2007). Mortality and randomized trials of antioxidant supplements for primary and secondary prevention: Systematic review and meta-analysis. *Journal of the American Medical Associatiion*, 297, 842-857.

Blazar, B. A. (1986). Suppression of natural killer-cell function in humans following thermal and traumatic injury. *Journal of Clinical Immunology*, 6, 26-32.

Block, G., Patterson, B., Subar, A. (1992). Fruit, vegetable, and cancer prevention: a review of the epidemiological evidence. *Nutrition in Cancer*, Vol. 18, 1-29.

Blot, W.J., Li, J.-Y., Taylor, P.R., Guo, W., Dawsey, S., Wang, G.-Q., et al. (1993). Nutrition intervention trials in Linxian, China: Supplementation with specific vitamin/mineral combinations, cancer incidence, and disease-specific mortality in the general population. *Journal of the National Cancer Institute*, 85, 1483-1491.

Boehnke-Michaud, L., Phillips-Karpenski, J., Jones, K. L., and Espirito, J. (2007). Dietary supplements in patients with cancer: risks and key concepts, part 2. *American Journal of Health-System Pharmacies*, 64, 467-480.

Bohlke, K., Cramer, D. W., Trichopoulos, D., and Manzoros, C. S. (1998). Insulin-like growth factor—I in relation to pre menopausal ductal carcinoma in situ of the breast. *Epidemiology*, 9, 570-573.

Boice, J. D. (1979). Risk of breast cancer following low-dose radiation exposure. *Radiology* 131, 589-597.

Bonakdar, R.A. (2006). Herbal and dietary supplements: An evidence-based update. Program and abstracts of the American

Academy of Family Practitioners (AAFP) Annual Scientific Assembly; September 26-October 1, 2006; Washington, D.C. Sessions 389,390,391. Retrieved October 3 2008 from http.//www.medscape.com/viewarticle/549067

Bonneterre, J., Peyrat, J. B., Beuscart, R., and Demaille, A. (1990). Prognostic significance of insulin-like growth factor-I receptors in human breast cancer. *Cancer Research,* 50, 6931-6935.

Boon, H., Stewart, M., Kennard, M. A., Gray, R., Sawkac, C., Brown, J. B., et al. (2000). The use of complementary/alternative medicine by breast cancer survivors in Ontario: Prevalence and perceptions. *Journal of Clinical Oncology,* 18, 2515-2521.

Boon, H., and Wong, J. (2004). Botanical medicine and cancer: A review of the safety and efficacy. *Expert Opinion*, 5, 2485-2501.

Boon, H. S., Olatunde, F., and Zick, S. M. (2007). Trends in complementary/alternative medicine use by breast cancer survivors: Comparing survey data from 1998 and 2005. *BMC Women's Health,* 7, 1472-1478.

Boquete, H. R., Sovradop. G. V., Fideleff. H. L., Sequeram, A. M., Giaccio, A. V., Suarez, M. G., et al. (2003). Evaluation of diagnostic accuracy of insulin-like growth factor (IGF)-I and IGF-Binding Protein-3 in growth hormone-deficient children and adults using ROC plot analysis. *Journal of Clinical Endocrinology and Metabolism,* 88, 4702-4708.

Borst, P. (2008). Mega-dose vitamin C is therapy for human cancer? *Proceedings of the National Academy of Science,* 105, E95.

Bouchayer, F. (1990). Alternative medicines. *Complementary Medicine Research,* 4, 4-8.

Brabant, G., von zur Muhlen, A., Wuster, C., Ranke, M. B., Kratzsch, J., Kiess, W., et al. (2003). Serum insulin-like growth factor I reference values for an automated chemiluminescence immunoassay system: Results from a multi center study. *Hormone Research,* 60, 53-60.

Brandi, G., Schimvano, G-F, Zaffaroni, N., De Marco, C., Paiardini, M., Cervasi, B., et al. (2005). Mechanisms of action and antiproliferative properties of *brassica olerarea*_juice in human breast cancer cell lines. *Journal of Nutrition,* 135, 1503-1509.

Braverman, E. R. (1987). The religious medical model: holy mechanics and the spiritual behavior inventory. *Southern Medical Journal,* 80, 415-420, 425.

Brinton,L., Lacey, Jr., J., and Devesa, S. S. (2002). Chapter 7: Epidemiology of breast cancer. In Donegan, W. L. and Spratt, J. S. (Eds.), *Cancer of the breast,* (5th ed.). Philadelphia: Saunders.

Brooks, J. D., Ward, W. E., Lewis, J. E., Hilditch, J., Nickell, L, Wong, E. et al. (2004). Supplementation with flax seed alters estrogen metabolism in post-menopausal women to a great extent then does supplementation with an equal amount of soy. *American Journal of Clinical Nutrition,* 79, 318-325.

Browder, T., Butterfield, C. E., Kraling, B. M., Shi, B., Marshall, B., O'Reilly, M. S., et al. (2000). Antioangiogenic scheduling of chemotherapy improves efficacy against experimental drug-resistant cancer. *Cancer Research,* 60, 1878-1886.

Brubacher, D., Moser, U., and Jordan, P. (2000). Vitamin C concentrations in plasma as a function of intake: A meta-analysis. *International Journal of Vitamin and Nutritional Research,* 70, 226-37.

Bruning, B. F, Van Doorn, J., Bonfrer, J. M., Van Noord, P. A., Korse, C. M., Linders, T. C., et al. (1995). Insulin-like-growth-factor-binding protein 3 is decreased in early-stage operable premenopausal breast cancer. *International Journal of Cancer,* 62, 266-270.

Bruyere, R. L. (1989). *Wheels of light.* New York: Simon and Schuster.

Bruzzi, P., Green, S. B., Byar, D. P., Brinton, L. A. and Schairer, C. (1985). Estimating the population attributable risk for multiple risk factors using case-Controlled data. *American Journal of Epidemiology*, 122, 904-914.

Bryan, T. M., and Redde, R. M. (1997). Telomere dynamics and telomerase activity in "invitro" immortalized human cells. *European Journal of Cancer*, 33, 767-773.

Bryan, T. M., Englecou, A., Gupta, J., Bacchetti, S., Reddell, R. R. (1995). Telomere elongation in immortal human cells without detectable telomerase activity. *EMBO Journal*, 17, 4240-4248.

Buckbinder, L., Talbott, R., Seizinger, B. R., and Kley, N., (1994). Gene regulation by temperature-sensitive p53 mutants: identification of p53 response genes. *Proceedings of the National Academy of Science, USA*, 91, 10640-10644.

Buckbinder, L., Talbott, R., Zelasco-Miguel, S., Gakenaga, I., Faha, B., Seizinger, B.R., et al (1995). Induction of the growth inhibitor IGF-binding protein-3 by p 53. *Nature*, 377, 646-649.

Bunne, M. (1989). Qualitative research methods in otorhinolaryngology. *International Journal of Pediatric Otorhinolaryngology*, 61, 1-10.

Burke, B. K. (1993). Wellness in the human ministry. *Health Progress*, 74, 34-37.

Burstein, H. J., Gelver, S., Guadagnolie, E., and Weeks, J. C. (1999). Use of alternative medicine by women with early stage breast cancer. *New England Journal of Medicine*, 340, 1733-1759.

Butt, A. J., Fraley, K. A., Firth, S. M., and Baxter, R.C. (2002). IGF-binding protein-3-induce growth inhibition and apoptosis do not require cell surface binding and nuclear translocation in human breast cancer cells. *Endocrinology*, 143 2693-2696.

Butt, A. J., Firth, S. M., and Baxter, R. C., (1999). The IGF axis and programmed cell death. *Immunology and Cell Biology*, 77, 256-262.

Byrd, R. C. (1988). Positive therapeutic effects of intercessory prayer in the coronary care unit population. *Southern Medical Journal*, 81, 826-829.

Cabanes, A., Wang, M., Olivo, S., de Assis, S., Gustafsson, J. A., Khan, G., et al. (2004). Prepubertal estradiol and genistein exposure up regulates BRCA 1 m RNA and reduce mammary tumorigenesis. *Carcinogenesis*, 25, 741-748.

Cade J., Thomas, E., and Vail, A. (1998). Case control study of breast cancer in southeast England: Nutritional factors. *Journal of Epidemiology and Community Health*, 52, 105-110.

Cadenas, S., Rojas, C., and Varga, G. (1998). Endotoxin increased oxidative injury to proteins in guinea pig liver: Protection by dietary vitamin C. *Pharmacology and Toxicology*, 82, 11-18.

Cameron, E., and Campbell, A. (1974). The orthomolecular treatment of cancer. II. Clinical trial of high-dose ascorbic acid supplements in advanced human cancer. *Chemistry and Biology Interactions*, 9, 285-315.

Cameron, E., Campbell, A., and Jack, T. (1975). The orthomolecular treatment of cancer. III. Reticulum cell sarcoma: Double complete regression induced by high-dose ascorbic acid therapy. *Chemistry and Biology Interactions*, 11, 387-393.

Cameron, E., and Pauling, L. (1976). Supplemental ascorbate in the supportive treatment of cancer: Prolongation of survival times in terminal human cancer. *Proceedings of the National Academy of Science USA*, 73, 3685-3689.

Cameron, E., and Pauling, L. (1978). Supplemental ascorbate in the supportive treatment of cancer: Re-evaluation of prolongation of survival times in terminal human cancer. *Proceedings of the National Academy of Science USA, 75,* 4538-4542.

Cameron, E. (1991). Protocol for the use of vitamin C in the treatment of cancer. *Medical Hypotheses, 36,* 190-194.

Cameron, J. L. (1997). William Stewart Halsted. Our surgical heritage. *Annals of Surgery, 225,* 445-458.

Campsi, J. (1997). The biology of replicative senescence. *European Journal of Cancer, 33,* 703-709.

Carlston, M., Pedigo, M. D., Sergeant, M.J., Tsuruoka, Y., Kajii, E., Wetzel, M. S., et al. (1999). Medical school courses in alternative medicine. *Journal of the American Medical Association, 281,* 609-611.

Carroll, P. V., Christ, E. R., Bengtsson, V. A., Carlsson, L, Christiansen, J. S., Clemmons, D., et al. (1998). Insulin-like growth factor family. *Journal of Clinical Endocrinology and Metabolism, 83,* 382-395.

Cassidy, A. (2003). Are herbal remedies and dietary supplements safe and effective for breast cancer patients? *Breast Cancer Research, 5,* 300-302.

Cassileth, B. R. (1999). Evaluating complementary and alternative therapies for cancer patients. *Ca: Cancer Journal for Clinicians, 49,* 362-375.

Cassileth, B. R., and Deng, G. (2004). Complementary and alternative therapies for cancer. *The Oncologist, 9,* 80-89.

Catani, M. V., Costanzo, A., Savini, I., Levrero, M., DeLaurenzi, V., Wang, J.Y.J., et al. (2002). Ascorbate up-regulates MLH1 (Mut L homologue-1) and p73: implications for the cellular response to DNA damage. *Biochemistry Journal, 364,* 441-447.

Catley, L., and Anderson, K. C. (2006). Velcade and vitamin C: Too much of a good thing? *Clinical Cancer Research, 12,* 3-4.

Boon, H. S., Olatunde, F., and Zick, S. M. (2007). Trends in complementary/alternative medicine use by breast cancer survivors: Comparing survey data from 1998 and 2005. *BMC Women's Health*, 7, 1472-1478.

Cauley, J. A., Lucas, F. L., Kuller, L. H., Stone, K., Browner, W., and Cummings, R. (1999). Elevated estradiol and testosterone concentrations are associated with a high risk for breast cancer: Study of Osteoporotic Fractures Research Group. *Annals of Internal Medicine*, 130, 270-279.

Cavalieri, E., Frenkel, K., Liehr, J. G., Rogan, E., and Roy, D. (2000). Estrogens as endogenous genotoxic agents-DNA adducts and mutations. *Journal of National Institute Monogram*, 27, 75-94.

Cavalieri E. L. and Rohan, E. G. (1992). The approach to understanding aromatic hydrocarbon carcinogenesis: The role of radical cations in metabolic activation. *Pharmacologic Therapies*, 55, 183-199.

Cawthorn, R. M., Smith, K. R., O'Brien, D., Sivatchenko, A., and Kerver. R. A. (2003). Association between telomere length in blood and mortality in people aged 60 years or older. *Lancet*, 361, 393-395.

Chagpar, A., Meric-Bernstam, F., Hunt, K. K., Ross, M. I., Cristofanilli, M., Singletary, E., et al. (2003). Chest wall recurrence after mastectomy does not always portend a dismal outcome. *Annals of Surgical Oncology*, 10, 628-634.

Chakravarthy, B., and Pietenpol, J. A. (2003). Combined modality management of breast cancer: Development of predictive markers through proteomics. *Seminars in Oncology*, 30 (supplement 9), 23-36.

Charefare, H., Limongelli, S., and Purshotham, A. D. (2005). Neoadjuvant chemotherapy and breast cancer. *British Journal of Surgery*, 92, 14-23.

Cheblowski, R.T. (2003). Editorial. *CA: A Cancer Journal for Clinicians*, 53, 292.

Cheblowski, R. T., Hendrix, S. L., Langer, R. D., Stefanick, M. L., Gass, M., Lane, D., et al. (2003). From the WHI Investigators.—Influence of estrogen plus progestin on breast cancer and mammography in healthy post menopausal women: The Women's Health Initiative randomized trial. *Journal of the American Medical Association*, 289, 3243-3253.

Chen, A. M., Meric-Bernstam, F., Hunt, K. K., Thames, H. D., Oswald, M. J., E. D., et al. (2004). Breast conservation after neoadjuvant chemotherapy: The M.D. Anderson Cancer Center experience. *Journal of Clinical Oncology*, 22, 2303-2312.

Chen, H., Karne, R.J., Hall, G., Campia, U., Panza, J.A., Cannon III, R.O., et al. (2005). High-dose oral vitamin C partially replenishes vitamin C levels with type 2 diabetes and low vitamin C levels but does not improve endothelial dysfunction or insulin resistance. *American Journal of Physiology: Heart and Circulatory Physiology*, 290, H137-H145.

Chen, J. C., Shao, Z. M., Sheikh, M. S., Hussin, A., LeRoith, D., Roberts, Jr., J. T., et al. (1994). Insulin-like growth-factor binding protein enhancement of insulin-like growth factor-I (IGF-I)-mediated DNA synthesis and IGF-I binding in a human breast carcinoma cell life. *Journal of Cell Physiology*, 158, 69-78.

Chen, J., Lin, H., and Hu, M. (2003). Metabolism of flavonoids via enteric recycling: Role of intestinal disposition. *Journal of Pharmacology and Experimental Therapeutics*, 304, 1228-1235.

Chen, L., Jia, R. H., Qui, C. T., and Ding, G. H. (2005). Hyperglycemia inhibits uptake of dehydroascorbate in tubular epithelial cells. *American Journal of Nephrology*, 25, 459-465.

Chen, Q., Espey, M. G., Krishna, M., Mitchell, J. B., Corpe, C. P., Buettner, G. R., et al. (2005). Pharmacologic ascorbic acid concentrations selectively kill cancer cells: Action as a pro-drug to deliver hydrogen peroxide to tissues. *Proceedings of the National Academy of Science USA,* 102, 13604-13609.

Chen, Q., Espey, M.G., Sun, A.Y., Lee, J.-H., Krishna, M.C., Shacter, E., et al. (2007). Ascorbate in pharmacologic concentrations selectively generates ascorbate radical and hydrogen peroxide in extracellular fluid in vivo. *Proceedings of the National Academy of Science,* 104, 8749-54.

Cheung, B., Yan, J., Smith, S. A., Nguyen, T., Lee, M., Kavallaris, M., et al. (2003). Growth inhibitory retinoid effects after recruitment of retinoid X receptor beta to the retinoid acid receptor beta promoter. *International Journal of Cancer,* 105, 856-867.

Cho, E., Spiegelman, D., Hunter, D. J., Chen, W. Y., Stampfer, M. J., Colditz, G. A., et al. (2003). Premenopausal fat intake and risk of breast cancer. *Journal of the National Cancer Institute,* 95, 1079-1085.

Cho, E., Spiegelman, D., Hunter, D. J., Chen, W. Y., Zhang, S. M., Colditz, G. A., et al. (2003). Premenopausal intakes of vitamins A, C, and E, folate, and carotenoids and risk of breast cancer. *Cancer Epidemiology Biomarkers and Prevention,* 12, 713-720.

Cho, E., Chen, W. Y., Hunter, D. J., Stampfer, M. J., Colditz, G. A., Hankinson, S. E., et al. (2006). Red meat intake and risk of breast cancer among premenopausal women. *Archives of Internal Medicine,* 166 2253-2259.

Christante, D., Pommier S., Garreau, J., Muller, P. P., LaFleur, B., and Pommier, R. (2008). Improved breast cancer survival among hormone replacement therapy users is durable after 5 years of additional follow-up. *American Journal of Surgery,* 96, 505-511.

Christensen, L. H., LAndersson, M., and Storm, H. H. (2001). Untreated breast cancer in Denmark 1978-1995. *Ugeskr Laeger,* 163, 2774-2778.

Chu, A. M., Cope, O., Russo, R., and Lew, R. (1984). Patterns of local-regional recurrence and results in stage I and II breast cancer treatment by irradiation following limited surgery: An update. *American Journal of Clinical Oncology*, 7, 221-229.

Chustecka, Z. (2007). Shark cartilage extract has no effect in cancer. Presented as abstract 7527 at the American Society of Clinical Oncology, 43rd Annual Meeting, June 2 2007, Chicago, Ill. Retrieved September 29 2008 from http.//www.medscape.com/viewarticle/557811

Clarke, R. V., Howell, A., and Anderson, E. (1997). Type I insulin-like growth factor receptor gene expression in normal human breast tissue treated with oestrogen and progesterone. *British Journal of Cancer*, 75, pp. 251-257.

Clemons, M., and Rea, D. (2004). Perspectives on the future of biphosphonate use in breast cancer patients. *Seminars in oncology*, 31, (supplement 10), 87-91.

Clemmons, D. R., Camacho-Hubner, C., Coronado, E., and Osborne, C. K. (1990). Insulin-like growth factor binding protein secretions by breast carcinoma cell lines: correlation with estrogen receptor status. *Endocrinology*, 127, 2679-2686.

Cmich, D. E. (1984). Theoretical perspectives of holistic health. *Journal of the School of Health*, 54, 30-32.

Cohen, P. (2006). Insulin-like growth factor binding protein-3: Insulin-like growth factor independence comes of age. *Endocrinology*, 147, 2109-2111.

Cokun, U., Gunel, N., Yamac, D., and Altinova, A.E. (2001). Effect of cisplatin on skin metastasis in breast cancer patients. *Onkologie*, 24, 576-579.

Collett-Solberg, P. F., and Zohen, P. (1996). The role of the insulin-like growth factor-binding proteins and the IGFBP proteases in modulating IGF action. *Endocrinology and Metabolism Clinics of North America,* 25, 591-614.

Collipp, P. J. (1969). The efficacy of prayer: a triple-blind study. *Medical Times,* 97, 201-204.

Colomer, et al (1997), Low levels of basic fibroblast growth factor (bFGF) are associated with a poor prognosis in human breast carcinoma. *British Journal of Cancer,* 76, 1215-1220.

Cooke, P. S., Selvaraj, V., Yellayi, S. (2006). Genistein, estrogen receptors, and the acquired immune response. *Journal of Nature,* 136, 704-708.

Coon, J. T., Vittler, M. H., and Ernst, E. (2007). Trifolium pretense isoflavones in the treatment of menopausal hot flushes: A systematic review and meta-analysis. *Phytomedicine,* 14 187-193.

Cooper, C. L., Cooper, R., and Faragher, E. B. (1989). Incidents and perception of psychosocial stress: The relationship with breast cancer. *Psychology and Medicine,* 19, 415-422.

Coughlin, S. S., and Piper, M. (1999). Genetic polymorphism and risk of breast cancer. *Cancer Epidemiology Biomarkers and Prevention,* 8, 1023-1032.

Creagan, C. T., Moertel, C. G., O'Fallon, J. R., Schutt, A. J., O'Connell, M. J., Rubin, J., et al. (1979). Failure of high-dose vitamin C (ascorbic acid) therapy to benefit patients with advanced cancer. A controlled study. *New England Journal of Medicine,* 301, 687-680.

Crespi, B., and Summers, K. (1971). The evolutionary biology of cancer. *Cell,* 10, 545-552.

Crocetti, E., Crott, N., Feltrin, A., Ponton, P., Geddes, M., and Buiattie, E. (1998). The use of complementary therapies by breast cancer patients attending conventional treatment. *European Journal of Cancer,* 34, 324-328.

Crowe, J. P., Gordon, N. H., Antunez, A. R., Shenk, R. R., Hubay, A. and Shuck, J. M. (1991). Local-regional breast cancer recurrence following mastectomy. *Archives of Surgery,* 126, 429-432.

Crown, J., Dieras, V., Kaufman, M., von Minckwitz, G., Kaye, S., Leonard, R., et al. (2002). Chemotherapy for metastatic breast cancer-report of A European Expert Panel. *Lancet Oncology,* 3, 719-727.

Cui, Y., Shikany, J.M., Liu, S., Shagufta, Y., and Rohan, T.E. (2008). Selected antioxidants and risk of hormone receptor-defined invasive breast cancers among postmenopausal women in the Women's Health Initiative Observational Study. *American Journal of Clinical Nutrition,* 87, 1009-1018.

Curcio, L.D., Chu, D.J., Ahn, C., Williams, W.L., Pal, B., Riihimaki, D., et al. (1997). Local recurrence in breast cancer: Implications for systemic disease. *Annals of Surgical Oncology,* 4, 24-27.

Cushing, H.L. (May 16 1919). Presidential address and introduction: To the old humanities and the new science. Retrieved November 21 2008 from www.medicalarchives.jhml.edu/osler/oldhum.htm

Dahl, C., Weiss, R., and Issel, L. V. (1985). Mitomycin: 10 years after approval for marketing. *Journal of Clinical Oncology,* 3, 276-286.

Damkier, A., Paludan-Muller, C., and Knoop, A. S. (2007). Use of complementary and alternative medicine (CAM) in breast cancer patients. Efficacy and interactions. *Ugeskr Laege,* 169, 3111-3114.

Dampier, K., Hudson, E. A., Howells, L. M., Manson, N. M., Walker, R. A., and Gescher, A. (2001). Difference between human breast cancer cell lines and susceptibility towards growth inhibition by genistein. *British Journal of Cancer,* 85, 618-624.

Daniells, S. (2009). Soy and breast cancer-isoflavones don't affect breast density, soy trial. Retrieved March 22 2009 from http://www.nutraingredients-usa.com/Research/Soy-and-breast-cancer

D'arcangelo, D., Facchiano, F., and Barlucchi, L. M. (2000). Acidosis inhibits endothelia apoptosis and function and induces fibroblast growth factor and vascular endothelial growth factor expression. *Circulation Research,* 86, 312-318.

Dave, B., Eason, R. R., Till, S. R., Geng, M., Velarde, M. C., Badger, T. M., et al. (2005). The soy isoflavone genistein promotes apoptosis in mammary epithelial cells by inducing tumor suppressor PTEN. *Carcinogenesis,* 26, 1793-1803.

Davis, V. L., Couse, J. F., Goulding, E. H., Power, S. G., Eddy, E. M., and Korach, K. S. (1994). Abberant reproductive phenotypes evident in transgenic mice expressing the wild-type mouse estrogen receptor. *Endocrinology,* 135, 379-386.

de Boer, H., Blok, G. J., Popp-Snijders, C., Stuurman, L., Baxter, R. C., and van der Veen, E. (1996). Monitoring of growth hormone replacement therapy in adults, based on measurement of serum markers. *Journal of Clinical Endocrinology and Metabolism,* 81, 1371-1377.

DeBuis, D. S., et al. (2001). Bone mineral density and endogenous hormones and increase of breast cancer in postmenopausal women (United States). *Cancer Causes and Control,* 12, 213-262.

Decroos, K., Eeckhaut, E., Possemiers, S., and Verstraete, W. (2006). Administration of equol-producing bacteria alters the equol production status in the simulator of the gastrointestinal microbial ecosystem (SHIME). *Journal of Nutrition,* 136, 946-952.

de Kleijn, M. J. J., van der Schouw, Y. T., Wilson, P. W. F., Aldercreutz, H., Mazur, W., Grobee, D. E., et al. (2001). Intake of dietary phytoestrogens is low in post menopausal women in the United States: The Framingham Study. *Journal of Nutrition,* 131, 1826-1832.

Del Guidice, M. E., Fantus, I. G., Ezzat, S., McKeown-Eyssen, G., Page, D., and Goodwin, P. J. (1998). Insulin and related factors in premenopausal breast cancer risk. *Breast Cancer Research and Treatment*, 47, 111-120.

Delafontaine, B., Song, Y-H., and Li, Y. (2004). Expression, regulation, and function of IGF-1, IGR-1R, and IGF-1 binding proteins in blood vessels. *Arteriosclerosis, Thrombosis, and Vascular Biology*, 24, 435-444.

Demarec, E. W. (1951). Local recurrence following surgery for cancer of the breast. *Annals of Surgery*, 134, 863-867.

DePacheco, M. R., and Hutti, M. H. (1998). Cultural beliefs and health care practices of childbearing Puerto Rican American women and Mexican American women: a review of the literature. *Mother Baby Journal*, 3, 14-23.

Deutsch, M., Land, S.R., Begovic, M., Weigand, H.S., Wolmark, N. and Fisher, B. (2003). The incidence of lung cancer after surgery for breast carcinoma with and without postoperative radiotherapy. Results of National Surgical Adjuvant Breast and Bowel Project (NSABP) clinical trials B-04 and B-06. *Cancer*, 98, 1352-1368.

DeVita, Jr., V. T., Hellman, S., and Rosenberg, S. A. (2003). (Eds.) *Cancer: principles and practice of oncology* (6th ed.). Philadelphia: J. B. Lipincott.

DiGianni, L. M., Garber, J. E., and Winer, E. P. (2002). Complementary and alternative medicine use among women with breast cancer. *Journal of Clinical Oncology*, 20, 34S-38S.

Diorio, C., Brisson, J., Berube, S., and Pollack, M. (2008). Genetic polymorphism involved in insulin-like growth factor (IGF) pathway in relation to mammographic breast density and IGF levels. *Cancer Epidemiology Biomarkers and Prevention*, 17, 880-887.

Djuric, Z., Depper, J. B., Uhley, V., Smith, D., Lababidi, S., Martino, S., et al. (1998). Oxidative DNA changes in blood from women at high risk for breasr cancer or associated with dietary intakes of meats, vegetables and fruits. *Journal of the American Dietetics Association*, 98, 524-526.

Donahue,L. R., Hunter, S. J., Sherbolm, A. P., and Rosen, C. (1990). Age-related changes in serum insulin-like growth factor-binding proteins in women. *Journal of Clinical Endocrinology and Metabolism*, 71, 575-579.

Donegan, W. L., and Spratt, J. S. (Eds.). (2002). *Cancer of the breast* (5th ed). Philadelphia: Saunders.

Dossey, L. (1993). *Healing words: the power of prayer and the practice of medicine.* New York: Harper.

Dossey, L. (1996). *Prayer is good medicine.* San Francisco: Harper Collins.

Drake, W. M., Howell, S. J., Monson, J. P., and Shalet, S. M. (2001). Optimizing growth hormone therapy in adults and children. *Endocrine Reviews*, 22, 422-450.

Drisko, J. A., Chapman, J., and Hunter, V. J. (2003). The use of antioxidants with first-line chemotherapy in two cases of ovarian cancer. *Journal of the American College of Nutrition*, 22, 118-123.

Drisko, J. A., Chapman, J., and Hunter, V. J. (2003). The use of antioxidant therapies during chemotherapy. *Gynecologic Oncology*, 88, 434-439.

Drivdahl, C., and Miser, W. (1998). The use of alternative health care by a family practice population. *Journal of the American Board of Family Practice*, 11, 193-199.

Duckro, P. N. and Magaletta, P. R. (1994). The effect of prayer on physical health: experimental evidence. *Journal of Religion and Health,* 33, 221-229.

Duconge, J., Miranda-Massari, J. R., Gonzalez, M. J., Jackson, J. A., Warnock, W., and Riordan, N.H. (2008). Pharmacokinetics of vitamin C: Insights into the oral and intravenous administration of ascorbate. *Proceedings of Royal Health Sciences,* J 27, 7-19.

Duffy, C., Perez, K., and Partridge, A. (2007). Implications of phytoestrogen intake for breast cancer. *CA: Cancer Journal for Clinicians*, 57, 260-277.

Dunne Boggs, N. and Mittman, P. (2004). Naturopathic medicine is an emerging field in one of medicine's most dynamic eras. Posted March 24 2004 *Medscape General Medicine* 6: e42. Retrieved September 12 2008 from http://www.medscape.com/viewarticle/470702/

Dunning, A. M., Heakyt, C. S., Pharoah, P. D. P., Teare, D., Ponder, B. A. J., and Easton, D. F. (1999) A systemic review of genetic polymorphis and breast cancer risk. *Cancer Epidemiology Biomarkers and Prevention*, 8, 843-854.

Early Breast Cancer Trialists' Collaborative Group (1992). Systemic treatment of early breast cancer by hormonal, cytotoxic, or immune therapy. *Lancet*, 339, 2-85.

Early Breast Cancer Trialists Collaborative Group (1995). Effects of radiotherapy and surgery in early breast cancer. An overview of the randomized trials. *New England Journal of Medicine*, 333, 1444-1451.

Early Breast Cancer Trialists' Collaborative Group (1998). Tamoxifen for early breast cancer. Overview of the randomized study 1998. *Lancet*, 351, 1451-1467.

Eddy, E. M., Washburn, T. F., LBunch, D. O., Goulding, E. H., Gladen, B. C., Lubhan, D. B., et al. (1996). Targeted disruption of the estrogen receptor gene in male mice causes alteration of spermatogenesis and infertility. *Endocrinology*, 137, 4796-4805.

Eisenberg, D. M., Kessler, R. C., Foster, C., Norlock, F. E., Calkins, D. R., and Delbanco, T. L. (1993). Unconventional medicine in the

United States: prevalence, cost and patterns of use. *New England Journal of Medicine,* 28, 246-252.

Eisenberg, D. M., Davis, R. B., Ettner, S. L., Appel, S., Wilkey, S., and Van Rompay, M. (1998). Trends in alternative medicine used in the United States 1990 to 1997. *Journal of the American Medical Association,* 280, 1569-1575.

Eisenberg, D. M., Kessler, R. C., Von Rompay, M. I., Kaptchuk, T. J., Wilkey, S. A., Appel, S., et al. (2001). Perception about complementary therapies relative to conventional therapies among adults who use both: Results from a national survey. *Annals of Internal Medicine,* 135, 344-351.

Elgin, R. G., Busby, Jr. W. H., and Clemmons, D. R. (1987). An insulin-like growth factor (IGF) binding protein enhances the biologic response to IGF-I. *Proceedings of the National Academy of Science, USA,* 84, 3254-3258.

Elkin, E. B., Weinstein, M. C., Winer, E. P., Kuntz, K. M., Schnitt, S. J., and Weeks, J. C. (2004). HER-2 testing and trastuzumab therapy for metastatic breast cancer: A cost-effectiveness analysis. *Journal of Clinical Oncology,* 22, 858-863.

Ellison, C. G., (1991). Religious involvement and subjective wellbeing. *Journal of Health and Social Behavior,* 32, 80-99.

Ellison, C. G. (1995). Race, religious involvement, and depressive symptomology in a southeastern US community. *Social Science in Medicine,* 40, 1561-1572.

Emblen, J. D. and Halstead, L. (1993). Spiritual needs and interventions: Comparing the views of patients, nurses, and chaplains. *Clinical Nurse Specialist,* 7, 175-182.

Emens, L. A. and Davidson, N. E. (2003). Follow-up of breast cancer. *Seminars in* Oncology, 30, 338-348.

Epel, D. S., Blackburn, E. H., Lin, J., Dhabhar, F. S., Adler, N. E., Morrow, J. E., et al. (2004). Accelerated telomere shortening in response to life's stress. *Proceedings of the National Academy of Science,* 101 17312-17315.

Erdman, J. W., Badger, T. M., Lampe, J. W., Setchell, K. D. R. and Messina, M. (2004). Not all soy products are created equal: Caution needed in interpretation of research Results. *Journal of Nutrition,* 134 1229S-1233S.

Ernst, E., and Cassileth, B. R. (1998). The prevalence of complementary/ alternative medicine in cancer: A systematic review, *Cancer,* 83, 777-782.

Eunyoung, C., Chen, W. Y., Hunter, D. J., Stampfer, M. J., Colditz, G. A., Hankinson, S. E., et al. (2006). Red meat intake and risk of breast cancer among premenopausal women. *Archives of Internal Medicine,* 2253-2259.

Evidence-Based Medicine Working Group. (1992). Evidence-based medicine. A new approach to tracking the practice of medicine. *Journal of the American Medical Association,* 268, 2420-2425.

Fabian C. J., and Kimler, B. F. (2005). Selective estrogen-receptor modulators for primary prevention of breast cancer. *Journal of Clinical Oncology,* 23, 1644-1655.

Fabian, C. J., Kimler, B. F., Mayo, M. S., and Khan, S. A. (2005). Breast-tissue sampling for risk assessment and prevention. *Endocrine Related Cancer,* 12, 185-213.

Fairfield, K. M., and Fletcher, R. H. (2002). Vitamins for chronic disease prevention in adults. Scientific review. *Journal of the American Medical Association,* 287, 3116-3126.

Falk, R. T., Dorgan, J. F., Kahle, L., Potischman, N., and Longcope, C. (1997). Assay reproducibility of hormone measurements in postmenopausal women, *Cancer Epidemiology Biomarkers and Prevention,* 6, 429-432.

Falk, R. T., Gail, M. H., Fears, T. R., Rossi, S. C., Stanczyk, F., Aldercreutz, H., et al. (1999). Reproducibility and validity of radioimmunoassays for urinary hormones and metabolites of pre and postmenopausal women. *Cancer Epidemiology Biomarkers and Prevention*, 8, 567-577.

Farrar, W. B., and Walker, M. J. (2000) Chapter 4, in Donegan, W. L., and Spratt, J. S. (Eds). *Cancer of the breast* (5th ed.). Philadelphia: Saunders.

Favero, A., Papinel, M., and Montella, M. (1999). Energy sources and risk of cancer of the breast and colon-rectum in Italy. *Advances in Experimental Medical Biology*, 472, 51-57.

Favoni, R. E., de Cupis, A., Perotta, A., Sforzini, S., Amoroso, D., Pensa, F., et al. (1995). Insulin-like growth factor-I (IGF-I) and IGF-binding proteins blood serum levels in women with early-and-late-stage breast cancer: Mutual relationship and possible correlations with patients' hormonal status. *Journal of Cancer Research and Clinical Oncology*, 121, 674-682.

Feldman, A. L., and Libutti, S. K. (2000). Progress in angiogenic gene therapy of cancer. *Cancer*, 89, 1181-1194.

Feldman, D. S., Novack, D. H., and Gracely, E. (1998). Effects of managed care on physician-patient relationships, quality of care, and the ethical practice of medicine: A physician survey. *Archives of Internal Medicine,* 158, 1626-1632.

Fentiman, I. S., Matthews, P. N., Davison, O. W., Mills, R. R., and Hayward, J. L. (2005). Survival following local skin recurrence after mastectomy. *British Journal of Surgery*, 72, 14-16.

Ferrara, J. J., Raiches, N. A., and Minton, J. P. (2006), Endocrine ablation in breast cancer patients who have failed cytotoxic therapy. *Journal of Surgical Oncology,* 18 231-235.

Ferrara, N. and Davis-Smith, T. (1997). The biology of vascular endothelia growth factor. *Endocrine Reviews,* 18, 4-11.

Ferraroni, M. (1998). Alcohol consumption and risk of breast cancer: A multicentre Italian case-control study. *European Journal of Cancer*, 34, 1403-1409.

Ferry, D. R., Smith, A., Malkhandi, J., Fyfe, D. W., deTakats, P. G., Anderson, D., et al. (1996). Phase I clinical trial of the flavonoid quercetin: Pharmacokinetics and evidence for in vivo tyrosine kinase inhibition. *Clinical Cancer Research*, 2, 659-668.

Fidler, I. (2003), The pathogenesis of cancer metastases: The 'seed and soil' hypothesis revisited. *Nature Reviews in Cancer*, 3, 453-458.

Figueroa, J. A., Jackson, J. G., McGuire, W. L., Krywicki, R. F., and Yee, D. (1993). Expression of insulin-like growth factor binding proteins by human breast cancer correlates with estrogen receptor status. *Journal of Cell Biochemistry*, 52, 196-205.

Finstad, H. S., Kolset, S. O., Holme, J. A., Wiger, R., Farrants, A. K., Blomhoff, R., et al. (1994). Effective n-3 and n-6 fatty acids on cell proliferation and differentiation of pro-myelocytic leukemic HL-60 cells. *Blood*, 84, 3799-3809.

Firth, S. M., and Baxter, R. C. (2002). Cellular actions of the insulin-like growth factor finding protein. *Endocrinology Reviews*, 23, 824-854.

Fisher, B. (1999). National Surgical Adjuvant Breast and Bowel Project Breast Cancer Prevention trial: A reflective commentary. *Journal of Clinical Oncology*, 17, 1632-1639.

Fisher, B., Redmond, C., Fisher, E. R., and Caplan, R. (1988). Relative worth of estrogen or progesterone receptors and pathologic characteristics of differentiation as indicators of prognosis in node negative breast cancer patients: Findings from National Surgical Adjuvant Breast and Bowel Project Protocol, B-06. *Journal of Clinical Oncology*, 6, 1076-1087.

Fisher, B., Anderson, S., Fisher, E. R., Redmon, C., Wickerham, D. L., Wolmark, N., et al. (1991). Significance of ipsilateral breast tumour recurrence after lumpectomy. *Lancet,* 338, 327-331.

Fisher, B., Dignam, J., Wolmark, N., Wickerham, D. L., Fisher, E. R., Mamounas, E., et al. (1999). Tamoxifen in treatment of intraductal breast cancer. National Surgical Adjuvant Breast and Bowel Project B-24 Randomized Control Trial. *Lancet,* 353, 1993-2000.

Fisher, P. and Ward, A. (1994). Complementary medicine in Europe. *British Medical Journal,* 309, 107-111.

Fitzgerald, F. T. (1999). Curiosity. On being a doctor. *Annals of Internal Medicine,* 130, 70-72.

Foekens, J. A., Eortengen, H., van Putten, W. L. Trapman, A. M., Reubi, J. C., Alexieva-Figusch, J., et al. (1989). Prognostic value of receptors for insulin-like growth factor-I, somatostatin, and epidermal growth factor in human breast cancer. *Cancer Research,* 49, 7002-7009.

Fogel, J. (2006). Conference report from the 27th Annual Meeting of the Society of Behavioral Medicine, March 22nd to 25th 2006. MedScape Psychiatry and Mental Health 11. Retrieved September 30 2008 from http.//www.medscape.com/viewarticle/531764_2

Folkman, J. (1989). What is the evidence that tumors are angiogenesis dependent? *Journal of the National Cancer Institute,* 82, 4-6.

Folkman, J. (1975). Tumor angiogenesis: A possible control point in tumor growth. *Annals of Internal Medicine,* 82, 96-100.

Forbes, G. B., Brown, M. R., Well, S. R., and Underwood, L. E. (1989). Hormonal response to over feeding. *American Journal of Clinical Nutrition,* 49, 608-611.

Forouhi, N. G., Luan, J., Cooper, A., Boucher, A. J., and Wareham, N. J. (2005). Baseline serum 25-hydroxy vitamin D is predictive of future glycemic status and insulin resistance: The Medical

Research Counsel Prospective Study 1990-2000. *Diabetes*, 57, 2619-2625.

Fowke, J. H., Longcope, C., and Hebert, J. R. (2000). *Brassica* vegetable consumption shifts estrogen metabolism in healthy postmenopausal women. *Cancer Epidemiology Biomarkers and Prevention*, 9, 773-779.

Fowke, J. H., Chung, F-L., Jin, F., Qi, Q., Cai, C., Conaway, J-R., et al. (2003). Urinary isothiocyanate levels, brassica and human breast cancer. *Cancer Research*, 63, 3980-3986.

Fox, S. B., Generali, D. G., and Harris, A. L. (2007). Breast tumour angiogenesis. *Breast Cancer Research*, 9. Retrieved September 20 2008 from http.//www.medscape.com/viewarticle/577631_1

Freedman, B. (1987). Equipoise and the ethics of clinical research. *New England Journal of Medicine*, 317, 141-145.

Freedman, L. S., Prentice, R. L., Clifford, C., Harlan, W., Hendersen, M. and Rossouw, J. (1993). Dietary fat and breast cancer: Where we are. *Journal of the National Cancer Institute*, 85, 764-765.

Freidmen, V., Humblet, C., Ponjean, K., and Boniver, J. (2000). Assessment of tumour angiogenesis in invasive breast carcinoma: Absence of correlation with the prognosis and pathologic factors. *Virchows Archives*, 437, 611-617.

Fromigue, O., Kheddoumi, N. I., and Body, J. J. (2003). Biphosphonates antagonize bone growth factors' effects in human breast cancer cell survival. *British Journal of Cancer*, 89, 178-184.

Frost, R. A., Fuhrer, J., Steigbigel, R., Mariuz, P., Lang, C. H., and Gelato, M. C. (1996). Insulin-like growth factors. *Clinical Endocrinology*, 44, 501-514.

Fujiki, H. (1999). Two stages of cancer prevention with green tea. *Journal of Cancer Research and Clinical Oncology*, 125, 589-597.

Gage, I., Shnitt, S. J., Recht, A., Abner, A., Come, S., Shulman, L. N., et al. (1998). Skin recurrences after breast-conserving therapy for early stage breast cancer. *Journal of Clinical Oncology*, 16, 480-486.

Gago-Dominguez, M., Yuan, J.-M., Sun, C.-L., Lee, H.-P., and Yu, M. C. (2003). Opposing effects of dietary n-3 and n-6 fatty acids on mammary carcinogenesis: The Singapore Chinese Health Study. *British Journal of Cancer*, 89, 1686-1692.

Galantar, M. (1997). Spiritual recovery movement in contemporary medical care. *Psychiatry*, 60, 211-223.

Gandini, S., Merzenich, H., Robertson, C., and Boyle, P. (2000). Meta-analysis of studies on breast cancer risk and diet: The role of fruit and vegetable consumption and the intake of associated micronutrients. *European Journal of Cancer*, 36, 636-646.

Gansler, T., Kaw, C., Crammer, C., and Smith, T. (2008). A population-based study of prevalence of complementary methods used by cancer survivors: A report from the American Cancer Society Studies of Cancer Survivors. *Cancer*, 113, 1048-1057.

Garvin, S., Ollinger, K., and Dabrosin, C. (2006). Resveratrol induces apoptosis and inhibits angiogenesis in human breast cancer xenografts *in vivo*. *Cancer Letters*, 231, 131-122.

Gasparini, G. (1992). Progesterone receptor determined by immunocyto chemical and biochemical methods in human breast cancer. *Journal of Cancer Research and Clinical Oncology*, 118, 557-563.

Gaudet, M. M., Britton, J. A., Kabat, G. C., Steck-Scott, S., Eng, S. M., Teitelbaum, S. L., et al. (2004). Fruits, vegetables and micronutrients in relation to breast cancer modified by menopause and hormone receptor status. *Cancer Epidemiology Biomarkers and Prevention*, 13, 1485-1494.

Gellert, G. C., Dikman, Z. G., Wright, W. E., Gryaznov, S., and Shay, J. W. (2006). Effects of a novel telomerase inhibitor, GRN 163 L, in human breast cancer. *Breast Cancer Research and Treatment, 96,* 73-81.

Genazzani, A. R., and Gambacciniani, L. (1999). Hormone replacement therapy: the perspectives of the 21st century. *Maturitas, 32,* 11-17.

Gerber, B., Cholz, C., Reimer, T., Briese, V., and Janni, W. (2006). Complementary and alternative therapeutic approaches in patients with early breast cancer: A systematic review. *Breast Cancer Research and Treatment,* 95, 199-209.

Gholam, D., Chebib, A., Hauteville, D., Bralet, M. P., and Jasmin, C. (2007). Combined paclitaxel and cetuximab achieved a major response in the skin metastasis of a patient with epidermal growth factor receptor-positive estrogen receptor-negative, progesterone receptor-negative and human epidural growth factor receptor-2-negative (triple-negative) breast cancer. *Anticancer Drugs,* 18, 835-837.

Giancotti, F. G. (1999). Integrin signaling. *Science,* 285, 1028-1032.

Gillenwater, J. Y., and Gray, N. (2003). Evidence: What is it, where do we find it, and how do we use it? *European Urology, 2* (supplement 2), 3-9.

Gimbrone, M. A., Leapman, S. B., Cotran, R. S., and Folkman, J. (1972). Tumor dormancy invivo by prevention of neovascularization. *Journal of Experimental Medicine,* 136, 261-276.

Glickman-Simon, R. (2005). Introduction and complementary and alternative medicine: An evidence-based approach. Retrieved October 4, 2008 from *http://www.medscape.com/viewarticle/507242*

Glik, D. C. (1990). Participation in spiritual healing, religiosity, and mental health. *Sociological Inquiry,* 60, 158-176.

Goldbeck-Wood, S., Dorozynski, A., Lie, L. G., Yamaguchi, M., Zinn, C., Josefson, D., et al. (1996), Complementary medicine is booming worldwide. *British Medical Journal*, 313, 131-133.

Gomez-Millan, J., Goldblatt, E.M., Gryaznov, S. M., Mendonca, M. S., and Herbert, B-S. (2007). Specific telomere dysfunction induced by GRN 163 L increases radiation sensitivity in breast cancer cells. *International Journal of Radiation Oncology, Biology, Physics,* 67, 897-905.

Gonzalez, M. J. (2005). Orthomolecular oncology review: ascorbic acid in cancer 25 years later. *Integrative Cancer Therapies,* 4, 32-44.

Gooch, J. L., Van Den Berg, C. L., and Yee, D. (1999). Insulin-like growth factor (IGF)-I rescues breast cancer cells from chemotherapy-induced cell death—proliferative and anti-apoptotic effects. *Breast Cancer Research and Treatment,* 56, 1-10.

Gotay, C. C., and Dumitriu, D. (2000). Health food store recommendations for breast cancer patients. *Archives of Family Medicine*, 9, 692-699.

Grabrick, D. M., Hartmann, L. C., Cerhan, J. R., Vierkant, R. A., Therneau, T. M. Vachon, C. M., et al. (2000). Risk of breast cancer with oral contraceptive use in women with a family history of breast cancer. *Journal of the American Medical Association,* 284, 1791-1798.

Grace, S. (2009). Evidence-based medicine. *Physician's Practice,* April 2009, 26-31.

Grasad, K. N. (2004). Multiple dietary antioxidants enhance the efficacy of standard and experimental cancer therapies and their toxicity. *Integrative Cancer Therapies*, 3, 310-322.

Gray, M. (2008, August). Evidence-based decision making for the wound care clinician: What is the process, where are the resources? *Ostomy and Wound Management, Supplement,* 3-6.

Green, M. C. (2003, October). Evolving management of metastatic disease. *M. D. Anderson Breast Medical Oncology-Classical Issues and Therapeutic Advances,* 6-8.

Greenberg, P. A., Hortobagyi, G. N., Smith, T. L., Ziegler, L. D., Frye, D. K., and Buzoar, A. U. (1996). Long-term followup of patients with complete remission following combination chemotherapy for metastatic breast cancer. *Journal of Clinical Oncology,* 14, 2197-2205.

Greenlee, H., Atkinson, C., Stanczyk, F. Z., and Lampe, J. W. (2007). A pilot and feasibility study on the effects of naturopathic botanical and dietary intervention on sex steroid hormone metabolism in premenopausal women. *Cancer Epidemiology Biomarkers and Prevention,* 16, 1601-1609.

Greenlee, R. T., Murray, T., Bolden, S., and Wingo, P. A. (2000) Cancer statistics 2000. *Cancer Journal for Clinicians,* 50, 7-11.

Greger, J. L. (2001). Dietary supplement use: Consumer characteristics and interests. *Journal of Nutrition,* 131, 1339S-1443S.

Groopman, J., and Hartzband, P. (2009). Why 'quality" care is dangerous. *The Wall Street Journal,* April 8 2009, A-13.

Gupta, M. (2003). A critical appraisal of evidence based medicine: Some ethical considerations. *Journal of Evaluation of Clinical Practice,* 9, 111-121.

Haas, E. M. with Levin, B. (2006). *Staying healthy with nutrition.* Berkeley, Ca: Celestial Arts.

Haffty, B. G., Reiss, M., Beinfield, M., Fischer, D., Ward, B., and McKhann, C. (1996). Ipsilateral breast tumor recurrence as a predictor of distant disease: Implications for systemic therapy at the time of local relapse. *Journal of Clinical Oncology,* 14, 52-57.

Hall, T. C. (1974). Predictive tests and cancer. *British Journal of Cancer,* 30, 191-199.

Halliwell, B. (1992). Free radicals, anti-oxidants, and human disease: curiosity, cause, or consequence. *Lancet,* 344, 721-724.

Halsted, William. Biography retrieved September 22 2008 from Answers.com

Halverson, K.J., Perez, C. A., Kuske, R. R., Garcia, D. M., Simpson, J. R. and Fineberg, B. (1992). Survival following locoregional recurrence of breast cancer: Univariate and multivariate analysis. *International Journal of Radiation Oncology Biology and Physics,* 23, 285-291.

Hamberg, K., Johansson, E., Lindgren, G., and Westman, G. (1994). Scientific rigour in qualitative research-examples from a study of women's health and family practice. *Family Practice,* 11, 176-181.

Hampshire, S. (1989). *Innocence and experience.* Cambridge, Ma: Harvard University Press.

Hanahan, D. (2000). Cancer: Benefit of bad telomeres. *Nature,* 406, 573-574.

Hanahan, D. and Folkman, J. (1986). Patterns and emerging mechanisms of angiogenic switch during tumorigenesis. *Cell,* 86, 353-364.

Hanahan, D., and Weinberg, R. A. (2000). The hallmarks of cancer. *Cell,* 100, 57-70.

Hanahan, D., Burgers, G., and Bergsland, E. (2000). Less is more, regularly: Metranomic dosing of cytotoxic drugs can target tumor angiogenesis in mice. *Journal of Clinical Investigation,* 105, 1045-1047.

Hankinson, S. E., Manson, J. E., Spiegelman, D., Willett, N. C., Loncope, C., and Speizer, F. E. (1995). Reproducibility of plasma hormone levels in postmenopausal women over a 2-3 year period. *Cancer Epidemiology Biomarkers and Prevention,* 4, 649-650.

Hankinson, S. E. (1997). A prospective study of oral contraceptive use and risk of breast cancer. (Nurses' Health Study, United States). *Cancer Causes and Control*, 8, 65-72.

Hankinson, S. E., Willett, W. C., Colditz, G. A., Hunter, D. J., Michaud, D. S., Deroo, B. et al. (1998). Circulating concentrations of insulin-like growth factor-I and risk of breast cancer. *Lancet*, 351, 1393-1396.

Hankinson, S. E., Willett, W. C., Michaud, D. S., Manson, J. E., Colditz, G. A., Loncope, C.,et al. (1999). Plasma prolactin levels and subsequent risk of breast cancer in postmenopausal women. *Journal of the National Cancer Institute*, 91, 629-634.

Harley, C. B. (2008). Telomerase and cancer therapeutics. *Nature Reviews Cancer*, 8, 167-179.

Harley, C. B. (2002). Telomerase is not an oncogene. *Oncogene*, 21, 494-502.

Hart, J. K. (2009). Health insurers and medical-imaging policy-a work in progress. *New England Journal of Medicine*, 360, 1030-1037.

Harwood, A. (1971). The hot/cold theory of disease, *Journal of the American Medical Association*, 216, 1153-1158.

Hebert, J. A., and Rosen, A. (1996). Nutritional, socioeconomic and reproductive factors in relation to female breast cancer mortality: Findings from a cross-national study. *Cancer Detection and Prevention*, 20, 234-239.

Hedley, D. W., Clark, G. M., Cornelisse, Cees J., Killander, D., Kute, T. and Merkel, D. (1993). Concensus review of the clinical utility of DNA cytometry in carcinoma of the breast: Report of the DNA Cytometry Concensus Conference. *Cytometry*, 14, 482-485.

Heldet, J. M. (1992). Poor advice from double talk: a probe of 'health food' store chains in centralized Ohio. *Nutition Forum*, 9, 6-9.

Hennipman, A. et al. (1989). Tyrosine kinase activity in breast cancer, benign breast disease, and normal breast tissue. *Cancer Research*, 49, 516-521.

Heppner, G. H., and Miller, F. R., (1997). The cellular basis of tumor progression. *International Review of Cytology*, 177, 1-56.

Hicks, C. (1995). The shortfall in published research: a study of nurses' research and publication activities. *Journal of Advances in Nursing*, 21, 594-604.

Hilakivi-Clarke, L., Rowland, J., Clarke, R. and Lippman, M. E. (1994). Psychosocial factors in the development and progression of breast cancer. *Breast Cancer Research and Treatment*, 29, 141-160.

Hilakivi-Clarke, L., Wang, C., Kalil, M., Riggins, R., and Pestell, R.G. (2004). Nutritional modulation of the cell cycle in breast cancer. *Endocrine Related Cancer*, 11, 603-622.

Hillner, B. E., Ingle, J. N., Chlebowski, R. T., Gralow, J., Yee, G. C., Janjan, N. A., et al (2003). American Society of Clinical Oncology update on the role of Biphosphonates and bone health issues in women with breast cancer. *Journal of Clinical Oncology*, 21, 4042-4057.

Hirayama, T. (1990). *Lifestyle and mortality*. Basel: Karger.

Hoey, B. M., and Butler, J. (1984). The repair of oxidized amino-acids by anti-oxidants. *Biochimica Biophysica Acta*, 791, 212-218.

Hoffer, L. J. (2003). Investigating CAM. *Canadian Medical Association Journal*, 168, 1527-1528.

Hoffer, L. J., Levine, M., Assouline, S., Melnychuk, D., Padayatty, S. J., Rosadiuk, K., et al. (2008). Phase I clinical trial of I.V. ascorbic acid and advanced malignancy. *Annals of Oncology*, 19, 1969-1974.

Holmberg, L. (1994).Diet and breast cancer risk. Results from a population-based, case-control study in Sweden. *Archives of Internal Medicine,* 154, 1805-1812.

Holmes, S. (2004). The potential risks of alternative therapies and treatment of cancer. *Journal of the Royal Society of Health,* 124, 63-64.

Holt, S. E., Wright, W. E., and Shay, J. W. (1997). Multiple pathways for the regulation telomerase activity. *European Journal of Cancer,* 33, 761-766.

Horwitz, K. B., Maguire, W. L., Pearson, O. H., and Segaloff, A. (1975). Predicting response to endocrine therapy and human breast cancer: A hypothesis. *Science,* 189, 726-757.

Hough, H., Dower, C., and O'Neil, E. (2001). *Profile of a profession: naturopathic practice.* San Francisco: Center for Health Professions, University of California.

Howard, B. (2009, May). Spotlight on a hidden cancer risk. *Readers Digest,* 75-76.

Howe, G., Rohan, T., Decarli, A., Iscovic, J., Kaldor, J., Katsouyanni, K., et al. (1990). The association between alcohol and breast cancer risk: Evidence from the combined analysis of six dietary case-control studies. *International Journal of Cancer,* 47, 707-710.

Howe, G. R., Hiruata, T., Hislop, G., Iscovich, J. M., Yuan, J-M., Katsouyanni, K., et al. (1990). Dietary factors and risk of breast cancer: Combined analysis of 12 case-control studies. *Journal of the National Cancer Institute,* 82, 561-569.

Hrushesky, W. J. (1988). Natural killer cell activity is age, esterase and circadian, stage dependent and correlates inversely with metastatic potential. *Journal of the National Cancer Institute,* 80, 1232-1238.

Hu, Y. (1997). Association of body mass index, physical activity, and reproduction histories with breast cancer: a case control study in Gifu, Japan. *Breast Cancer Research and Treatment,* 43, 65-72.

Huang, Z., Hankinson, E., Colditz, G. A., Stampfer, M. J., Hunter, D. J., Manson, J. E., et al. (1997). Dual effects of weight and weight gain on breast cancer risk. *Journal of the American Medical Association,* 278, 1407-1411.

Hudson, M. J., Humphrey, L. J., Mantz, F. A., and Morse, P. A. (1974). Correlation of circulating serum antibody to the histologic findings in breast cancer. *American Journal of Surgery,* 128, 756-759.

Hughes, E. G. (1996). Systematic literature review and meta-analyses. *Seminars in Reproductive Endocrinology,* 14 161-169.

Huggins, C. B., Stevens, R. B., and Hodges, C. V. (1941). The effects of castration on advanced carcinoma of the prostate gland. *Archives of Surgery,* 43, 209-214.

Huinink, ten Bokkel, W., and van Leeuwenhoek Ziekenhuis, A. (1999). Treatment of skin metastasis with breast cancer. *Cancer Chemotherapy and Pharmacology,* 44 (supplement), S31-33.

Hulley, S., Grady, D., Bush, T., Furberg, C., Herrington, D., Riggs, B. et al for the Heart and Estrogen/progesterone Replacement Study Research Group. (1998). Randomized trial of estrogen plus progestin for secondary prevention of coronary heart disease in post menopausal women. Heart and estrogen/progestin replacement study (HERS) research group. *Journal of the American Medical Association,* 280, 605-613.

Hummer, R. A., Rogers, R. G., Nam, C. V. and Ellison, C. G. (1999). Religious involvement in US adult mortality. *Demography,* 36, 273-285.

Hunter, D. J., Morris, J. S., Stampfer, M. J., Colditz, G. A., Speizer, F. E., and Willett, W. C. (1990). A prospective study of selenium status and breast cancer risk. *Journal of the American Medical Association,* 264, 1128-1131.

Huseby, R. A., Ownby, H. E., Brooks, S., Russo, J., (1990). Evaluation of the predictive power of progesterone receptor levels in primary breast cancer: A comparison with other criteria in 559 associated with amine follow-up of 74.8 months. *The Breast Cancer Prognostic Study Associates, Henry Ford Hospital Medical Journal,* 38, 79-84.

Hyunh, H., Yang, X., and Pollack, M. (1996). Estradiol and antiestrogens regulate a growth inhibitory insulin-like growth factor binding protein-3 autocrine loop in human breast cancer cells. *Journal of Biochemistry and Molecular Biology,* 271, 1016-1021.

Iglehart, J. K. (2009). Health insured medical-imaging policy-a work in progress. *New England Journal of Medicine,* 360, 1030-1037.

Ikawa, S., Nakagawara, A., and Ikawa, Y. (1999). p 53 family genes: Structural comparison, expression and mutation. *Cell Death and Differentiation,* 6, 1154-1161.

Ingall, J. N. (1984). Additive hormonal therapy in women with advanced breast cancer. *Cancer,* 53, 766-777.

Ingehom, P., Pedersen, L., and Holek, S. (1999). Quantification of microvessel density of breast carcinoma: An assessment of the inter-and intraobserver variation. *Breast,* 8, 251-256.

Ingle, J. N., Suman, V. J., Cardinal, C. G., Krook, J. E., Maillard, J. A., Veeder, M. H., et al. (1999). A randomized trial of tamoxifen alone or in combination octreodide in the treatment of women with metastatic breast cancer. *Cancer,* 85, 1284-1289.

Ingram, D. M. (1990). Prolactin and breast cancer risk. *Medical Journal of Australia,* 153-159.

Inositol Hexaphosphate retrieved September 13 2008 from http://www.cancer.org/documnent/ETO/content?ETO_5_3X_Inositol_H

Inoue. M, Roblin, K., Wang, R., van den Berg, D. J., Kohy-P, and Yu, M. C. (2008). Green tea intake MTHFR/TYMS genotype and breast cancer risk: The Singapore Chinese Health Study. *Carcinogenesis,* 29, 1967-1972.

Irie, M., Asami, S., Nagata, S., Miyata, M., and Kasai, H. (2001). Relationships between perceived work load, stress, and oxidative DNA damage. *International Archives of Occupation and Environmental Health,* 74, 153-157.

Irie, M., Asami, S., Ikeda, M., and Kasai, H. (2003). Depressive state relates to female oxidative DNA damage via neutrophil activation. *Biochemistry and Biophysiology Research Communications,* 311, 1014-1018.

Isaacs, D. (1999). Seven alternatives to evidence-based medicine. *British Medical Journal,* 319, 16-18.

Izzo, A. A., and Ernst, E. (2002). Interactions between herbal medicines and prescribed drugs: A systematic review. *Drugs,* 61, 2163-2175.

Jackson, D. (2008, September). Health threat. *Glamour,* 355.

Jacobson, J. S., Rokman, S. B., and Kronenberg, F. (2000). Research on complementary/alternative medicine for patients with breast cancer. A review of the biomedical literature. *Journal of Clinical Oncology,* 18, 668-683.

Janjan, N. A., McNeese, M. D., Buzdar, A. U., Montague, E. D. and Oswald, M. J. (1986). Management of locoregional recurrent breast cancer. *Cancer,* 58, 1552-1556.

Jarvis, G. K and Northcott, H. C. (1987). Religion and differences in mobidity and mortality. *Social Science in Medicine* 25, pp. 813-824.

Jariwalla, R. J. (1999). Inositol hexaphosphate (IPG) as an antineoplastic and lipid-lowering agent. *Anticancer Research*, 19, 3699-3702.

Jensen, E.V. (2005). The contribution of "alternative approaches" to understanding steroid hormone action. *Molecular Endocrinology*, 19,1439-1442.

Jiang, W., Zhu, N., and Thompson, H. J. (2003). Effective energy restriction on cell cycle machinery in 1-methol-1-nitrosourea-induced mammary carcinogenesis in rats. *Cancer Research*, 53, 12128-12134.

Jiang, X., Patterson, N. M., Ling, Y., Xie, F., Helferich, W. G., and Shapiro, D. J. (2008). Low concentrations of the soy phytoestrogen genistein induce proteinase inhibitor 9 and block killing of breast cancer cells by immune cells. *Endocrinology*, 149, 5366-5373.

Johns, A., Freay, A. D., Fraser, N., Korach, K. S., and Rubanyi, G. M. (1996). Disruption of estrogen receptor gene prevents 17 beta estradiol-induced angiogenesis in transgenic mice. *Endocrinology*, 137, 4511-4513.

Jones, J. I., and Clemmons, D. R. (1995). Insulin-like growth factors and their binding proteins: Biological actions. *Endocrinology Reviews*, 16, 3-9.

Juul, A., Holm, K. Kastrup, K. W., Pedersen, S. A., Michaelsen, K. F., Scheike, T., al, (1997). Free insulin-like growth factor I serum levels in 1430 healthy children and adults and its diagnostic value in inpatients suspected of growth hormone deficiency. *Journal of Clinical Endocrinology and Metabolism*, 82, 2497-2502.

Kabuto, M., Akiba, S., Stevens, R. G., Neriishi, K., and Land, C. E. (2000). The prospects of study of estradiol and breast cancer in Japanese women. *Cancer Epidemiology Biomarkers and Prevention*, 9, 575-579.

Kadowaki, J., Hamkyama, U., Chi, T., Terauchi, Y., Tobe, K., and Nagai, R. (2003). Molecular mechanism of insulin resistance in obesity. *Experimental Biology and Medicine,* 228, 1111-1117.

Kaegl, E. (1998). Unconventional therapies for cancer: 1. Essiac. The task force on alternative therapies of the Canadian breast cancer research initiative. *Canadian Medical Association Journal,* 158, 897-902.

Kamen, B., Rubin, E., and Asiner, J. (2000). High-time for low dose chemotherapy. *Journal of Clinical Oncology,* 18, 2935-2937.

Kano, M., Takayanagit, T., Harada, K., Sawada, S., and Ishikawa, F. (2006). Bioavailability of isoflavones after ingestion of soy beverages in healthy adults. *Journal of Nutrition,* 136, 2291-2296.

Kaptchuk, T. J. (2000). *The web that has no weaver.* New York: McGraw-Hill.

Kaptchuk, T. J. (2003). Effective interpretive bias on research evidence. *British Medical Journal,* 326, 1453-1455.

Karashima, A. T., and Schally, A. V. (1997). Inhibitory effects of somatostatin analogs on prolactin secretion in rats pretreated with estrogen or haloperidol (42518). *Proceedings of the Society of Experimental Biology and Medicine,* 185, 69-72.

Katsouyanni, K., Trichopoulos, D., Boyle, P., Xirouchaki, E., Trichopoulou, A., Lisseos, B., et al. (1994). Ethanol and breast cancer: an association that may be both confounded and causal. *International Journal of Cancer,* 58, 356-361.

Kavanaugh, C. J., Trumbo, P. R., and Ellwood, K. C. (2007). The U.S. Food and Drug Administration's evidence-based review for qualified health claims: Tomatoes, lycopene, and cancer. *Journal of the National Cancer Institute,* 99, 1074-1085.

Kelley, K. M., Ohygargosky, S. E., Gucev, Z., Matsumoto, T., Hwa, V., et al (1996). Insulin-like growth factor-binding proteins (IGFBPs) and their regulatory dynamics. *International Journal of Biochemistry and Cell Biology,* 28, pp. 619-637.

Kay, J. and Robinson, K. M. (1994). Spirituality among caregivers. *Journal of Nursing Schools,* 1994 218-221.

Kelley, K. M., Ohygargosky, S. E., Gucev, Z., Matsumoto, T., Hwa, V., et al. (1996). Insulin-like growth factor-binding proteins (IGFVPs) and their regulatory dynamics. *International Journal of Biochemistry and Cell Biology,* 28, 619-637.

Kelsey, J. L. (1993). Breast cancer epidemiology: Summary and future directions. *Epidemiology Reviews,* 15, 356-363.

Kelsey, J. L. and Bernstein, L. (1996). Epidemiology and prevention of breast cancer. *Annual Reviews of Public Health,* 17, 47-67.

Kennedy, M. J. and Abeloff, M. D. (1993). Management of locally recurrent breast cancer. *Cancer,* 71 2395-2409.

Khandwala, H. M., McCutcheon, I. E., Flyvbjerg, A., and Friend, K. E. (2000). The effects of insulin-like growth factors on tumorigenesis and neoplastic growth. *Endocrine Reviews,* 21 215-244.

Khaw, K.T., Bingham, S., Welch, A., Luben, R., Wareham, N., Oakes, S., et al. (2001). Relation between the plasma ascorbic acid and mortality in men and women in EPIC-Norfolk prospective study. A prospective population study. European Prospective Investigation Into Cancer And Nutrition. *Lancet,* 357, 657-63.

Kiene, H. and von Schon-Angeror, T. (1998). Single-case causality assessment as a basis for clinical judgment. *Alternative Therapies in Health and Medicine,* 4, 41-47.

Kim, E. M. H., Lobocki, C., Dubay, L., and Mittal, B. K. (2009). A specific vascular endothelial growth factor receptor tyrosine kinase inhibitor enhances the anti-proliferative effect of trastuzumab in human epidermal growth factor receptor 2 over expressing breast cancer cell life. *American Journal of Surgery,* 197, 331-336.

Kim, H., Peterson, T. G., and Barnes, S. (1998). Mechanisms of action of the soy isoflavone genistein: Emerging role for its effects via transforming growth factor beta signaling pathways. *American Journal of Clinical Nutrition*, 68, 1418S-1425S.

Kim, N. W. (1997). Clinical implications of telomerase activity in cancer. *European Journal of Cancer*, 33, 781-786.

King, D. E., Sobil, J., Haggerty, J., Dent, M., and Patton, D. (1992). Experiences and attitudes about faith healing among family physicians. *Journal of Family Practice*, 35, 158-162.

Kirchfield, F., and Boyle, W. (1994). *The nature doctors: pioneers in naturopathic medicine*. Portland, Or: Medicina Biologica.

Koenig, H. G., Bearon, L. B., and Dayringer, R. (1989). Physician perspectives on the role of religion in the physician-older patient relationship. *Journal of Family Practice*, 28, 441-448.

Korach, K. S., Couse, J. F., Curtis, J. W., Washburn, T. F., Lindzy, J., Kimbro, K. S., et al. (1996). Estrogen receptor gene disruption: Molecular characterization and experimental and clinical phenotypes. *Recent Progress in Hormone Research*, 51, 159-186.

Kouloulias, V. E., Plataniotis, G. A., Kouvaris, J. R., Dardoufaf, C. E., Gennatas, C., Landuy, T. W., et al; (2003). Re-irradiation in conjunction with liposomal doxorubicin for the treatment of skin metastasis of recurrent breast cancer: a radiobiological approach and 2 year follow-up. *Cancer Letters*, 193, 33-40.

Kritchesky, D. (1992). Caloric restrictions and experimental carcinogenesis. *Advances in Experimental and MolecularBiology*, 322, 134-141.

Krone, C. A. (2005). Controlling hyperglycemia as an adjunct to cancer therapy. *Integrative Cancer Therapies*, 4, 25-31.

Krywicki, R. F., and Yee, D. (1992). The insulin-like growth factor family of ligands, receptors, and binding proteins. *Breast Cancer Research and Treatment, 22*, 7-19.

Kurtz, J. M., Amalric, R., Brandone, H., Ayme, Y., Jackquemier, J., Pietra, J. C., et al. (1989). Local recurrence after breast-conserving surgery and radiotherapy. Frequency time course and prognosis. *Cancer, 63*, 1912-1917.

LaCour, F. (1982). A new adjuvant treatment with polyadenylic-polyuridylic acid in operable breast cancer. *Recent Results in Cancer Research, 80*, 200-204.

Lad, V. (2004). Ayurveda. The science of self-healing. A practical guide. Twin Lakes, Wi: Lotus Press.

Lajous, M., Boutron-Ruault, M.-C., Fabre, A., Clavel-Chapelon, F., and Romieu, I. (2008). Carbohydrate intake, glycemic index, glycemic load, and risk of postmenopausal breast cancer in a prospective study of French women. *American Journal of Clinical Nutrition, 87*, 1384-1391.

Lam, D. (1998). Paclitaxel: an angiogenesis antagonist in the metastatic breast cancer model. *Proceedings of the American Society of Clinical Oncology, 17*, 107-111.

Lamartiniere, C. A., Moore, J. B., Brown, M. N., Thompson, R., Hardin, M. J., and Barnes, S. (1995). Genistein suppresses mammary cancer in rats. *Carcinogenesis, 16*, 2833-2840.

Lampe, J. W., and Peterson, S. (2002). *Brassica*, biotransformation and cancer risk: Genetic polymorphism after the preventive effects of cruciferous vegetables. *Journal of Nutrition, 132*, 2991-2994.

Lampe, J. W., Nishino, Y., Ray, R. M., Wu, C., Li, W., Lin, M.-G., et al. (2007). Plasma isoflavones and fibrocystic breast conditions and breast cancer among women in Shang Hai, China. *Cancer Epidemiology Biomarkers and Prevention, 16*, 2579-2586.

Lan, C. E. (1995). Studies of cancer and radiation dose among atomic bomb-survivors: The example of breast cancer. *Journal of the American Medical Association,* 274, 402-407.

Larson, D. B., Pattison, E. M., and Blazer, D. G. (1986). Systematic analysis of research on religious variables in four major psychiatric journals 1978-1982. *American Journal of Psychiatry,* 143, 329-334.

Lathaby, A. E., Brown, J., Marjoribawks, J., Kronenberg, F., Roberts, H., and Eden, J. (2007). Phytoestrogens for vasomotor menopausal symptoms. *Cochrane Data Base System Review:* cdoo 1395.

Lau, C. B., Ho, T. C., Chan, T. W., and Kim, S. C. (2005). Use of dong quai (angelica sinensis) to treat peri- or postmenopausal symptoms in women with breast cancer: Is it appropriate? *Menopause,* 12, 734-740.

LaVecchia, C. (2002). Tomatoes, lycopene intake, and digestive tract and female hormone-related neoplasms. *Experimental and Biological Medicine,* 227, 860-863.

La Vecchia, C. Favero, A., and Francheschi, S. (1998). Monounsaturated and other types of fat, and the risk of cancer. *European Journal of Cancer Prevention,* 7, 461-464.

Lawenda, B. D., Kelly, K. M., Ladas, E. J., Sagar, S. M., Vickers, A., and Blumberg, J. B. (2008). Should supplemental antioxidant administration be avoided during chemotherapy and radiation? *Journal of the National Cancer Institute,* 100, 773-783.

Le, M. G., Arriagada, R., Spielman, M., Guinebretriere, J-M., and Richard, F. (2002). Prognostic factors for death after an isolated local recurrence in patients with early-stage breast cancer. *Cancer,* 94, 2813-2820.

Lee, A. V., Hilgenbeck, S. G., and Yee, D. (1998). IGF system components are prognostic markers in breast cancer. *Breast Cancer Research and Treatment,* 47, 295-302.

Lee, F. Y., Borzilleri, I., Fairchild, C. R., Kim, S_H., Long, B. H., Reventos-Suarez, C., et al. (2001). A novel epothilone analog with a mode of action similar to paclitaxel but possessing superior antitumor efficacy. *Clinical Cancer Research,* 7, 1429-1437.

Lee, M. M., Lin, S. S., Wrench, M.R., Adler, S. R. and Eisenberg, D. (2000). Alternative therapies used by women with breast cancer in four ethnic populations. *Journal of the National Cancer Institute,* 92, 42-47.

Lee, Y-T. N. (1984). Delayed cutaneous hypersensitivity, lymphocyte count, and blood tests in patients with breast carcinoma. *Journal of Surgical Oncology,* 27, 135-140.

Lengacher, C. A., Bennett, M. P., Kipp, K. E., Gonzales, L., Jacobsen, P., and Cox, C. E. (2006). Relief of symptoms, side effects, and psychological distress through the use of complementary and alternative medicine in women with breast cancer. *Oncology Nursing Forum,* 33, 97-104.

Lennox, E. S. (1985). What are tumor antigens? In Reif, A. E., Mitchell, M. S. (Eds.), *Immunity to cancer,* Orlando, Florida: Academic Press.

Le Roith, D. (1997). Insulin-like growth factors. *New England Journal of Medicine,* 336, 633-640.

LeRoith, D., Baserga, R., Helman, L., and Roberts, Jr. C. T. (1995). Insulin-like growth factors in cancer. *Annals of Internal Medicine,* 122, 54-59.

LeRoith, D., Werner, H., Beitner-Johnson, D., and Roberts, Jr., C. T. (1995). Molecular and cellular aspects of the insulin-like growth factor-I receptor. *Endocrinology Reviews,* 16, 143-163.

Levin, J. S., and Banderpool, H. Y. (1987). Is frequent religions attendance really conducive to better health? Toward an epidemiology of religion. *Social Science and Medicine,* 24, 589-600.

Levin, J. S. and Schiller, P. C. (1987). Is there a religious factor in health? *Journal of Religion and Health*, 26, 9-36.

Lewis, J. S., Osipo, C., Meeke, K., and Jordan, V.C. (2005). Estrogen-induced apoptosis in a breast cancer model resistant to long-term estrogen withdrawal. *Journal of Steroid Biochemistry and Molecular Biology*, 94, 131-141.

Li, A. V., Hilsenbeck, S. G., and Yee, D. (1998). IGF system components as prognostic markers in breast cancer. *Breast Cancer Research and Treatment*, 47, 295-302.

Li, Y., and Schellhorn, H. E. (2007). New developments in novel therapeutic perspectives for vitamin C. *Journal of Nutrition*, 137, 2171-84.

Li, Y., and Schellhorn, H. E. (2007). Can ageing-related degenerative diseases be ameliorated through administration of vitamin C at pharmacological levels? Med Hypotheses, 68, 1315-17.

Lie, D. (2006). AAFP 2006—evidence-based complementary and alternative medicine (CAM): what should physicians know? Presented at the Academy of Family Physicians 2006 scientific assembly. Retrieved October 4 2008 from *http://www.medscape.com/viewarticle/549067*

Linos, E., Willett, W. C., Cho, E., Colditz, G., and Frazier, L. A. (2008). Red meat consumption during adolescence among premenopausal women and the risk of breast cancer. *Cancer Epidemiology and Biology Prevention*, 17, 2146-2151.

Lins, S., Rensch, M. R., Adler, S. R., and Eisenberg, D. (2000). Alternative therapies used by women with breast cancer in four ethnic Populations, *Journal of the National Cancer Institute*, 92, 42-47.

Lipton, A., Santner, S. J., Santen, R. J., Harvey, H. A., Fell, P. D., White-Hershey, D., et al. (1987). Aromatase activity in primary and metastatic breast cancer. *Cancer*, 59, 779-789.

Loewy, E.H. (1998). Curiosity, imagination, compassion, science and ethics: do curiosity and imagination serve a central function? *Health Care Analysis*, 6, 286-294.

Loewy, E. H. (2007). Ethics and evidence-based medicine: is there a conflict? *Medscape General Medicine*, 9, 30. Retrieved September 14, 2008 from *http://www.medscape.com/viewarticle/559977*

Lodovico, B. (2000). Evidence-based management of cancer in the elderly. *Cancer Control: Journal of the Moffitt Cancer Center*, 7, 368-376.

Longnecker, M. P., Newcomb, P. A., Mittendorf, R., Greenberg, E. R., Clapp, R. W., Bogdaw, F., et al. (1995). Risks of breast cancer in relation to lifetime alcohol consumption. *Journal of the National Cancer Institute*, 87, 923-929.

Loria, C. M., Klag, M. J., Caulfield, L. E., and Whelton, P. K. (2000). Vitamin C status and mortality in U.S. adults. *American Journal of Clinical Nutrition*, 72, 139-145.

Love, S. B. (2000). *Dr. Susan Love's breast book*. New York: Harper Collins.

Lukaczer, D., Darland, G., and Tripp, M. (2005). Clinical effects of a proprietary combination isoflavone nutritional supplement in menopausal women: A pilot trial. *Alternate Alternative Therapy in Health and Medicine*, 11, 60-65.

Lutsenko, E. A., Carcamo, J. M., and Golde, D. W. (2002). Vitamin C prevents DNA mutation induced by oxidative stress. *Journal of Biology and Chemistry*, 277, 16895-16899.

Lyons, W. R., Li, C. H., and Johnson, R. E. (1958). The hormonal control of mammary growth and lactation. *Recent Progress in Hormone Research*, 14, 219-227.

Lyons, A. S., and Petrucelli, II, R. J. (1978). *Medicine. An illustrated history*, New York : Harry Abrams.

MacKenzie, E., Taylor, L., and Bloom, B. (2003). Ethnic minority use of complementary and alternative medicine (CAM): A national probability survey of CAM utilizers. *Alternative and Therapies in Health and Med,* 9, 50-56.

Magno, L., Bignardi, M., Micheletti, E., Bardelli, D., and Pleban, I. F. (1987). Analysis of prognostic factors in patients with isolated chest wall recurrence of breast cancer. *Cancer,* 60, 240-244.

Maguire, W. L., Horwitz, K. B., Pearson, O. H., and Segaloff, A. (1977), Current status of estrogen and progesterone receptors in breast cancer. *Cancer,* 39 (supplement 6), 2934-2947.

Mahady, G. B. (2005). Do soy isoflavones cause endometrial hyperplasia? *Nutritional Reviews,* 63, 392-397.

Mallenrude, K. (1993). Shared understanding of the qualitative research process. Guidelines for the medical researcher. *Family Practice,* 10, 201-206.

Manach, C., Scalber, T. A., Morand, C., Remesy, C., and Jimenez, L. (2204). Polyphenols: Food sources and bioavailability. *American Journal of Clinical Nutrition,* 79, 727-747.

Martinez, M. E., Thomson, C. A., and Smith-Warner, S. A. (2006). Soy and breast cancer: The controversy continues. *Journal of the National Cancer Institute,* 98, 430-431.

Maskarinec, G., Franke, A. A., Williams, A. E., Hebshi, S., Oshiro, C., Murphy, S., et al. (2004). Effects of two-year randomized soy intervention on sex hormone levels in premenopausal women. *Cancer Epidemiology Biomarkers and Prevention,* 13, 1736-1744.

Maskarinec, G., Verheus, M., Steinberg, F. M., Amato, P., Cramer, M. K., Lewis, R. D., et al. (2009). Various doses of soy isoflavones do not modify mammographic density in postmenopausal women. *Journal of Nutrition,* 139, 981-986.

Matsuyama, R., Reddy, S., and Smith, T. J. (2006). Why do patients choose chemotherapy near the end of life? A review of the perspective of those facing death from cancer. *Journal of Clinical Oncology*, 24, 3490-3496.

Mattson, A. (1980). Dose- and time-response for breast cancer risks after radiation therapy for benign breast disease. *Journal of the National Cancer Institute*, 72 1054-1061.

Maugans, T. A. and Wadland, W. C. (1991). Religion and family medicine: a survey of physicians and patients. *Journal of Family Practice*, 32 210-213.

McCarty, Jr., K. S. (1989). Proliferative stimuli in a normal breast: Estrogens or progestins. *Human Pathology*, 20, 1137-1138.

McCaulay, Z. M. (1992). Insulin-like growth factors in cancer. *British Journal of Cancer*, 65, 311-320.

McGoldric, M., Pearce, J. K., and Giordano, J. (1996). *Ethnicity and family therapy*. NY: The Guilford Press.

McGuire, W. L., Carbone, P. P., and Vollmer, E. (Eds.), (1975). *Estrogen receptors in human breast cancer*. New York: Raven Press.

McGuire, W. L., Horwitz, K. B., Pearson, O. H., and Segaloff, A. (1977). Current status of estrogen and progesterone receptors in breast cancer. *Cancer*, 39 (*supplement 6*), 2934-2947.

McMahon, G. (2000). VEGF receptor signaling in tumor angiogenesis. *The Urologist*, 5, 3-10.

McManus, R. J., Wilson, S., and Delaney, V. C. (1998). Review of the usefulness of contacting other experts when conducting a literature search for systematic reviews. *British Medical Journal*, 317, 1562-1563.

Medina, D. (2005). Mammary developmental fate and breast cancer risk. *Endocrine Related Cancer*, 12, 483-495.

Memorial Sloan-Kettering Cancer Center. (2004). About herbs: Inositol hexaphosphate. Retrieved May 22 2009 from *http://www.mskcc.org/mskcc/html/11571.cfm?Record* ID=459&tab=HC

Merlo, L. M. F., Pepper, J. W., Reid, B. J., and Maley, C. C. (2006). Cancer is an evolutionary and ecological process. *Nature Reviews Cancer,* 6, 924-935.

Messina, M. (1999). Soy, soy phytoestrogens (isoflavones), and breast cancer. *American Journal of Clinical Nutrition,* 70, 574-575.

Messina, M., McCaskill-Stevens, W., Lampe, J. W., (2006). Addressing the soy and breast cancer relationship: Review, commentary and workshop proceedings. *Journal of the Nation Cancer Institute,* 98, 1275-1274.

Meyer, K. K. (1970). Cellular immune response to mastectomy and radiation. *Guthrey Clinical Bulletin,* 40, 48-50.

Michna, H., Nishino, Y., Neef, G., McGuire, W. L., and Schneider, N. (1992). Progesterone antagonist: Tumor-inhibiting potential and mechanism of action. *Journal of Steroid Biochemistry and Molecular Biology,* 41, 339-348.

Migliaccio, A., DiDomenico, M., Castoria, G., de Falco, A., Bontempo, P., Nola, E., et al. (1996). Tyrosine kinase/p21ras/MAP-kinase pathway activation by estradiol-receptor complex in MCF-7 cells. *EMBO,* 15, 1292-1300.

Miller, D. R., Anderson, G. T., Stark, J. J., Granick, J. L., and Richardson, D. (1998). Phase I/II trial of the safety and efficacy of shark cartilage in the treatment of advanced cancer. *Journal of Clinical Oncology,* 16, 3649-3655.

Mills, E., Ernst, E., Singh, R., Grass, C., and Wilson, K. (2003). Health food store recommendations: Implications for breast cancer patients *Breast Cancer Research,* 5, R170-174.

Mincey, A. (2000). Prevention and treatment of osteoporosis in women with breast cancer. *Mayo Clinic proceedings, 75*, 821-829.

Minchinton, A. I., Fryer, K. H., Wendt, K. R., Clow, K. A., and Hayes, M. M. M. (1996). The effect of thalidomide on experimental tumors and metastases. *Anticancer Drugs, 7*, 339-343.

Moertel, C. G., Fleming, T. R., Creagan, E. T., Rubin, J., O'Connell, M. J., et al. (1979). High dose vitamin C versus placebo in the treatment of patients with advanced cancer who have had no prior chemotherapy. A randomized double-blind comparison. *New England Journal of Medicine, 312*, 137-141.

Mohan, S., Daylink, D. J., and Pettis, J. L. (1996). Editorial: Insulin-like growth factor (IGF)-binding proteins in serum—do they have additional roles besides modulating the endocrine IGF actions. *Journal of Clinical Endocrinology and Metabolism, 81*, 3817-3824.

Moorman, P. G., and Terry, P. D. (2004). Consumption of dairy products and the risk of breast cancer: A review of the literature. *American Journal of Clinical Nutrition, 80*, 5-14.

Mora, E. M., Singletary, S. E., Buzdar, A. U., and Johnston, D. A. (1996). Aggressive therapy for local regional recurrence after mastectomy in stage II and stage III breast cancer patients. *Annals of Surgical Oncology, 3*, 162-168.

Moran, M. S. and Hafty, B. G. (2002). Local-regional breast cancer recurrence and prognostic groups based on patterns of failure. *Breast Journal, 8*, 81-87.

Morgentaler, A. (2008, December). Destroying the myth about testosterone replacement and prostate cancer. *Life Extension*, 49-62.

Morgentaler, A., Bruning, C. O., and DeWolf, W. C. (1996). Incidence of occult prostate cancer among men with low total or free serum testosterone. *Journal of the American Medical Association, 276*, 1904-1906.

Moritz, A. (2008). *Cancer is not a disease—it's a survival mechanism.* Landrum, S.C.: Ener Chi Wellness Center.

Morris, K.T., Johnson, N., Holmer, L., and Walts, D. (2000.) Comparison of complementary therapy used between breast cancer patients and patients with other primary tumor sites. *American Journal of Surgery,* 179, 474-511.

Moschen, R., Kemmler, G., Schweigkofler, H., Holzner, B., Dunsar, M., Richter, R., et al. (2001). Use of alternative/complementary therapy in breast cancer patients—a psychological perspective. *Supportive Care in Cancer.* 9, 267-274.

Moshin, S. K., Weiss, H. L., and Gutierrez, M. C. (2005). Neoadjuvant trastuzumab induces apoptosis in primary breast cancers. *Journal of Clinical Oncology,* 23, 22460-22468.

Moss, R. W. (2006). Should patients undergoing chemotherapy and radiotherapy be prescribed antioxidants? *Integrative Cancer Therapies,* 5, 63-82.

Mouridsen, H. T., Rose, C., Brodie, A. H., and Smith, I. E. (2003). Challenges in the endocrine management of breast cancer. *Breast,* 12(*Supplement* 2), S2-19.

Mueller, C. B., and Ammers, F. (1978). Bilateral carcinoma of the breast: Frequency and mortality. *Canadian Journal of Surgery,* 21, 459-464.

Nakachi, K. (1998). Influence of dietary green tea on breast cancer malignancy among Japanese patients. *Japanese Journal of Cancer Research,* 89, 254-259.

Nahin, R.L. (2002). Use of the best case series to evaluate complimentary and alternative therapies for cancer: A systematic review. *Seminars in Oncology,* 29, 552-562

Nahleh, Z., and Tabbara, I. A. (2003). Complementary and alternative medicine in breast cancer patients. *Palliative and Supportive Care,* 1, 267-273.

Naidu, K. A., Tang, J.L., Naidu, K. A., Prockop, L. D., Nigosia, S. V., and Coppola, D. (2001). Anti-proliferative and apoptotic effect of ascorbyl stearate in human gliobalstoma multiforme cells. Modulation of insulin-like growth factor-I receptor (IGF-IR) expression. *Journal of Neuro Oncology,* 54, 15-22.

Naidu, K. A., Karl, R. C., Naidu, K. A., and Coppola, D. (2003). Anti-proliferative and pro-apoptotic effect of ascorbyl stearate in human pancreatic cells: Association with decreased expression of insulin-like growth factor-I receptor. *Digestive Disease Science,* 48, 230-237.

Narod, S. A. and Offit, K. (2005). Prevention and management of hereditary breast cancer. *Journal of Clinical Oncology,* 23, 1656-1663.

Nass, S.J. (1996). Role for Bcl-xL in the regulation of apoptosis by EGF and TGF beta in c-myc over expressing mammary epithelial cells. *Biochemistry and Biophysiology Research Communication,* 227, 248-256.

National Center for Complementary and Alternative Medicine: National Institutes of Health. The use of complementary and alternative medicine in the United States. September 2004. Retrieved October 1 2008, from http://nccam.nih.gov/news/camsurvey_fs1.htm#spend

National Council on Radiation Protection and Measurement. (1987). Ionizing radiation exposure of the population of the United States. *NCRP report # 93.*

Nattleton, J. A., Greany, K. A., Thomas, W., Wangen, K. E., Aldercreutz, H., and Kurzer, M. S. (2005). The effect of soy consumption on the urinary 2: 16 hydroxyestrone ratio in postmenopausal women depends on equol production status but is not influenced by probiotic consumption. *Journal of Nutrition,* 135, 603-608.

Nespeira, B., Perez-Ilzarbe, M., Fernandez, P., Fuentess, A. M., Baramo, J. A., and Rodriguez, J. A. (2003). Vitamins C and E down-regulate vascular VEGF and VEGF-2 expression in apolipoprotein-E-dificient mice. *Atherosclerosis,* 171, 67-73.

Neville-Webbe, H. L., Holen, I., and Coleman, R. E. (2002). Anti-tumour activity of biphosphonates. *Cancer Treatment Reviews,* 28, 305-319.

Newman, L. A., and Sabel, M. (2003). Advances in breast cancer detection and management. *Medical Clinics of North America,* 87, 997-1028.

Newman, L. A. and Washington, T. A. (2003). New trends in breast conservation therapy. *Surgical Clinics of North America,* 83, 841-883.

Nicosia, R. F., Nicosia, R. V., and Smith, M. (1994). Vascular endothelial growth factor, platelet-derived growth factor, and insulin-like growth factor-1 promote rat aortic angiogenesis in vitro. *American Journal of Pathology,* 145, 1023-1029.

Nowell, P. C. (1976). The clonal evolution of tumor cell populations. *Science,* 194, 23-28.

O"Hara, D. P. (2002). Is there a role for prayer and spirituality in healthcare? *Medical Clinics of North America,* 86, 33-46.

O'Sullivan, A.J., Cramton, L.J., Freund, J., and Ho, K.K. (1998). The route of estrogen replacement therapy confers divergent effects on substrate oxidation and body composition in postmenopausal women. *Journal of Clinical Investigation,* 102, 1035-1040.

Ohlen, J., Balneaves, L. G., Bottorff, J. L., and Brazier, A. S. (2006). The influence of significant others in complementary and alternative medicine decisions by cancer patients. *Social Science and Medicine*, 63, 1625-1636.

Ohmuller, H. L., Pham, H., and Rosenfeld, R. G. (1993). Demonstration of receptors for insulin-like growth factor binding protein-3 on Hs578T human breast cancer cells. *Journal of Biology and Chemistry*, 268, 26045-26048.

Old, L. J. (1985). *Tumor necrosis factor (TNF) science*, 230, 630-637.

Oppel, L. B. (2003). Investigating CAM. *Canadian Medical Association Journal*, 168, 1527.

Orr, R. D. and Isaac, G. (1992). Religious variables are infrequently reported in clinical research. *Family Medicine*, 24, 602-606.

Ortiz, B., Shields, K. M., Clauson, K. A., and Clay, P. G. (2007). Complementary and alternative medicine use among Hispanics in the United States. *Annals of Pharmacotherapeutics*, 41, 994-1004.

Osborne, C. K., Boldt, D. H., Clark, G. M., and Trent, J. M. (1983). Effects of tamoxifen on human breast cancer cells kinetics. Accumulation of cells in early G-1 phase. *Cancer Research*, 43, 3583-3585.

Oshimura, M., and Varrett, J. C. (1997). Multiple pathways to cellular senescence: role of telomerase repressors. *European Journal of Cancer*, 33, 710-715.

Osler, William. Biography retrieved September 22 2008 from Answers. com.

Osler, William. Biography retrieved September 29, 2008 from Wikipedia

Ovaskainen, M-L., Torronen, R., Koponen, J. M., Sinkko, H., Hellstrom, J., Reinivuo, H., et al. (2008). Dietary intake and major food sources of polyphenols in Finnish adults. *Journal of Nutrition*, 138, 562-566.

Owens, P. C., Gill, P. G., DeYoung, N. J., Weger, M. A., Knowles, S. S., and Moyse, K. J. (1993). Estrogen and progesterone regulates the increasing of Insulin-like growth factor binding proteins by human breast cancer cells. *Biochemistry and Biophysiology Research Communication*, 193, 467-473.

Pachter, L. (1994). Culture and clinical care. Folk illness beliefs and behaviors and their implications for health care delivery, *Journal of the American Medical Association*, 271, 690-694.

Padayatty, S. J., and Levine, M. (2000). Reevaluation of ascorbate in cancer treatment: Emerging evidence, open minds and serendipity. *Journal of the American College of Nutrition*, 19, 423-425.

Padayatti, S.J., and Levine, M. (2001). New insights into the physiology and pharmacology of vitamin C. *Canadian Medical Association Journal*, 164, 353-5.

Padayatty, S. J., Katz, A., Wang, Y., Eck, P., Kwon, O., Lee, J.-H., et al. (2003). Vitamin C as antioxidant: Evaluation of its role in disease prevention. *Journal of the American College of Nutrition*, 22 18-35.

Padayatty, S. J., Sun, H., Wang, Y., Riordan, H. D., Hewitt, S. M., Katz, A., et al. (2004). Vitamin C pharmacokinetics: Implications for oral and intravenous use. *Annals of Internal Medicine*, 140, 533-537.

Padayatti, S. J., Riordan, H. D., Hewitt, S. M., Katz, A., Hoffer, L. J., and Levine, M. (2006). Intravenously administered vitamin C as cancer therapy: Three cases. *Canadian Medical Association Journal*, 174, 937-942.

Padayatty, S. J., Doppman, J. L., Chang, R., Wang, Yaohui, Gall, J., Papanicolaou, D. A., et al. (2007). Human adrenal glands secrete vitamin C in response to adrenal corticotrophic hormone. *American Journal of Clinical Nutrition*, 86, 145-149.

Page, L. (2002). *Detoxification*. Carmel Valley, Ca: Traditional Wisdom.

Palmer, M. E., Haller, C., McKinney, P. E., and Klein-Schwartz, W. (2003). Adverse events associated with dietary supplements: An observational study. *Lancet*, 361, 101-106.

Pandian, R., and Nakmoto, J. M. (2004). Rational use of the laboratory for childhood and adult growth hormone deficiency. *Clinical Laboratory Medicine*, 24, 141-174.

Papa, V., Gliozzo, B., Clark, G. M., McGuire, W. L., Moore, D., Fugaita-Yamaguchi, Y., et al. (1993). Insulin-like growth factor-I receptors are over expressed and predict a low risk in human breast cancer. *Cancer Research*, 53, 3736-3740.

Papatestas, A. E. (1977). Thymus and breast cancer-plasma androgens, thymic pathology and peripheral lymphocytes in breast cancer. *Journal of National Cancer Institute*, 59, 1583-?

Papatestas, A. E. and Kark A. E. (1974). Peripheral lymphocyte counts in breast carcinoma. *Cancer*, 34, 2014-2017.

Papetti, M., and Herman, I. M., (2002). Mechanisms of normal and tumor-derived angiogenesis. *American Journal of Physiology and Cell Physiology* 282, c947-c970.

Parodi, P. W. (2005). Dairy product consumption and the risk of breast cancer. *Journal of the American College of Nutrition*, 24, 556S-568S.

Patterson, R., Neuhouser, M. L., Hedderson, M. M., Schwartz, S. M., Standish, L. G., Bowen, D. J., et al. (2002). Types of alternative medicine used by patients with breast, colon or prostate cancer: predictors, motives and costs. *Journal of Alternative and Complementary Medicine*, 8, 477-485.

Pawlias, K. T., Dockerty, M. B. and Ellis, Jr., F. H. (1958). Late local recurrent carcinoma of the breast. *Annals of Surgery*, 148, 192-198.

PDRHealth.com: Inositol hexaphosphate retrieved May 22, 2009.

PDRHealth.com: MGN III retrieved May 22, 2009.

Pearlman, A. W. (1976). Breast cancer—influence of growth rate on prognosis and treatment evaluation: A study based on mastectomy scar recurrences. *Cancer*, 38, 1826-1833.

Pekonen, F., Partanen, S., Makinen, T., and Rutanen, E-M. (1988). Receptors for epidermal growth factor and insulin-like growth factor-I and their relation to steroid receptors in human breast cancer. *Cancer Research*, 48, 1343-1347.

Pekonen, F., Nyman, T., Ilvesmaki, V., and Partanen, S. (1992). Insulin-like growth factor binding proteins in human breast cancer tissue. *Cancer Research*, 52, 5204-5207.

Perkin, M. R., Pearcy, R. M., and Fraser, J.S. (1994). A comparison of the attitudes shown by general practitioners, hospital doctors and medical students towards alternative medicine. *Journal of the Royal Society of Medicine*, 87, 523-525.

Petersen, L. A., Woodard, L. D. Urech, T., Daw, C., and Sookanan, S. (2006). Does pay-for-performance improve the quality of health care? *Annals of Internal Medicine*, 145, 265-278.

Peterson, G. and Barnes, S. (1991). Genistein inhibition of the growth of human breast cancer cells: Independence from estrogen receptors and the multi-drug resistance gene. *Biochemistry and Biophysiology Research Communications*, 179, 661-667.

Peyrat, J-P, Bonneterre, J., Beuscart, R., Dijane, J., and Demaille, A. (1988). Insulin-like growth factor-I receptors in human breast cancer and the relation to estradiol and progesterone receptors. *Cancer Research*, 48, 6429-6433.

Pflaum-Kielbassa, C., Garmyn, M., and Epe, B. (1998). Oxidative DNA damage induced by visible light in mammalian cells: Extent, inhibition by anti-oxidants and genotoxic effects. *Mutation Research*, 408, 137-146.

Phillips, K. A., Milne, R. L., Friedlander, M. L., Jenkins, M. A., McRedie, M. R. E., Giles, G., et al. (2004). Prognosis of postmenopausal breast cancer and child birth prior to diagnosis. *Journal of Clinical Oncology*, 22, 699-705.

Phillipe, E., and Le Gal, Y. (1968). Growth of seventy-eight recurrent mammary cancers; quantitative study. *Cancer* 21, 461-467.

Piao, W., Wang, Y., Adachi, Y., Yamamoto, H., Li, R., Insumran, A., et al. (2008). Insulin-like growth factor-1 receptor blockade by a specific tyrosine kinase inhibitor for human gastrointestinal carcinoma. *Molecular Cancer Therapeutics*, 7, 1483-1489.

Pike, M. C., Spicer, D. V., Dahmdush, L., and Press, M. F. (1993). Estrogens, progesterones, normal breast cell proliferation, and breast cancer risk. *Epidemiology Reviews*, 15, 17-35.

Pisani, P., Park, D. M., Bray, F., and Ferlay, J. (1999). Eratum: Estimates of the worldwide mortality from 25 cancers in 1990. *International Journal of Cancer*, 83, 18-29.

Poloma, M. M. and Pendleton, B. F. (1991). The effects of prayer and prayer experiences on measures of general well-being. *Journal of Psychology and Theology*, 19, 71-83.

Poehlman, E. T., and Copeland, K. C. (1990). Influence of physical activity on insulin-like growth factor-I in healthy younger and older men. *Journal of Clinical Endocrinology and Metabolism*, 71, 1468-1473.

Potischman, N., Weiss, H. A., Swanson, C. A., Coates, R. J., Gammon, M. D., Malone, K. E., et al. (1998). Diet during adolescence and risk of breast cancer among young women. *Journal of the National Cancer Institute*, 9, 226-233.

Powles, T. (2004). Isoflavones and women's health. *British Cancer Research*, 6, 140-142.

Prasad, K. N. (2004). Multiple dietary antioxidants enhance the efficacy of standard and experimental cancer therapies and their toxicity. *Integrative Cancer Therapies,* 3, 310-322.

Prehn, R. T. (1993). Two competing influences that may explain breast tumor resistance. *Cancer Research,* 53, 3266-3269.

Pritchard, R. S., Hill, A. D. K., Dijkstra, B., McDermott, E. W., and O'Higgins, N. J. (2003). The prevention of breast cancer. *British Journal of Surgery,* 90, 772-783.

Propst, L. R., Ostrom, R., and Watkins, P. (1990). Comparative efficacy of religious and non-religious cognitive-behavioral therapy for the treatment of clinical depression in religious individuals. *Journal of Consulting and Clinical Psychology,* 60, 94-103.

Rajaram, S., Baylink, D. J., and Mohan, S. (1997). Insulin-like growth factor-binding protein in serum and other biological fluids: regulation and function. *Endocrinology Reviews,* 18, 801-813.

Ramana, B. (2008, October). The Indo-American surgical intercourse. *General Surgery News,* 42-43.

Ratajczak, H. B., Sothern, R. B., and Hrushesky, W. J. (1988). Esterase influence on Surgical care of metastatic breast cancer. *Journal of Experimental Medicine,* 168, 88-93.

Recht, A., Gray, R., Davidson, N. E., Fowble, B. L., Solin, L. J., Cummings, F., et al. (1999). Locoregional failure 10 years after mastectomy and adjuvant chemotherapy with or without tamoxifen without irradiation: Experience of the Eastern Cooperative Oncology Group. *Journal of Clinical Oncology,* 17, 1689-1695.

Reddy, V. G., Khanna, N., and Singh, N. (2001). Vitamin C augments chemo-therapeutic response of cervical carcinoma HeLa cells by stabilizing p53. *Biochemistry and Biophysiology Research Communications,* 282, 409-415.

Rees, R., Feigel, I., Vickers, A., Zollman, C., McGurk, R., and Smith, C. (2000). Prevalance of complementary therapy use by women with breast cancer: a population based survey. *European Journal of Cancer*, 36, 1359-1364.

Resnicoff, M., Abraham, D., Yutanawiboonchai, W., Rothman, H. L., Kajstura, J., Rubin, R., et al. (1995). The insulin-like growth factor I receptor protects tumor cells from apoptosis "invivo". *Cancer Research*, 55, 2463-2469.

Rhoden, E. L., and Morgentaler, A. (2004). Risks of testosterone-replacement therapy and recommendations for monitoring. *New England Journal of Medicine*, 350, 482-492.

Rice, S., and Whitehead, S. A. (2006). Phytoestrogens and breast cancer-promoters are protectors? *Endocrine Related Cancer*, 13, 995-1015.

Richards, J. A. and Bruegemeier, R. W. (2003). Prostaglandin E2 regulates aromatase activity and expression in human adipose stromal cells via 2 distinct receptor subtypes. *Journal of Clinical Endocrinology and Metabolism*, 88, 2810-2816.

Richardson, M. A., Sanders, T., Palmer, J. L., Greisinger, A., and Singletary, S. E. (2000). Complementary/alternative medicine use in comprehensive cancer center and the implications for oncology. *Journal of Clinical Oncology*, 18, 2505-2514.

Ries, L. A., Melbert, D., Krapcho, M., Stinchcomb, D. G., Howlader, N., and Homer, M. J. (2000). SEER cancer statistics review 1973-1997. Bethesda, Md: National Cancer Institute.

Rocha, R. L., Hilsenbeck, S. G., Jackson, J. G., Van Den Berg C. L., Weng, C., Lee, V., et al. (1997). Insulin-like growth factor binding protein-3 and insulin receptor substrate-I in breast cancer: Correlation with classical perimeters and disease-survival. *Clinical Cancer Research*, 3, 103-109.

Rochefort, H. (1984). Chemical basis of breast cancer treatment by androgens and progestins. In Gurpide, E (ed.), *Hormones in Cancer* (*pp.* 79-96). New York: Alan, R. Liss.

Rodriguez, J. A., Nespeira, B., Terez-Ilzarbe, M., Eguinda, E., and Paramo, J. A. (2005). Vitamins C and E prevent endothelial VEGF and VEGFR-II over-expression induced by porcine hypercholecterolemic LOL. *Cardiovascular Research,* 65, 665-673.

Roizen, M. F., and Oz, M. C. (2008, November). Detenga su reloj. *Selecciones (Readers Digest),* 59-63.

Ronco, A. (1999). Vegetable, fruits, and related nutrients, and risk of breast cancer: A case-controlled study in Uruguay. *Nutrition and Cancer,* 35, 111-117.

Rosen, C. J., and Conover, C. (1997). Growth hormone/insulin-like growth factor-I axis in aging: A summary of a National Institutes of Aging-sponsored symposium. *Journal of Clinical Endocrinology and Metabolism,* 82, 3919-3922.

Rosenberg, W., and Donald, A. (1995). Evidence-based medicine: An approach to clinical problem solving. *British Medical Journal,* 310, 1122-1126.

Rosenfeld, R. G., Hwa, Z., Wilson, L., Lopez-Bermego, A., Buckway, C., Burren, C., et al. (1999). The insulin-like growth factor binding protein super family: new perspectives. *Pediatrics,* 104, 1018-1021.

Ross, J. (2006). Soy and coat color: Another changing of the guard. *Cancer Epidemiology Biomarkers and Prevention,* 15, 1057-1058.

Rossouw, J. E., Anderson, G. L., Perentice, R. L., LaCroix, A. Z., Kooberver, G. C., and Stefanick, M. L. (2002). Risks and benefits of estrogen plus progestin in healthy post menopausal women: Principle results from Women's Health Initiative randomized health study. *Journal of the American Medical Association, 288,* 321-333.

Rowe, J.W. (2006). Pay-for-performance and accountability: Related themes in improving health care. *Annals of Internal Medicine, 145,* 695-699.

Ruan, W., Catanese, V., Wiezzorek, R., Feldman, M., and Kleinverg, D. L. (1995). Estradiol enhances the stimulatory effect of insulin-like growth factor-I (IGF-I) on mammary development and growth-hormone induced IFG-I messenger ribonucleic acid. *Endocrinology, 136,* 1296-1302.

Rudolph, I. L., Kelley, D. S., Clasing, K. C., and Erickson, K. L. (2001). Regulation of cellular differentiation and apoptosis by fatty acids and their metabolites. *Nutrition Research, 21,* 381-393.

Rush, Jr., B. F. (1982). Chapter 15: Breast. In Shires, T. G., Spencer, F. C. and Storer, E. H. (Eds.), *Principles of surgery* (2nd ed.). New York: McGraw-Hill.

Sa Couta, J. (2003). An objectivist's view on the ethics of evidence-based medicine: commentary on 'A critical appraisal of evidence-based medicine: some ethical considerations'(Gupta 2003; *Journal of Evaluation in Clinical Practice,* 9: 111-121). *Journal of Evaluation in Clinical Practice,* 9, 137-139.

Sage, W. M., and Kalyn, D. N. (2006). Horses or unicorns: can paying for performance make quality competition routine? *Journal of Health Politics and Policy Law,* 31, 531-556.

Salganick, R. I. (2001). The benefits and hazards of antioxidants: controlling apoptosis and other protective mechanisms in cancer patients and the human population. *Journal of the American College of Nutrition,* 20, 464S-472S.

Sanderson, A. A. (2006). Pay-for-performance programs in the United Kingdom. *New England Journal of Medicine,* 355 1832-1833.

Saphner, T., Tormey, D. C., and Gray, R. (1996). Annual hazard rates of recurrence for breast cancer after primary therapy. *Journal of Clinical Oncology,* 14, 2738-2746.

Sariego, J. (2008). Regional variation in breast cancer treatment throughout the United States. *American Journal of Surgery,* 196, 572-574.

Sarkar, F. H., and Li, Y. (2003). Soy isoflavones and cancer prevention. *Cancer Investigation,* 21, 744-757.

Schally, A. V. (1986). Endocrine, gastrointestinal, and anti-tumor activity of somatostatin analogs. In Moody, T. W. (ed.), *Neuroendocrine peptides and receptors.* New York: Plenum.

Schmoor, C., Sauerbrei, W., Bastert, G., and Schumacher, M. (2000). Role of isolated local regional recurrence of breast cancer: Results of four prospective studies. *Journal of Clinical Oncology,* 18, 1696-1708.

Schwaibold, F., Fowble, B. L., Solin, L. J., Schultz, D. J., and Goodman, R. L. (1991).The results of radiation therapy for isolated locoregional recurrence after mastectomy. *International Journal of Radiation Oncology Biology and Physics,* 21, 299-310.

Schwartzs' Principles of Surgery. (2005) (8th ed.). Brunicardi, F. C., Anderson, D., K., Billiar, T. R., Dunn, D. L. Hunter, J. G. and Pollard, R. E. (Eds.), New York: McGraw-Hill.

Seewaldt, V. L., Kim, J. H., Taldwell, L. E., Johnson, B. S., Swisshelm, K., and Collins, S. J. (1997). All-trans-retinoic acid mediates G1 arrest but not apoptosis of normal human mammary epithelial cells. *Cell Growth and Differentiation,* 8, 631-641.

Seewaldt, V. L., Dietz, E. C., Johnson, B. S., Collins, S. J., and Parker, M. B. (1999). Retinoic acid-mediated G1-S-phase arrest of normal human mammary epithelial cells is independent of the level of small p53 protein expression. *Cell Growth and Differentiation,* 10, 49-59.

Sener, S. F., Winchester, D. J., Winchester, D. P., Du, H., Varrera, E., Bilimoria, M., et al. (2009). The effects of hormone replacement therapy on postmenopausal breast cancer biology and survival. *American Journal of Surgery,* 197, 403-407.

Sered, S., and Agigiani A. (2008). Holistic sickening: breast cancer in the discursive worlds of complementary and alternative practitioners. *Sociology in Health and Illness,* 30, 616-631.

Setchell, K. D. R. (2001). Soy isoflavones-benefits and risks from nature's selective estrogen receptor modulators (SERMs). *Journal of the American College of Nutrition,* 26, 354S-362S.

Setchell, K. D., Borriello, S. P. Hulme, P., Kirk, D. N., and Axelson, M. (1984). Non-steroidal estrogens of dietary origin: Possible roles in hormone-dependent disease. *American Journal of Clinical Nutrition,* 40, 569-578.

Setchell, K. D. R., Brown, N. M., Zimmer-Nechemias, L., Brashear, W. T., Wolfe, E., Kirschner, A. S., et al. (2002). Evidence for lack of absorption of soy isoflavone glycosides in humans supporting the crucial role of intestinal metabolism for bioavailability. *American Journal of Clinical Nutrition,* 76, 447-453.

Setchell, K. D. R., Brown, N. M., Desai, P. B., Zimmer-Nech, I., Mias, L. Wolfe, B., Jakate, A. S., et al. (2003). Bioavailability, disposition, and dose-response effects of soy isolflavones when consumed by healthy women at physiologically typical dietary intakes. *Journal of Nutrition,* 133 1027S-1035S.

Sepp-Lorenzino, L. (1998). Structure and function of the insulin-like growth factor I receptor. *Breast Cancer Research and Treatment,* 47, 235-253.

Shanon, J., Ray, R., Wu, C., Nelson, Z., Gao, D. L., Li, W., Hu, W., et al. (2005). Food in botanical groupings and risk of breast cancer: A case-controlled study in Shang Hai, China. *Cancer Epidemiology Biomarkers and Prevention,* 14, 81-89.

Shay, J. W., and Baddhetti, S.(1997). A survey of telomerase activity in human cancer. *European Journal of Cancer,* 33, 787-791.

Sheikh, M. S., Shad, Z. M., Clemmons, D. R., LeRoith, D., Roberts, Jr., C. T., and Fontana, J. A. (1992). Identification of the insulin-growth factor binding proteins 5 and 6 (IGFBP 5 and 6) in human breast cancer cells. *Biochemistry and Bio-physiology Research Communications,* 183 1003-1010.

Shi, Ye. (1994). Progestins and anti-progestins in mammary tumor growth and metastases. *Human Reproduction,* 9, 162-173.

Shiang, E., and Li, F. P. (1971). The yin-yang (hot-cold) theory of diseases. *Journal of the American Medical Association,* 217, 1108.

Shiu, R. P., and Friesen, H. G. (1980). Mechanism of prolactin in the control of mammary gland function. *Annals of Reviews in Physiology,* 42, 83-89.

Sicat, B.L., and Brokaw, D.K. (2004). Non-hormonal alternatives for the treatment of hot flushes. *Pharmacotherapy,* 24, 79-93.

Siegel, B.S. (1986). *Love, medicine, and miracles.* New York: Harper and Row.

Sigdestad, C. P., Spratt, J. S. and Connor, A. M. (2002). Chapter 8;Ionizing radiation and the breast. In Donegan, W. L., and Spratt, J. S. (Eds.), *Cancer of the breast,* (5th ed.). Philadelphia: Saunders.

Simon, H-U, Haj-Y, Ehia, A., and Levi-Schaffer, F. (2000). Role of reactive oxygen species (ROS) in apoptotic induction. *Apoptosis,* 5, 415-418.

Singh, R. P., Agarwal, C., and Agarwal, R., (2003). Inositol hexaphosphate inhibits growth and induces G1 arrest and apoptotic death of prostate carcinoma DU145 cells: modulation of CDKl-CDK-CYCLIN and pRb-related protein-E2F complexes. *Carcinogenesis,* 24, pp. 555-563.

Slamon, D. J., Leyland-Jones, B., Shak, S., Fucas, H., Paton, V., Bajamonde, A., et al. (2001). Use of chemotherapy plus monoclonal antibody against HER2 for metastatic breast cancer that over expresses HER2. *New England Journal of Medicine,* 344, 783-792.

Slaton, J. W., Perrotte, P., Inoue, K., Dinney, C. P. N., and Fidler, I. J. (1999). Interferon-alpha-mediated down-regulation of angiogenesis-related gene and therapy of bladder cancer are dependent on optimization of biological dose and schedule. *Clinical Cancer Research,* 5, 2726-2734.

Sledge, Jr. G.W., Loehrer, P. J., Roth B. J., and Einhorn, L. H. (1988). Cisplatin as first-line therapy for metastatic breast cancer. *Journal of Clinical Oncology,* 6, 1811-1814.

Smith, W. J., Underwood, L. E., and Clemmons, D. R., (1995). Effects of caloric or protein restriction on insulin-like growth factor I and its receptor. Effects of on gene expression and binding. *Journal of Clinical Endocrincology and Metabolism,* 80, pp. 43-49.

Smith-Warner, S. A., Spiegelman, D., Yaun, S.-S., Adama, H.-O., Beeson, W. L., van den Brandt, P. A., et al. (2001). Intake of fruits and vegetables and risk of breast cancer. A pooled analysis of cohort studies. *Journal of the American Medical Association,* 285, 769-776.

Sowers, M. R., Crawford, S., McConnell, D. S., Randolvh, Jr., J. F., Gold, E. B., Wilkin, M. K., et al (2006). Selected and lifestyle factors are associated with estrogen metabolites in a multi racial/ethnic population of women. *Journal of Nutrition,* 136, 1588-1595.

Spector, R. (2004). *Cultural diversity in health and illness.* Sixth edition. Upper Saddle River, NJ: Prentice Hall.

Spratt, J. S. and Donegan, W. L. (2002). Chapter 28: Surgical techniques. In Donegan, W. L., and Spratt, J. S. (Eds.), *Cancer of the breast,* (5th edition). Philadelphia: Saunders.

Spratt, J. A. (1993). Decelerating growth in human breast cancer. *Cancer*, 71, 213-219.

Stanner, S. A., Hughes, J., Kelly, C. N. M., and Buttriss, J. (2004). A review of the epidemiological evidence for the 'antioxidant hypothesis.' *Public Health Nutrition*, 7, 407-422.

Stasburger, C. (2001). Normal values of insulin-like growth factor-1 and their clinically utility in adults. *Hormone Research*, 55 (supplement 2) 100-105.

Steeg, P. S., and Theodorescu, D. (2008). Metastasis: A therapeutic target for cancer. *Nature Clinical Practice of Oncology*, 5, 206-219.

Steele-Perkins, G., Turner, J., Edman, J. C., Hari, J., Pierce, S. B., Stover, C., et al. (1988). Expression and characterization of a functional human insulin-like growth factor-I receptor. *Journal of Biology and Chemistry*, 23, 11486-11492.

Steinmetz, K. A., and Hunter, J. D. (1996). Vegetable, fruit, and cancer prevention: A review. *Journal of the American Medical Association*, 96, 1027-1039.

Stewart, A. J., Johnson, M. D., May, F. E., and Westley, V. R. (1990). Role of insulin-like growth factor and the type I insulin-like growth factor receptor in estrogen-stimulated proliferation of human breast cancer cells. *Journal of Biology and Chemistry*, 34, 21172-21178.

Stewart, C., and Ratain, M. (1997). Topoisomerase interactive agents. In DeVita, V., Hellman, S., and Rosenberg, S. (Eds), *Cancer: principles and practice of oncology* (pp. 461-465). Philadelphia: Lippincott Ravens.

Stewart, C. E., and Rotwein, P. (1996). Growth, differentiation, and survival: Multiple physiological functions for insulin-like growth factor. *Physiological Reviews*, 76, 1005-1026.

Stierer, M., Rosen, H., Weber, R., Hanak, H., Auerbach, L., Spona, J., et al. (1995). A prospective analysis of immunohystochemically hormone receptor and nuclear factors as predictors of early recurrence in primary breast cancer. *Breast Cancer Research and Treatment*, 36, 11-21.

Stoffer, S., Szpunar, W., Coleman, B., and Mellos, P. (1980). Advice from some health food stores. *Journal of the American Medical Association*, 244, 2044-2046.

Stoll, B. A.(1999). Western nutrition and ther insulin-resistance syndrome: A link to breast cancer. *European Journal of Clinical Nutrition*, 53, 83-87.

Su, S. J., Yeh, T. M., Chuang, W. J., Ho, C. L., Chang, K. L., Cheng, H. L., et al. (2005). The novel targets of anti-angiogenesis of genistein on human cancer cells. *Biochemistry and Pharmacology*, 69, 307-318.

Sun, C-L, Yuan, J-M., Koh, W-P, Yu, M. C. (2006), Green tea, black tea, and breast cancer risk: Meta-analysis of epidemiologic studies. *Carcinogenesis*, 27, 1310-1315.

Surmz, E., Guvakova, M. A., Nolaw, M. K., Nicosia, R. F., and Sciarra, L. (1998). Type I insulin-like growth factor receptor function in breast cancer. *Breast Cancer Research and Treatment*, 47, 255-267.

Symonds, H., Karll, L., Remington, L., Saenz-Robles, M., Lowes, C., Jacks, T., et al. (1994). p 53-dependent apoptosis suppresses tumor growth and progression in vivo. *Cell*, 78, 703-711.

Tagliaferri, M., Cohen, I., and Tripathy, D. (2001). Complementary and alternative medicine in early-stage breast cancer. *Seminars in Oncology*, 28, 121-134.

Talamini, R., Franceschi, S., Favero, A., Negri, E., Parazzini4, F., and La Vecchia, C. (1997). Selected medical conditions and risk of breast cancer. *British Journal of Cancer*, 75, 1699-1703.

Tessier, D. and Bash, D. S. (2004). A surgeon's guide to herbal supplements. *Journal of Surgical Research*, 114, 30-36.

Thangapazham, R. L., Gaddipati, J. P., Rajeshkumar, N. V., Sharma, A., Singh, A. K., Ives, J. A., et al. (2006). Homeopathic medicines do not alter growth and gene expression in prostate and breast cancer cells in vitro. *Integrative Cancer Therapeutics*, 5, 356-361.

Thissen, J. B., Ketelslegers, J. M., Underwood, L. E. (1994). Nutritional regulation of the insulin-like growth factors. *Endocrine Reviews*, 15, 80-101.

Thomas, H. V., Reeves, G. K., and Key, T. J. (1997). Endogenous estrogen in post-menopausal breast cancer: A quantitative review. *Cancer Causes Control*, 8, 922-928.

Thorsen, T., Lahoot, I., Hrasmussen, M., and Aakvaag, A. (1992). Oestradiol treatment increases the sensitivity of MCL-7 cells for the growth stimulatory effect of IGF-I. *Journal of Steroid Biochemistry and Molecular Biology*, 41, 53740-53747.

Tokunaga, M. (1987). Instances of female breast cancer among atomic bomb-survivors: Hiroshima and Nagasaki. *Radiation Research*, 11, 243-272.

Tomin, R., and Donegan, W. L. (1987). Screening for recurrent breast cancer: Its effectiveness and prognostic value. *Journal of Clinical Oncology*, 5, 62-67.

Tomolo, P., Bruning, P. F., Akhmedkhanov, A., Bonfrer, J. M., Koenig, K. L., Lukanova, A., et al. (2000). Serum insulin-like growth factor-I and breast cancer. *International Journal of Cancer*, 88, 828-832.

Tonner, E. (2000). Insulin-like growth factor binding protein-5 (IGFBP-5) potentially regulates programmed cell death and plasminogen activation in the mammary gland. *Advances in Experimental Medicine and Biology*, 480, 45-53.

Tonnesen, E., Brinkley, M. M., Schou Olesen, A. and Christensen, N. J. (1985). Natural killer cell activity in a patient undergoing open-heart surgery complicated by an acute myocardial infarction. *Acta Pathologica Microbiologica Immunologica Scandinavica*, 93, 229-231.

Touillaud, M. S., Thiebaut, A. C. M., Niravong, M., Boutron-Ruault, M.-C., and Clavel-Chapelon, F. (2006). No association between dietary phytoestrogens and risk of premenopausal breast cancer in a French cohort study. *Cancer Epidemiology Biomarkers and Prevention*, 15, 2574-2576.

Trentham-Dietz, A., Newcomb, P. A., Storer, B. E., Longnecker, M. P., Baron, J., Greenberg, E. R., et al. (1997). Body size and risk of breast cancer. *American Journal of Epidemiology*, 145, 1011-1019.

Trindle H. A., Davis, R. B., Phillips, R. S., and Eisenberg, D.M. (2005). Trends in use of complementary and alternative medicine by US adults. *Alternative Therapies in Health and Medicine*, 11, 42-49.

Trock, B. J., Hilakivi-Clark, L., and Clarke, R. (2006). Meta-analysis of soy intake and breast cancer risk. *Journal of the National Cancer Institute*, 98, 459-471.

Tseng, M. (1999). Calculation of population attributable risk for alcohol and breast cancer (United States). *Cancer Causes and Control*, 10, 119-123.

Tsumoda, N., Pomeroy, S., and Nestel, P. (2002). Absorption in humans of isoflavones from soy and red clover is similar. *Journal of Nutrition*, 132, 2199-22201.

U. S. Food and Drug Administration. (1993). Unsubstantiated claims and documented health hazards in the dietary supplement marketplace. Rockville, Md: Food and Drug Administration.

Vachon, C. M., Kushi, L. H., Cerhan, J. R., Kuni, C. C., and Sellers, T. A. (2000), Association of diet and mammographic density in

Minnesota Heart Cancer Family Cohort, *Cancer Epidemiology Biomarkers and Prevention*, 9, 151-160.

Vadgama, J. V., Wu, Y., Datta, G., Khan, H., and Chillar, R. (1999). Plasma insulin-like growth factor-I and serum IGF-binding protein-3 can be associated with the progression of breast cancer, and predict the risk of recurrence and the probability of survival in African-American and Hispanic women. *Oncology*, 57, 330-340.

Valtuena, S., Pellegrini, N., Franzini, L., Pianchi, M. A., Ardigo, D., Del Rio, D., et al. (2008). Food selection based on total antioxidant capacity can modify antioxidant intake, systemic inflammation, and liver function without altering markers of oxidative stress. *American Journal of Clinical Nutrition*, 87, 1290-1297.

val Krischnan, R.; Dugan, E.; Camacho, F.T. and Hall, M.A. (2003). Trust and satisfaction with physicians, insurers, and the medical profession. *Medical Care*, 41, 1058-1064.

Vanchieri, C. (2000). Alternative therapies getting noticed through best case series program. *Journal of the National Cancer Institute*, 92, 1558-1560.

VandeCreek, L., Rogers, E., and Lester, J. (1999). Use of alternative therapies among breast cancer outpatients compared to the general population. *Journal of Alternative and Complementary Medicine*, 5, 71-76.

van der Weg, F., and Streulie, R. A. (2003). Use of alternative medicine by patients with cancer in a rural area of Switzerland, *Swiss Medical Weekly*, 133, 233-240.

van der Weijer, P. H., and Barensten, R. (2002). Isoflavones from red clover (promensil) significantly reduce menopausal hot flush symptoms compared with placebo. *Maturitas*, 42, 187-193.

van Gils, C. H., Peeters, P. H. M., Bueno-DeMesquita, B., Boshuizen, H. C., Lahmann, P. H., Clavel-Chapelon, F., et al. (2005).

Consumption of vegetables and fruits and risk of breast cancer. *Journal of the American Medical Association,* 293, 183-93.

Vena, J. E., Graham, S., Hellman, R., Swanson, M., and Brasure, J. (1991). Use of electric blankets and risk of postmenopausal breast cancer. *American Journal of Epidemiology,* 134, 180-185.

Verheul, H. M. W., Panigrahy, D., Yuan, J., and D'Amato, R. J. (1999). A combination of oral and antiangiogenic therapy with thalidomide and sulindac inhibits tumour growth in rabbits. *British Journal of Cancer,* 79, 114-118.

Veronesi, U., Marubini, E., del Vecchio, M., Manzari, A., Andreola, S., Greco, M., et al. (1995). Local recurrences and distal metastases after conservative breast cancer treatments: Partly independent events. *Journal of the National Cancer Institute,* 87, 19-27.

Veronesi, U., Boyle, P., Goldhirsch, A., Orrchia, R., and Viale, G. (2005). Breast cancer. *Lancet,* 365, 1724-1741.

Walker, L. G., Anderson, J. (1999). Testing complementary and alternative therapies within a research protocol. *European Journal of Cancer,* 35, 1614-1618.

Wang, W., Higuchi, C. M., and Zhang, R. (1997). Individual and combinatory effects of soy isoflavones in the in vitro potentiation of lymphocyte activation. *Nutrition and Cancer,* 29, 29-34.

Warner, J. (2006). Vitamin D may fight prostate cancer. Web MD Health News. Retrieved September 22 2008 from http.//www.medscape.com/viewarticle/523406

Watzl, B. (2005). Consumption of vegetables and fruits and risk of breast cancer. *Journal of the American Medical Association,* 293, 2209-2210.

Wefel, J. S., Lenzi., R., Theriault, R., Buzdar, A. U., Cruikshanks, S., and Meyer, C. A. (2003). "Chemobrain" in breast carcinoma. *Cancer,* 101, 466-475.

Weidner, N., Semple, J. P., Welch, W. R., and Folkman, J. (1991). Tumor angiogenesis and metastasis-correlation in invasive breast carcinoma. *New England Journal of Medicine, 324*, 1-8.

Weiger, W. A., Smith, M., Boone, H., Richardson, M. A., Kaptchuk, T. J., and Eisenberg, D.M. (2002). Advising patients who seek complementary and alternative therapies for cancer. *Annals of Internal Medicine, 137,* 889-903.

Weinberg, R. A. (1996). How cancer arises. *Scientific American, 275,* 62-77.

Weindruck, R. (1992). Effect of caloric restriction on age-associated cancers. *Experimental Gerontology, 27,* 575-581.

Weinstein, B. S., and Ciszek, C. (2002). The reserve-capacity hypothesis: Evolutionary origins and modern implications of the trade-off between tumor-suppression and tissue-repair. *Experimental Gerontology, 37,* 615-627.

Weinzimer, S. A., Beers Gibson, T., Collett-Solberg, P. F., Khare, A., Liu, B., and Cohen, P. (2001). Transferrin is an insulin-like growth factor-binding protein-3 binding protein. *The Journal of Clinical Endocrinology and Metabolism, 86,* 1806-1812.

Wells, M., Sarna, L., Cooley, M. E., Brown, J. K., Chernecky, C., Williams R.D., et al. (2007). Use of complementary and alternative medicine therapy to control symptoms in women living with lung cancer. *Cancer Nursing, 30,* 45-55.

Welsch, C. W. (1987). Enhancement of mammary turmorigenesis by dietary fat: Review of potential mechanisms. *American Journal of Clinical Nutrition, 25* 192-202.

Wetterau, L. A., Francis, M. J., Ma, L., and Cohen, P. (2003). Insulin-like growth factor I stimulate telomerase activity in prostate cancer cells. *Journal of Clinical Endocrinology and Metabolism, 88,* 3354-3359.

Whelan, T., Clark, R., Roberts, R., Levine, M. and Foster, G. (1994). Ipsilateral breast tumor recurrence post-lumpectomy is predictive of subsequent mortality: Results from a randomized trial. Investigators of the Ontario Clinical Oncology Group. *International Journal of Radiation Oncology Biology and Physics*, 30, 11-16.

Wheler, J. (2005). Treatment for metastatic breast cancer: Novel approaches. Presented at 28th Annual San Antonio Breast Cancer Symposium. Retrieved September 22 2008 from *http://www. medscape.com/viewarticle/522230*

White, A., and Ernst, E. (2001). The case of uncontrolled clinical trials: A starting point for the evidence based for CAM. *Complimentary Therapies in Medicine, 9*, 111-116.

White, J. D. (2002). Complementary and alternative medicine research: A National Cancer Institute perspective. *Seminars in Oncology, 29*, 546-551.

White, M. F., and Khan, R. (1994). The insulin signaling system. *Journal of Biological Chemistry, 269*, 1-4.

Whittiker, M. G., and Clark, C. G. (1971). Depressed lymphocyte function in carcinoma of the breast. *British Journal of Surgery, 58*, 717-720.

Willett, W. C. (2007), Soy consumption, markers of inflammation, and endothelial function. *Diabetes Care, 30*, 967-973.

Williams, J. E. (2003). *Prolonging health*. Charlottsville, Va: Hampton Roads.

Willner, J., Kiricuta, I. C., and Kolbl, O. (1997). Locoregional recurrence of breast cancer following mastectomy: Always a fatal event? Results of univariate and multivariate analysis. *International Journal of Radiation Oncology Biology and Physics*, 37, 853-863.

Willner, J., Kircuta, I. C., Kolbl, O., and Fletje, M. (1999). Long-term survival following post-mastectomy locoregional recurrence of breast cancer. *Breast*, 8, 200-204.

Wilson, J. X. (2005). Regulation of vitamin C transport. *Annual Reviews in Nutrition,* Vol. 25, 105-125.

Wolf, I., Sadetski, S., Catane, R., Karsik, A., and Kaufman, B. (2005). Diabetes mellitus and cancer. *Lancet Oncology,* 6, 103-111.

Wood, C. E., Register, T. C., Franke, A. A., Anthony, M. S., and Cline, J. M. (2006). Dietary soy isoflavones inhibit estrogen effects in the postmenopausal breast. *Cancer Research*, 66, 1241-1249.

Wu, A. H., Wan, P., Hankin, J., Tseng, C.-C., Yu, M. C., and Pike, M. C. (2002). Adolescent and adult soy intake and risk of breast cancer in Asian-Americans. *Carcinogenesis*, 23, 1491-1496.

Wu, A. H., Tseng, C.-C., Van Den Berg, D., and Yu, M. C. (2003). Tea intake, COMT genotype, and breast cancer in Asian-American women. *Cancer Research*, 63, 7526-7529.

Wu, A. H., Stanczyk, F. Z., Martinez, C., Tseng, C-C, Hendrich, S., Murphy, P., et al. (2005). A controlled 2-month dietary fat reduction and soy food supplementation study in post menopausal women. *American Journal of Clinical Nutrition,* 81, 1133-1141.

Wu, A. H., Pike, M. C., Williams, L. D., Spicer, D., Tseng, C-C, Churchwell, M. I. et al. (2007). Tamoxifen, soy, and lifestyle factors in Asian-American women with breast cancer. *Journal of Clinical Oncology,* 25, 3024-3030.

Wu, A. H., Yu, M. C., Tseng, C-C, Stanczyk, F. Z., and Pike, M. C. (2007). Diabetes and risk of breast cancer in Asian-American women. *Carcinogenesis*, 28, 1561-1566.

Wu, H., Mistry, J., Nicar, M. J., Ahosravi, M. J., Diamandis, A., van Doorn, J., et al. (1999). Insulin-like growth factors (IGF-I, free IGF-I, and IGF-II) and insulin-like growth factor finding proteins

(IGF-BP-2, IGFBP-3, and ALF) in blood circulation. *Journal of Clinical Laboratory Analysis,* 13, 166-172.

Wynford-Thomas, D. (1997). Proliferation life span check points: cell-type specificity and influence on tumour biology. *European Journal of Cancer,* 33, 716-726.

Yamamoto, S., Sobue, T., Kobayashi, M., Sasaki, S., and Tsugane, S. (2003). Soy, isoflavones, and breast cancer risk in Japan. *Journal of the National Cancer Institute,* 95, 906-913.

Yang, C. S. (1999). Tea and health. *Nutrition,* 15, 946-959.

Yarbro, J. W., (1985). Cancer research and the development of cancer centers. In Gross, S. C. and Gard, S. (Eds.), *Cancer treatment and research in humanistic perspective* (pp.3-15). New York: Springer.

Yee, D., Favoni, R. E., Lippman, M. C., Powell, D. R. (1991). Identification of insulin-like growth factor binding proteins in breast cancer cells. *Breast Cancer Research and Treatment,* 18, 3-10.

Yeager, J. D. (2000). Endogenous estrogens as carcinogens through metabolic activation. *Journal of the National Cancer Institute Monogram,* 27, 67-73.

Yeom, C. H., Jung, G. C., and Song, K. J. (2007). Changes of terminal cancer patients' health-related quality of life after high dose vitamin C administration. *Journal of Korean Medical Science,* 22, 7-11.

Yiangou, C. (1997). Fibroblast growth factor 2 in breast cancer: Occurrence of prognostic significance. *British Journal of Cancer,* 75, 28-33.

Yoder, K. M. (1987). Hot and cold in women's ethnotherapeutics: The American Mexican west, *Social Science in Medicine,* 25, 347-355.

Yong, G. J., and Conrad, D. A. (2007). Practical issues in the design and implementation of pay-for-quality programs, *Journal of Health Care Management*, 52, 10-18.

Yu, H. and Berkel, J. (1999). Do insulin-like growth factors mediate the effect of alcohol on breast cancer risk? *Medical Hypothesis*, 52, 491-496.

Yu, H., and Rohan, T. (2000). Role of the insulin-like growth factor family in cancer development and progression. *Journal of the National Cancer Institute*, 92, 1472-1484.

Yu, H., Levesque, M. A., Khosravi, M. J., Patanatasiou-Diamandi, A., Clark, G. M., and Diamandis, E. P. (1998). Insulin-like growth factor-binding protein-3 in breast cancer survival. *International Journal of Cancer*, 79, 624-628.

Yu, H., Jin, F., Shu, X-O, Li, Bdl, Dai, Q., Cheng, J-R, et al. (2002). Insulin-like growth factors and breast cancer risk in Chinese women. *Cancer Epidemiology Biomarkers and Prevention*, 11, 705-712.

Yuan, J.-M., Koh, W-P., Sun, C-L., Lee, H-P., and Yu, M. C. (2005). Green tea intake, *ACE* gene polymorphism and breast cancer risk among Chinese women in Singapore. *Carcinogenesis*, 26, 1389-1394.

Zaridze, D., Lifanova, Y., Maximovitch, D., Day, N. E. and Duffy, S. W. (1991). Diet, alcohol consumption and reproductive factors in case-controlled study in Moscow, *International Journal of Cancer*, 48, 493-501.

Zelen, M. (1979). A new design for randomized clinical trials. *New England Journal of Medicine*, 300, 1242-1245.

Zhang, M., Holman, C., d'Arcy, J., Huang, J., and Xie, X. (2007). Green tea and the prevention of breast cancer: A case-controlled study in Southeast China. *Carcinogenesis*, 28, 1074-1078.

Zhang, S., Hunter, D. J., Forman, M. R., Rosner, B. A., Speizer, F. E., Colditz, G. A., et al. (1999). Dietary carotenoids and vitamins A, C and E, and risk of breast cancer. *Journal of the National Cancer Institute*, 91, 547-556.

Zhu, Z., Jiang, W., and Thomson, H. J. (2002). An experimental paradigm for studying the cellular and molecular mechanisms of cancer inhibition by energy restriction. *Molecular Carcinogenesis*, 35, 51-56.

Zimmerman, D. (2009, Winter). The power of evidence-based medicine. *Creative Living*, 32.

Ziyaie, D. L., Hupp, T., R., and Thompson, A. M. (2000). P53 and breast cancer. *Breast*, 9, 239-246.

Zou, W., Yue, P., Lin, N., He, M., Zhou, Z., Lonial, S., et al. (2006). Vitamin C inactivates the proteasome inhibitor P.S.-341 in human cancer cells. *Clinical Cancer Research*, 12, 273-80.

Appendix A

Photographs of Mastectomy Site
(Chest Wall-Skin Metastases)

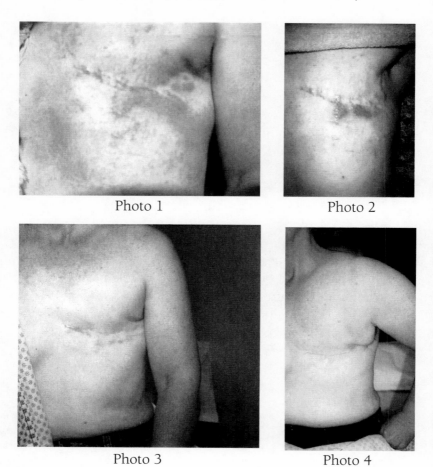

Photo 1

Photo 2

Photo 3

Photo 4

Appendix B

Health-Care Professional Questionnaire

Questionnaire used for personal interviews:

1.) What is your medical specialty?
2.) Are you board certified in this area?
3.) How many years of practice do you have in this field?
4.) Do you have any experience with natural health methods?
5.) Have your patients communicated their use of CAM in the treatment of their breast cancer?
6.) Do you feel that they volunteer information, or would they be honest if you directly questioned them?
7.) To what degree would your patient population be willing to use CAM, along with conventional treatment?
8.) To what degree would your patient population be willing to use CAM, *only* as a treatment?
9.) To what degree does this depend on the stage of disease at the time of treatment?
10.) In your experience, have you seen any results that were unusual or unexpected that may be related to CAM?
11.) What is your opinion on soy and its relationship to the development or treatment in breast cancer?

Edwards Brothers, Inc.
Thorofare, NJ USA
September 8, 2011